COMPLEX REGIONAL PAIN SYNDROME CAUSATION

An Evidence Based Medicine Approach

William Edward Ackerman III MD

COMPLEX REGIONAL PAIN SYNDROME CAUSATION

An Evidence Based Medicine Approach

This book is dedicated to my significant other who is also my best friend.

Acknowledgments

I wish to furthermore acknowledge Professor Gabor Racz , a world expert in the Complex Regional Pain Syndrome who taught me most of what I now know on CRPS when I was one of his Pain Fellows when I was at the Texas Tech Heal Sciences Center in Lubbock, Texas.

I wish to also acknowledge my staff and patients whose questions on pain management modalities including "What works?" and "What doesn't?" prompted me to write this book. I wish to thank my previous residents whose dedication and interest helped kindle my research on Reflex Sympathetic Dystrophy.

Foreword

Dr. William Ackerman is a pain management specialist who brings considerable expertise and experience to both the medical and legal communities. He has over 20 years of clinical medicine and litigation support experience. He is double-board certified in both Anesthesiology and in Pain Medicine. In the capacity of a medical expert witness, Dr. Ackerman has testified in injury causation, diagnosis, apportionment, reasonable medical care and treatment, need for future medical treatment, permanent damages, functional impairment, negligence, and standard of care issues.

Dr. Ackerman is an independent medical examiner and was the former medical director of pain management and was an associate professor at a university hospital. He has also been medical director of two private hospital pain centers. He has authored over 135 scientific articles in prestigious journals such as Anesthesia Analgesia, Canadian Journal of Anesthesia, Regional Anesthesia and Pain Management etc.

Dr. Ackerman maintains an active private practice. His practice consists of interventional and medical treatment of chronic pain and is considered an expert in Reflex Sympathetic Dystrophy. He has published chapters in multiple medical textbooks and has published nine books including coauthoring and editing the AMA best seller book the AMA Guides to Injury and Disease Causation (First and Second Editions).

Dr. Ackerman has been a Lt. Col. in the U.S. Army and Chief of Anesthesiology at two Army medical centers. He has had an extensive successful academic career and is now in private practice. He also has been an Associate Professor of three academic, universities, pain management departments and has been on the academy faculty at three medical schools. He has been on the Editorial Board of two peer reviewed medical journals. He was nominated previously for the Southern Medical Society Medical Research Award and the Bristol-Meyers Squibb award for distinguished achievement in Pain Research.

He was a past recipient of the prestigious Karl Koeller research grant from the American Society of Regional Anesthesia and Pain Medicine and was selected to "Who's Who in International Medicine".

GS

Table of Contents

1. Overview

The Complex regional pain syndrome condition currently known as CRPS was originally described during the American Civil War by Silas Weir Mitchell. Is the Complex Sympathetic Regional Pain Syndrome (CRPS) an inflammatory entity or an autoimmune disease? Because treatments can differ between these two entities it is important to understand what is the pathology of each entity so the proper treatment can be introduced.

The complex regional pain syndrome is an uncommon form of chronic pain that usually affects an arm or a leg. (CRPS) is a chronic pain condition that mainly affects the arms, legs, hands, and feet, but may involve the entire body. CRPS symptoms often begin after an injury. The main feature of CRPS is continuous, intense pain that is out of proportion to the severity of the injury.

The complex regional pain syndrome typically develops after an injury, surgery, stroke or heart attack, but the pain is out of proportion to the severity of the initial injury. CRPS occurs as a result of dysfunction in the central or peripheral nervous systems. It affects women more often than men. There is no cure for CRPS. With CRPS a patient's brain develops maladaptive neuroplasticity.

CRPS most likely does not have a single cause; rather, it results from multiple causes that produce similar symptoms.1 With injury-related CRPS, the syndrome may be caused by a triggering of the immune response.2 There is no specific diagnostic test for CRPS, but some tests can rule out other conditions.

An autoimmune disease, also known as autoimmune disorder, is one where the body initiates an immune response to healthy tissues, mistaking them for harmful pathogens or irritants. The immune response triggers an inflammatory response too.

Inflammation is the body's attempt at self-protection; the aim being to remove harmful stimuli, including damaged cells, irritants, or pathogens - and begin the healing process. When something harmful or irritating affects a part of a body, there is a biological response to try to remove it. The signs and symptoms of acute inflammation show that the body is trying to heal itself.

The involvement of the immune system in the pathophysiology of CRPS is appreciated for several reasons. First, CRPS shows several clinical characteristics of an inflammatory disease. Additionally, levels of proinflammatory cytokines are elevated in blister fluid from CRPS affected limbs. CRPS shows a beneficial response to treatment with inhibitors of inflammation, such as corticosteroids.

Triple-phase bone scans can be used to identify changes in the bone and in blood circulation. There are two similar forms of CRPS called CRPS-I and CRPS-II. CRPS-II is the term used for patients with confirmed nerve injuries. Individuals without confirmed nerve injury are classified as having CRPS-I. Because immunological functions can modulate CNS physiology, it has also been hypothesized that a variety of immune processes may contribute to the initial development and maintenance of peripheral and central sensitization.

The International Association for the Study of Pain (IASP) lists the diagnostic criteria for complex regional pain syndrome I (CRPS I) (RSDS) as follows: The presence of an initiating noxious event or a cause of immobilization, Continuing pain, allodynia (perception of pain from a nonpainful stimulus), or hyperalgesia (an exaggerated sense of pain) disproportionate to the inciting event.

Evidence at some time of edema, changes in skin blood flow, or abnormal sudomotor activity in the area of pain and the diagnosis is excluded by the existence of any condition that would otherwise account for the degree of pain and dysfunction. CRPS II is defined by a known nerve injury.

It is much more common in women. The average age of affected individuals is about age forty. CRPS also affects the immune system. High levels of cytokines have been found in the tissues of people with CRPS. These contribute to the redness, swelling, and warmth reported by many patients. CRPS is more common in individuals with other inflammatory and autoimmune conditions such as asthma.

Research has shown that CRPS-related inflammation is supported by the body's natural immune response. It may initially affect one limb and then spread throughout the body; 35% of people afflicted report symptoms throughout their whole body. Clinical features of CRPS have been found to be neurogenic inflammation, nociceptive sensitization, vasomotor dysfunction, and maladaptive neuroplasticity.

There are numerous etiological pathophysiological events that have been incriminated in development of CRPS, including inflammation, autoimmune responses, abnormal cytokine production, sympathetic-sensory disorders, altered blood flow and central cortical reorganization.3 Pro-inflammatory cytokines contribute to the nociceptive and vascular sequelae of fracture.4 It's not well-understood why injuries can trigger the complex regional pain syndrome, but it may be due to a dysfunctional interaction between the central and peripheral nervous systems and inappropriate inflammatory responses.

Autoimmunity has been suggested as one of the pathophysiologic mechanisms that may underlie complex regional pain syndrome. Screening for antinuclear antibodies (ANA) is one of the diagnostic tests, which is usually performed if a person is suspected to have a systemic autoimmune disease. Antineuronal antibodies are autoantibodies directed against antigens in the central and/or peripheral nervous system. Autoantibodies may be associated with the pathophysiology of CRPS, at least in a subset of patients.5 An autoimmune etiology of CRPS is a new pathophysiological concept and may have severe impact on the treatment of this often chronic disease.6

The complex Regional Pain Syndrome is a multifactorial and disabling disorder with complex etiology and pathogenesis. Goals of therapy in CRPS should be pain relief, functional restoration, and psychological stabilization, but early interventions are needed in order to achieve these objectives. An inflammatory reaction may cause the syndrome in which leukocytes may play an important role. Researchers have found a significantly increased accumulation of leukocytes in patients with CRPS I.7This is the first study to show a possible role for leukocytes in the pathophysiology of acute CRPS I.

Proinflammatory cytokines are increased in CRPS 1 affected extremities during the intermediate stage of the disease. This indicates that the initiation and sustained development of the disease are only partially affected by proinflammatory cytokines. Follow-up in the chronic stage is necessary to draw more definite conclusions about the existence of a supposed relation between clinical signs and symptoms and the level of proinflammatory cytokines.8

Several drugs have been used to reduce pain and to improve functional status in CRPS, despite the lack of scientific evidence supporting their use in this scenario. They include anti-inflammatory drugs, analgesics, anesthetics, anticonvulsants, antidepressants, oral muscle relaxants, corticosteroids, calcitonin, bisphosphonates, calcium channel blockers and topical agents.9 NSAIDs showed no value in treating CRPS. Glucocorticoids are the only anti-inflammatory drugs for which there is direct clinical trial evidence in early stage of CRPS.

Recent research has shown that some patients respond to treatment with immunoglobulins, and that a majority have IgG serum-autoantibodies directed against, and activating autonomic receptors. CRPS serum-IgG, when transferred to mice elicits abnormal behavior. These results suggest that CRPS is associated with an autoantibody-mediated autoimmune process in some cases.10

Further preliminary evidence for immune activation early in CRPS and, additionally, those patients with minimal trauma may comprise an autoimmune subgroup.11 The identification of functionally active autoantibodies in serum samples from CRPS patients supports an autoimmune pathogenesis of CRPS.12 Elevated IL-8 and sTNFR I/II levels indicate an association between CRPS I and an inflammatory process. Normal WBC, CRP, and IL-6 give evidence for localized inflammation. The hypothesis of neurogenic-induced inflammation mediated by neuropeptides is supported by elevated substance P levels.13

There are three stages of CRPS. Stage one is characterized by severe, burning pain at the site of the injury, muscle spasms, joint stiffness, restricted mobility, rapid hair and nail growth, and vasospasm. Magnetic resonance imaging or triple-phase bone scans sometimes identify CRPS-characteristic changes in the bone metabolism. There are changes in the color and temperature of the skin. Some patients may experience hyperhidrosis. In Stage two the extremity hair growth diminishes and joints thicken, and muscles atrophy. Stage three is characterized by irreversible changes in the skin and bones and the pain becomes inflexible and may involve the entire limb. There is marked muscle atrophy, severely limited mobility of the affected area, and flexor tendon contractions.

Some features of acute CRPS (vasodilatation, swelling, pain) indicate a localized inflammatory process.14 No specific test is available for CRPS, which is diagnosed primarily through observation of the symptoms. Thermography, sweat testing, x-rays, electro diagnostics, and sympathetic blocks can be used to build up a picture of the disorder. Good progress can be made in treating CRPS when CRPS treatment is begun early, ideally within three months of the first symptoms.

There is convincing evidence that inflammation plays a pivotal role in the pathophysiology of complex regional pain syndrome (CRPS). Besides inflammation, central sensitization is also an important phenomenon. Mast cells are known to be involved in the inflammatory process of

CRPS and also play a role (at least partially) in the process of central sensitization.15 On the other hand results furthermore support the hypothesis that autoantibodies may contribute to the pathophysiology of CRPS, and that autoantibody-removing therapies may be effective treatments for long-standing CRPS.16

Before speaking of clear evidence of a CRPS autoimmune etiology, Witebsky's criteria for an autoimmune disease should be considered. These criteria include (1) demonstration of a specific antigen, (2) circumstantial evidence of an autoimmune or inflammatory disorder from clinical clues, and (3) reproduction of clinical features in recipient animals by passive transfer of putatively pathogenic antibodies.17,18 In a study by Sieweke, anti-inflammatory agents had no effect on CRPS pain on human subjects. These results indicate a non-inflammatory pathogenesis in CRPS presumably central in origin.19

Clinical observations of patients with CRPS associated with patchy osteoporosis suggest that CRPS may have two distinct components: (1) neuropathic pain that includes severe spontaneous pain or severe persistent mechanical allodynia and (2) prolonged regional inflammation, the early phase of which could be indicated by positive inflammatory symptoms of pain (tenderness), heat, redness, swelling and loss of function and their alleviation with corticosteroids.

It is increasingly evident that there is a close connection between the generation of cutaneous inflammatory cytokines and elevated neuropeptide signaling in CRPS patients.20 Neuropeptides induce nociceptive sensitization by enhancing IL-1 beta production in keratinocytes. Neuropeptides rely on both caspase-1 and cathepsin B for this enhanced production. Neurocutaneous signaling involving neuropeptide activation of the innate immunity may contribute to pain in CRPS patients.

Inflammatory mediator production occurs acutely in CRPS, but central spinal changes may be more important for the persistent nociceptive changes in a CRPS model.21 At the time of this writing Witebsky's criteria for a CRPS autoimmune etiology has not been established. It is hypothesized that peripheral CRPS pain may be influenced by an inflammatory cause while central neurologic pain may be related to an autoimmune origin. Further research in this area is definitely indicated.

It is anticipated that this information presented will provoke discussion, interest and promote further empirical studies on the interactions between central and peripheral inflammatory pathways manifest in CRPS.

References

1. Watkins LR, Maier SF. Immune regulation of central nervous system functions: from sickness responses to pathological pain. J Intern Med. 2005;257(2):139-155.

2. Marinus J, Moseley GL, Birklein F, et al. Clinical features and pathophysiology of complex regional pain syndrome. Lancet Neurol. 2011;10(7):637-648.

3. Borchers AT, Gershwin ME. Complex regional pain syndrome: a comprehensive and critical review. Autoimmun Rev. 2014;13(3):242-265.

4. Wei T, Sabsovich I, Guo TZ, et al. Pentoxifylline attenuates nociceptive sensitization and cytokine expression in a tibia fracture rat model of complex regional pain syndrome. Eur J Pain. 2009;13(3):253-262.

5. Dirckx M, Schreurs MW, de Mos M, Stronks DL, Huygen FJ. The prevalence of autoantibodies in complex regional pain syndrome type I. Mediators Inflamm. 2015;2015:718201.

6. Blaes F, Tschernatsch M, Braeu ME, et al. Autoimmunity in complex-regional pain syndrome. Ann N Y Acad Sci. 2007;1107:168-173.

7. Tan EC, Oyen WJ, Goris RJ. Leukocytes in Complex Regional Pain Syndrome type I. Inflammation. 2005;29(4-6):182-186.

8. Munnikes RJ, Muis C, Boersma M, Heijmans-Antonissen C, Zijlstra FJ, Huygen FJ. Intermediate stage complex regional pain syndrome type 1 is unrelated to proinflammatory cytokines. Mediators Inflamm. 2005;2005(6):366-372.

9. Resmini G, Ratti C, Canton G, Murena L, Moretti A, Iolascon G. Treatment of complex regional pain syndrome. Clin Cases Miner Bone Metab. 2015;12(Suppl 1):26-30.

10. Goebel A, Blaes F. Complex regional pain syndrome, prototype of a novel kind of autoimmune disease. Autoimmun Rev. 2013;12(6):682-686.

11. Goebel A, Vogel H, Caneris O, et al. Immune responses to Campylobacter and serum autoantibodies in patients with complex regional pain syndrome. J Neuroimmunol. 2005;162(1-2):184-189.

12.   Kohr D, Singh P, Tschernatsch M, et al. Autoimmunity against the beta2 adrenergic receptor and muscarinic-2 receptor in complex regional pain syndrome. Pain. 2011;152(12):2690-2700.

13.   Schinkel C, Gaertner A, Zaspel J, Zedler S, Faist E, Schuermann M. Inflammatory mediators are altered in the acute phase of posttraumatic complex regional pain syndrome. Clin J Pain. 2006;22(3):235-239.

14.   Baron R. Mechanistic and clinical aspects of complex regional pain syndrome (CRPS). Novartis Found Symp. 2004;261:220-233; discussion 233-228, 256-261.

15.   Dirckx M, Groeneweg G, van Daele PL, Stronks DL, Huygen FJ. Mast cells: a new target in the treatment of complex regional pain syndrome? Pain Pract. 2013;13(8):599-603.

16.   Tekus V, Hajna Z, Borbely E, et al. A CRPS-IgG-transfer-trauma model reproducing inflammatory and positive sensory signs associated with complex regional pain syndrome. Pain. 2014;155(2):299-308.

17.   Zhang Y, Popovich P. Roles of autoantibodies in central nervous system injury. Discov Med. 2011;11(60):395-402.

18.   Sommer C. Anti-autonomic nervous system antibodies in CRPS. Pain. 2011;152(12):2675-2676.

19.   Sieweke N, Birklein F, Riedl B, Neundorfer B, Handwerker HO. Patterns of hyperalgesia in complex regional pain syndrome. Pain. 1999;80(1-2):171-177.

20.   Shi X, Wang L, Li X, Sahbaie P, Kingery WS, Clark JD. Neuropeptides contribute to peripheral nociceptive sensitization by regulating interleukin-1beta production in keratinocytes. Anesth Analg. 2011;113(1):175-183.

21.   Wei T, Guo TZ, Li WW, Kingery WS, Clark JD. Acute versus chronic phase mechanisms in a rat model of CRPS. J Neuroinflammation. 2016;13:14.

2. Inflammatory Cause?

Almost everyone experiences pain at some time. Pain can be a natural response to injury and disease in some instances. Pain is an unpleasant sensory and emotional experience following tissue injury. Pain occurs as a response to tissue irritation, injury, infection, ischemia or inflammation. Most pain however is a result of inflammation. Patients should try to avoid strong narcotic medications for any type of pain. Anti-inflammatory medications, anticonvulsants, steroid injections and mild pain medications may be of benefit.

Pain is a complex, idiosyncratic experience. When pain is the primary complaint for seeking medical attention, understanding of multiple factors is essential in guiding successful treatment. Behavioral medicine, a branch of psychology, has been an integral part of interdisciplinary/multidisciplinary care of pain patients. Prominent and distressing emotions, cognitions, and behaviors frequently accompany chronic pain. Chronic pain is a disease. Could the Complex Regional Pain Syndrome be an autoimmune disease? An autoimmune disease is a condition arising from an abnormal immune response to a normal body part. Women are found to be more commonly affected than men.

Americans spend over one hundred billion dollars annually on pain care. One-third of all adult Americans suffer from chronic pain. Over the counter annual analgesic cost of medical care is rapidly escalating. Employers may not be able to afford health insurance for their employees. The cost of pain management is contributing to the increase in health care costs and amounts to hundreds of thousands of dollars. As a result, there is considerable profit to be made by unethical health care providers that include hospitals as well as physicians.

Complex regional pain syndrome (CRPS) is a chronic pain condition. It causes intense pain, usually in the arms, hands, legs, or feet. It may happen after an injury, either to a nerve or to tissue in the affected area. Rest and time may only make it worse. The IASP (International Association for the Study of Pain) definition of the syndrome reads as follows: "CRPS Type I is a syndrome that usually develops after an initiating noxious event, is not limited to the distribution of a single peripheral nerve, and is apparently disproportioned to the inciting event. It is associated at some point with evidence of edema, changes in skin blood flow, abnormal sudomotor activity in the region of the pain, or allodynia or hyperalgesia".

The exact reason that reflex sympathetic dystrophy develops is not well understood, but generally it involves nerve trauma associated with a physical injury. CRPS is a rare complication of limb injury in biologically susceptible individuals. The pathogenesis of CRPS is due in part to central neuroimmune activation. The inflammatory response is a defense mechanism that evolved in higher organisms to protect them from infection and injury.

Its purpose is to localize and eliminate the injurious agent and to remove damaged tissue components so that the body can begin to heal. The response consists of changes in blood flow, an increase in permeability of blood vessels, and the migration of fluid, proteins, and white blood cells (leukocytes) from the circulation to the site of tissue damage. An inappropriate immune response may give rise to a prolonged and damaging inflammatory response. In some cases, chronic inflammation is not a sequel to acute inflammation but an independent response.

Peripheral nerve abnormalities found in individuals with CRPS usually involve the small unmyelinated and thinly myelinated nerve fibers (axons) that carry pain messages and signals to blood vessels. (Myelin is a mixture of proteins and fat-like substances that surround and insulate some nerve fibers.)

Because small fibers in the nerves communicate with blood vessels, small nerve fiber injuries may trigger the many different symptoms of CRPS. Molecules secreted from the ends of hyperactive injured small nerve fibers are thought to contribute to inflammation and blood vessel abnormalities. These peripheral nerve abnormalities in turn trigger abnormal neurological function in the spinal cord and brain, leading in some cases to complex disorders of higher cortical function.

Another abnormality in CRPS involves the blood vessels in the affected limb, which may dilate (open wider) or leak fluid into the surrounding tissue, causing red, swollen skin. The underlying muscles and deeper tissues can become starved of oxygen and nutrients, causing muscle and joint pain and damage. At times, the blood vessels may over-constrict (clamp down), causing cold, white, or bluish skin. The dilation and constriction of small blood vessels is controlled by small nerve fiber axons as well as chemical messengers in the blood.

CRPS also affects the immune system. High levels of inflammatory chemicals (cytokines) have been found in the tissues of people with CRPS. These contribute to the redness, swelling, and warmth reported by many patients. CRPS is more common in individuals with other inflammatory and autoimmune conditions such as asthma.

Activation of pain receptors, transmission and modulation of pain signals, neuro plasticity and central sensitization are all one continuum of inflammation and the inflammatory response. Irrespective of the characteristic of the pain, whether it is sharp, dull, aching, burning, stabbing, numbing or tingling, all pain arise from inflammation and the inflammatory response.

Corticosteroids have been used to treat CRPS-I, all of limited methodological quality. All the studies found corticosteroids to have a very pronounced beneficial effect. The inflammatory profile may have variations from one person to another and may have variations in the same person at different times.

The key to treatment of Pain Syndromes is an understanding of their inflammatory profile. Pain syndromes may be treated medically or surgically. The goal should be inhibition or suppression of production of the inflammatory mediators and inhibition, suppression or modulation of neuronal afferent and efferent (motor) transmission.

Other pro-inflammatory compounds include proteins called cytokines. Some of these cytokines, such as interleukin-6and C-reactive protein cause the formation of many pro-inflammatory compounds. Sensory testing showed a predominant loss of small fiber-related modalities in the patient group. The shift towards a pro-inflammatory cytokine profile in patients with CRPS suggests a potential pathogenic role in the generation of pain.

Eicosanoids are a group of biochemicals in a body that signal oxidation. Arachidonic acid is an example. These chemicals cause chronic pain. Prostaglandins, thromboxane leukotrienes etc. are also examples of eiconosoids. They cause pain, inflammation, allergy, hypertension, etc.

The origin of all pain is inflammation and the inflammatory response. The biochemical mediators of inflammation include cytokines, neuropeptides, growth factors and neurotransmitters. Irrespective of the type of pain whether it is acute or chronic pain, peripheral or central pain, nociceptive or neuropathic pain, the underlying origin is inflammation and the inflammatory response.

Sensory testing has shown a predominant loss of small fiber-related modalities in the patient group. The shift towards a pro-inflammatory cytokine profile in patients with CRPS suggests a potential pathogenic role in the generation of pain.

Cytokines are a broad and loose category of small proteins that are important in cell signaling. They are released by cells and affect the behavior of other cells. Cytokines have been classed as lymphokines, interleukins, and chemokines, based on their presumed function, cell of secretion, or target of action.

Cytokines are regulators of host responses to infection, immune responses, inflammation, and trauma. Some cytokines act to make disease worse (proinflammatory), whereas others serve to reduce inflammation and promote healing (anti-inflammatory). Interleukin (IL)-1 and tumor necrosis factor (TNF) are proinflammatory cytokines, and when they are administered to humans, they produce fever, inflammation, tissue destruction, and, in some cases, shock and death.

Proinflammatory cytokines are cytokines that are important in cell signaling and promote systemic inflammation. They are produced predominantly by activated macrophages and are involved in the upregulation of inflammatory reactions.

There is convincing evidence that inflammation plays a pivotal role in the pathophysiology of complex regional pain syndrome. Besides inflammation, central sensitization is also an important phenomenon. Mast cells are known to be involved in the inflammatory process of CRPS and also play a role (at least partially) in the process of central sensitization.

Complex regional pain syndrome type I (CRPS-I) can affect an extremity after minor trauma or operation. The pathogenesis of this syndrome is unclear. It has clinical signs of severe local inflammation as a result of an exaggerated inflammatory response, but neurogenic dysregulation is also a contributor.[1]

There appears to be a decentralization super sensitivity, as it is extended to different monoamines (5-HT, dopamine, noradrenaline, tyramine). This type of super sensitivity is compatible with the theory of a deficiency of neurotransmitters at the level of the anti-nociceptive and integrated systems, with subsequent central and peripheral super sensitivity. The severity of injury alone cannot be a determining factor for predicting the probability of RSD.[2]

The most important mediators for CRPS are the calcitonin gene-related peptide (CGRP) and substance P (SP). After peripheral trauma immune reaction (e.g. cytokines) and the attempts of the tissue to regenerate (e.g. growth factors) sensitize nociceptors and amplify neurogenic inflammation.3

Central sensitization is the physiologic manifestation of many severe peripherally induced pain states. It is maintained by nociceptive input and a physiologic change in the N-methyl-D-aspartate receptor.4

Mast cells are known to be involved in the inflammatory process of CRPS and also play a role (at least partially) in the process of central sensitization. In the development of a more mechanism-based treatment, influencing the activity of mast cells might be important in the treatment of CRPS.5

Mast cells could play a role in the production of cytokines. Furthermore, a significantly increased accumulation of leukocytes has been found in patients with CRPS I.6

CRPS I inflammation is localized. Elevated IL-8 and sTNFR I/II levels indicate an association between CRPS I and an inflammatory process. Normal WBC, CRP, and IL-6 give evidence for localized inflammation. The hypothesis of neurogenic-induced inflammation mediated by neuropeptides is supported by elevated substance P levels.7

The norepinephrine level is lower in the CRPS-affected than contralateral limb, but sympathetic sprouting and up-regulation of alpha-adrenoceptors may result in an adrenergic supersensitivity.8

The sympathetic nervous system and inflammation interact: norepinephrine influences the immune system and the production of cytokines. There is substantial evidence that this interaction contributes to the pathophysiology and clinical presentation of CRPS.

Vitamin K level decreases in the distal site of an injured extremity consequently result in patchy osteoporosis due to high level of under-carboxylated osteocalcin and unrestricted inflammation which are the cause for both initiation and progression of CRPS.9 Vitamin K was shown to suppress the inflammatory cytokines and NF-kappaB and prevent oxidative, hypoxic, ischemic injury (which have key role in both initiation and progression of CRPS) to oligodendrocytes and neurons.

In summary, Omoigui has hypothesized that the origin of all pain is inflammation and the inflammatory response.10 The biochemical mediators of inflammation include cytokines, neuropeptides, growth factors and neurotransmitters. Irrespective of the type of pain whether it is acute or chronic pain, peripheral or central pain, nociceptive or neuropathic pain, the underlying origin is inflammation and the inflammatory response. In both autoimmune and inflammatory diseases, the condition arises through aberrant reactions of the human adaptive or innate immune systems.

Immune system disorders cause abnormally low activity or over activity of the immune system. In cases of immune system over activity, the body attacks and damages its own tissues. In autoimmunity, the patient's immune system is activated against the body's own proteins.

Autoimmune diseases are chronic conditions with no cure. In chronic inflammatory diseases, neutrophils and other leukocytes are constitutively recruited by cytokines and chemokines, leading to tissue damage.

Imune system disorders cause abnormally low activity or over activity of the immune system. In cases of immune system over activity, the body attacks and damages its own tissues. With this in mind, it is hypothesized that CRPS is an inflammatory disease most probably caused by an injury in most cases. Furthermore, inflammatory diseases can be cured in many instances.

Neuropeptides induce nociceptive sensitization by enhancing IL-1 beta production in keratinocytes. 11Neuropeptides rely on both caspase-1 and cathepsin B for this enhanced production. Neurocutaneous signaling involving neuropeptide activation of the innate immunity may contribute to pain in CRPS patients.

Activation of pain receptors, transmission and modulation of pain signals, neuro plasticity and central sensitization are all one continuum of inflammation and the inflammatory response. Irrespective of the characteristic of the pain, whether it is sharp, dull, aching, burning, stabbing, numbing or tingling, all pain arises from inflammation and the inflammatory response.

In some cases, chronic inflammation is not a sequel to acute inflammation but an independent response. As previously mentioned, this could be an explanation for the development of CRPS.

References

1.   Schinkel C, Kirschner MH. Status of immune mediators in complex regional pain syndrome type I. Curr Pain Headache Rep. 2008;12(3):182-185.

2.   Bahador R, Mirbolook A, Arbab S, Derakhshan P, Gholizadeh A, Abedi S. The Relation Between Reflex Sympathetic

Dystrophy Syndrome and Trauma Severity in Patients With Distal Tibia Fracture. Trauma Mon. 2016;21(2):e25926.

3.   Birklein F, Schmelz M. Neuropeptides, neurogenic inflammation and complex regional pain syndrome (CRPS). Neurosci Lett. 2008;437(3):199-202.

4.   Schwartzman RJ, Grothusen J, Kiefer TR, Rohr P. Neuropathic central pain: epidemiology, etiology, and treatment options. Arch Neurol. 2001;58(10):1547-1550.

5.   Dirckx M, Groeneweg G, van Daele PL, Stronks DL, Huygen FJ. Mast cells: a new target in the treatment of complex regional pain syndrome? Pain Pract. 2013;13(8):599-603.

6.   Tan EC, Oyen WJ, Goris RJ. Leukocytes in Complex Regional Pain Syndrome type I. Inflammation. 2005;29(4-6):182-186.

7.   Schinkel C, Gaertner A, Zaspel J, Zedler S, Faist E, Schuermann M. Inflammatory mediators are altered in the acute phase of posttraumatic complex regional pain syndrome. Clin J Pain. 2006;22(3):235-239.

8.   Schlereth T, Drummond PD, Birklein F. Inflammation in CRPS: role of the sympathetic supply. Auton Neurosci. 2014;182:102-107.

9.   Ediz L, Hiz O, Meral I, Alpayci M. Complex regional pain syndrome: a vitamin K dependent entity? Med Hypotheses. 2010;75(3):319-323.

10.   Omoigui S. The biochemical origin of pain: the origin of all pain is inflammation and the inflammatory response. Part 2 of 3 - inflammatory profile of pain syndromes. Med Hypotheses. 2007;69(6):1169-1178.

11.   Shi X, Wang L, Li X, Sahbaie P, Kingery WS, Clark JD. Neuropeptides contribute to peripheral nociceptive sensitization by regulating interleukin-1beta production in keratinocytes. Anesth Analg. 2011;113(1):175-183.

3. Autoimmune Cause?

Complex Regional Pain Syndrome (CRPS) is associated with non-dermatomal patterns of pain, unusual movement disorders, and somatovisceral dysfunctions. These symptoms are viewed by some neurologists and psychiatrists as being psychogenic in origin.1

An autoimmune attack on self-antigens found in the peripheral and central nervous system may underlie a number of CRPS symptoms. Immune system disorders cause abnormally low activity or over activity of the immune system. In cases of immune system over activity, the body attacks and damages its own tissue.

CRPS is an etiologically unclear syndrome with the main symptoms being pain, trophic and autonomic disturbances, and functional impairment that develops after limb trauma or operation and is located at the distal site of the affected limb.

Acute CRPS I is considered an exaggerated inflammatory disorder but over time, because of altered function of the sympathetic nervous system, and maladaptive neuroplasticity, CRPS I evolves into a neurological disorder.2

Increased systemic CGRP levels in patients with acute CRPS suggest neurogenic inflammation as a pathophysiologic mechanism contributing to vasodilation, edema, and increased sweating. However, pain and hyperalgesia, in particular in chronic stages, were independent of increased neuropeptide concentration.3

A previous study reported that immobilization alone increased neuropeptide signaling and caused nociceptive and inflammatory changes similar to those observed after tibia fracture and casting, and that early mobilization after fracture with pinning inhibited these changes. Early limb mobilization after fracture may prevent the development of CRPS.4

In the complex regional pain syndrome (CRPS) patients exhibit multiorgan pathology and inflammatory changes after limb trauma. The role of inflammatory cytokines and other mediators in both the central and peripheral nervous systems that contribute to the development and progression of CRPS has been hypothesized. 5

In an animal study here was an up-regulation of inflammatory cytokine expression in the rat hind paw skin and in keratinocytes at 4 weeks post-fracture. These inflammatory mediators appear to play a crucial role in the development of pain behavior after fracture, as we have repeatedly demonstrated that inhibition of cytokine and NGF signaling prevents the allodynia and attenuates unweighting at 4 weeks post-fracture.6

Patients with CRPS may have the following two distinct components: neuropathic pain that includes severe spontaneous pain or severe persistent mechanical allodynia and prolonged regional inflammation, the early phase of which could be indicated by positive inflammatory symptoms of pain (tenderness), heat, redness, swelling and loss of function and their alleviation with corticosteroids.7

There are almost as many diagnostic criteria as there are names to this disorder. The term CRPS has been subdivided into type I and type II. CRPS I is intended to encompass reflex sympathetic dystrophy and similar disorders without a nerve injury; while CRPS II occurs after damage to a peripheral nerve.

There are numerous etiological pathophysiological events that have been incriminated in development of CRPS, including inflammation, autoimmune responses, abnormal cytokine production, sympathetic-sensory disorders, altered blood flow and central cortical reorganization.8

CRPS is currently considered to be a multi-system condition that includes interactions between the immune system, the Autonomic Nervous System (ANS) and the Central Nervous System (CNS). An autoimmune disorder is a condition that occurs when the immune system mistakenly attacks and destroys healthy body tissue.

There are more than 80 different types of autoimmune disorders. Autoimmunity, on the other hand, is the presence of self-reactive immune response with or without damage or pathology resulting from it. This may be restricted to certain organs or involve a particular tissue in different places.

Differential activity of endogenous pain modulating systems may play a pivotal role in the development of CRPS. Neuronal plasticity of the somatosensory cortex accounts for central sensory signs. Also the motor system is subject to central adaptive changes in patients with CRPS.

Additionally other proinflammatory cytokines involved in the inflammatory response in CRPS have been identified. In terms of the sympathetic nervous system, recent evidence rather points to a sensitization of adrenergic receptors than to increased efferent sympathetic activity.

Particularly the expression of alpha (1)-adrenoceptors on nociceptive C-fibers may play a major role. These pathophysiological ideas do not exclude each other. The variety of the involved systems may explain the versatile clinical picture of CRPS.9

CRPS patients exhibit changes which occur in somatosensory systems processing noxious, tactile and thermal information, in sympathetic systems innervating skin (blood vessels, sweat glands), and in the somatomotor system. This indicates that the central representations of these systems are changed and data show that CRPS is a systemic disease involving several neuronal systems.

The immune system is a complex organization within the body that is designed normally to "seek and destroy" invaders of the body, including infectious agents. Screening for antinuclear antibodies (ANA) is one of the diagnostic tests, which is usually performed if a person is suspected to have a systemic autoimmune disease. Antineuronal antibodies are autoantibodies directed against antigens in the central and/or peripheral nervous system.

CRPS is associated with limb-confined sensory, motor, skin, bone and autonomic abnormalities. Recent research has shown that some patients respond to treatment with immunoglobulins, and that a majority have IgG serum-autoantibodies directed against, and activating autonomic receptors.10

Patients with autoimmune diseases frequently have unusual antibodies circulating in their blood that target their own body tissues. Autoimmune diseases are more frequent in women than in men.

It is felt that the estrogen of females may influence the immune system to predispose some women to autoimmune diseases. Furthermore, the presence of one autoimmune disease increases the chance for developing another simultaneous autoimmune disease.

Patients with minimal preceding trauma had stronger nervous tissue-specific reactivity than other patients, regardless of disease duration. These results provide preliminary evidence for immune activation early in CRPS and, additionally, that patients with minimal trauma may comprise an autoimmune subgroup.11

A study demonstrated the presence of autoantibodies in a subset of CRPS patients with agonistic-like properties on the beta(2) adrenergic receptor and/or the muscarinic-2 receptor.12 The investigators identified these autoantibodies as immunoglobulin G directed against peptide sequences from the second extracellular loop of these receptors. The identification of functionally active autoantibodies in serum samples from CRPS patients supports an autoimmune pathogenesis of CRPS.

The human immune system typically produces both T-cells and B-cells that are capable of being reactive with self-antigens, but these self-reactive cells are usually either killed prior to becoming active within the immune system, placed into a state of anergy (silently removed from their role within the immune system to over-activation), or removed from their role within the immune system by regulatory cells.

When any one of these mechanisms fail, it is possible to have a reservoir of self-reactive cells that become functional within the immune system. The mechanisms of preventing self-reactive T-cells from being created takes place through Negative selection process within the thymus as the T-cell is developing into a mature immune cell.

The blood cells in the body's immune system help protect against harmful substances. Examples include bacteria, viruses, toxins, cancer cells, and blood and tissue from outside the body. These substances contain antigens. The immune system produces antibodies against these antigens that enable it to destroy these harmful substances.

When a patient has an autoimmune disorder, the immune system does not distinguish between healthy tissue and antigens. As a result, the body sets off a reaction that destroys normal tissues.

Tests that may be done to diagnose an autoimmune disorder include: Antinuclear antibody tests, Autoantibody tests, CBC, C-reactive protein (CRP) and the Erythrocyte sedimentation rate (ESR).

Sera of 12 patients with complex regional pain syndrome (CRPS) were previously tested for the occurrence of autoantibodies against nervous system structures.[13]

Immunohistochemistry revealed autoantibodies against autonomic nervous system structures in 5 of 12 (41.6%) of the patients. Western blot analysis showed neuronal reactivity in 11 of 12 (91.6%) patients. The authors hypothesize that CRPS can result from an autoimmune process against the sympathetic nervous system.

Because autoantibodies against nervous system structures have been described in CRPS patients, an autoimmune etiology of CRPS is hypothesized.[14]

These autoantibodies bind to the surface of peripheral autonomic neurons. Using a competitive binding assay, it can be shown that at least some of the CRPS sera bind to the same neuronal epitope. Autoimmune etiology of CRPS is a new pathophysiological concept.

Autoimmunity has been suggested as one of the pathophysiologic mechanisms that may underlie complex regional pain syndrome (CRPS).

Screening for antinuclear antibodies (ANA) is one of the diagnostic tests, which is usually performed if a person is suspected to have a systemic autoimmune disease. Autoantibodies may be associated with the pathophysiology of CRPS, at least in a subset of patients.15

Patients with longstanding CRPS have serum antibodies to alpha-1a receptors, and that measurement of these antibodies may be useful in the diagnosis and management of the patients.16 Preliminary evidence for immune activation early in CRPS and, additionally, patients with minimal trauma may comprise an autoimmune subgroup.11

Data show that about 30-40% of CRPS patients have surface-binding autoantibodies against an inducible autonomic nervous system autoantigen. These data support an autoimmune hypothesis in CRPS patients.17

In as IgG-transfer-trauma model for CRPS, serum IgG from chronic CRPS patients induced clinical and laboratory features resembling the human disease were studied. These results support the hypothesis that autoantibodies may contribute to the pathophysiology of CRPS, and that autoantibody-removing therapies may be effective treatments for long-standing CRPS.18

CRPS is associated with an autoantibody-mediated autoimmune process in some cases. CRPS has unusual features, including a non-destructive and regionally-confined course.

A previous study proposed that CRPS constitutes a prototype of a new kind of autoimmunity, which was termed injury-triggered, regionally-restricted autoantibody-mediated autoimmune disorder with minimally-destructive course.10

Screening for antinuclear antibodies (ANA) is one of the diagnostic tests, which is usually performed if a person is suspected to have a systemic autoimmune disease. Antineuronal antibodies are autoantibodies directed against antigens in the central and/or peripheral nervous system.15

The identification of functionally active autoantibodies in serum samples from CRPS patients supports an autoimmune pathogenesis of CRPS.12 An autoimmune etiology of CRPS is a new pathophysiological concept and may have severe impact on the treatment of this often chronic disease. Autoantibodies may contribute to the pathophysiology of CRPS, and that autoantibody-removing therapies may be effective treatments for long-standing CRPS.18

At early stages, complex regional pain syndrome (CRPS) is clinically characterized by damage of peripheral tissues and nerves (edema, activation of osteoblasts, hyperalgesia to blunt pressure). These signs are the result of a dysbalance of pro- and anti-inflammatory cytokines, which normalizes approximately 6 months after the beginning of the disease, independent from clinical outcome.

At the same time, evolving clinical signs such as allodynia, cold hyperalgesia, reduced tactile acuity or symptoms of disrupted body representation (e.g., neglect-like syndrome, impaired hand laterality recognition or shift of the body midline) suggest a crucial role of the CNS in the pathophysiology of this pain syndrome.[19]

The origin of all pain is inflammation and the inflammatory response. The biochemical mediators of inflammation include cytokines, neuropeptides, growth factors and neurotransmitters. Irrespective of the type of pain whether it is acute or chronic pain, peripheral or central pain, nociceptive or neuropathic pain, the underlying origin is inflammation and the inflammatory response.

Activation of pain receptors, transmission and modulation of pain signals, neuro plasticity and central sensitization are all one continuum of inflammation and the inflammatory response.[20]

References

1.   Cooper MS, Clark VP. Neuroinflammation, neuroautoimmunity, and the co-morbidities of complex regional pain syndrome. J Neuroimmune Pharmacol. 2013;8(3):452-469.

2.   Bussa M, Mascaro A, Cuffaro L, Rinaldi S. Adult Complex Regional Pain Syndrome Type I: A Narrative Review. PM R. 2016.

3.   Birklein F, Schmelz M, Schifter S, Weber M. The important role of neuropeptides in complex regional pain syndrome. Neurology. 2001;57(12):2179-2184.

4.   Guo TZ, Wei T, Li WW, Li XQ, Clark JD, Kingery WS. Immobilization contributes to exaggerated neuropeptide signaling, inflammatory changes, and nociceptive sensitization after fracture in rats. J Pain. 2014;15(10):1033-1045.

5.   Hauser J, Hsu B, Nader ND. Inflammatory processes in complex regional pain syndromes. Immunol Invest. 2013;42(4):263-272.

6.   Kingery WS. Role of neuropeptide, cytokine, and growth factor signaling in complex regional pain syndrome. Pain Med. 2010;11(8):1239-1250.

7.   Moriwaki K, Yuge O, Tanaka H, Sasaki H, Izumi H, Kaneko K. Neuropathic pain and prolonged regional inflammation as two distinct symptomatological components in complex regional pain syndrome with patchy osteoporosis--a pilot study. Pain. 1997;72(1-2):277-282.

8.   Borchers AT, Gershwin ME. Complex regional pain syndrome: a comprehensive and critical review. Autoimmun Rev. 2014;13(3):242-265.

9.   Nickel FT, Maihofner C. [Current concepts in pathophysiology of CRPS I]. Handchir Mikrochir Plast Chir. 2010;42(1):8-14.

10.   Goebel A, Blaes F. Complex regional pain syndrome, prototype of a novel kind of autoimmune disease. Autoimmun Rev. 2013;12(6):682-686.

11.   Goebel A, Vogel H, Caneris O, et al. Immune responses to Campylobacter and serum autoantibodies in patients with complex regional pain syndrome. J Neuroimmunol. 2005;162(1-2):184-189.

12.   Kohr D, Singh P, Tschernatsch M, et al. Autoimmunity against the beta2 adrenergic receptor and muscarinic-2 receptor in complex regional pain syndrome. Pain. 2011;152(12):2690-2700.

13.   Blaes F, Schmitz K, Tschernatsch M, et al. Autoimmune etiology of complex regional pain syndrome (M. Sudeck). Neurology. 2004;63(9):1734-1736.

14.   Blaes F, Tschernatsch M, Braeu ME, et al. Autoimmunity in complex-regional pain syndrome. Ann N Y Acad Sci. 2007;1107:168-173.

15.   Dirckx M, Schreurs MW, de Mos M, Stronks DL, Huygen FJ. The prevalence of autoantibodies in complex regional pain syndrome type I. Mediators Inflamm. 2015;2015:718201.

16.   Dubuis E, Thompson V, Leite MI, et al. Longstanding complex regional pain syndrome is associated with activating autoantibodies against alpha-1a adrenoceptors. Pain. 2014;155(11):2408-2417.

17.   Kohr D, Tschernatsch M, Schmitz K, et al. Autoantibodies in complex regional pain syndrome bind to a differentiation-dependent neuronal surface autoantigen. Pain. 2009;143(3):246-251.

18.   Tekus V, Hajna Z, Borbely E, et al. A CRPS-IgG-transfer-trauma model reproducing inflammatory and positive sensory signs

associated with complex regional pain syndrome. Pain. 2014;155(2):299-308.

19.   Reinersmann A, Maier C, Schwenkreis P, Lenz M. Complex regional pain syndrome: more than a peripheral disease. Pain Manag. 2013;3(6):495-502.

20.   Omoigui S. The biochemical origin of pain: the origin of all pain is inflammation and the inflammatory response. Part 2 of 3 - inflammatory profile of pain syndromes. Med Hypotheses. 2007;69(6):1169-1178.

4. Legal Causation

Physicians who treat nonspecific disease entities may be asked on occasion to give their expert opinions on causation of a particular pathologic entity. For example the cause of the Complex Regional Pain Syndrome (CRPS) has yet to be determined. Furthermore, there is no consensus on the diagnostic or treatment criteria for this entity. This results in controversies regarding the validity of both the diagnosis and the treatment of this disorder. Physicians must therefore attempt to assign causation of CRPS with attention to relevant evidence based medicine.

There is minimal consensus as mentioned among physicians with respect to the diagnosis of CRPS and the causation of CRPS. Unfortunately, it is a difficult entity to diagnose and treat. A gold standard in diagnosing CRPS has not been found yet, and diagnostics are based on the patients medical history and correlating clinical signs. The criteria for the diagnosis of CRPS are mainly based on the patient's history and physical examination and are determined by the patient's examining physician.

There is currently no imaging X ray or other tests that will diagnose CRPS. Because of the controversy concerning the manner in which the sympathetic nervous system is involved in reflex sympathetic dystrophy (RSD), its name was changed to one having no mechanistic connotations.1

Historically, there has been considerable controversy regarding CRPS as a specific disease entity. In particular, the precise mechanism of the sympathetic dysfunction as well as the nature of the psychological dysfunction commonly observed in patients with CRPS has been the subject of considerable debate.

Differences exist between states as well with reference to CRPS diagnosis and treatment with respect to causation in workman's compensation cases. Furthermore, some health insurance companies will not pay for stellate ganglion blockade which is a modality commonly used to treat CRPS.

There is a consensus that two types of CRPS exist. CRPS I does not involve a partial injury to a nerve or one of its branches but does involve a minor injury following a sprain or fracture. CRPS II on the other hand involves an injury to a nerve or one of its branches.

Complex regional pain syndrome (CRPS) most often follows injury to peripheral nerves or their endings in soft tissue. A combination of prostanoids, kinins and cytokines cause peripheral nociceptive sensitization. In time, these neurons undergo central sensitization that lead to a major physiological change of the autonomic, pain and motor systems.

The role of the immune system and the sickness response is becoming clearer as microglia are activated following injury and can induce central sensitization while astrocytes may maintain the process.2

There are two primary criteria for the diagnosis of CRPS, the ISAP and Budapest.

IASP diagnostic criteria for complex regional pain syndrome (CRPS): All four of the following criteria can be used for the diagnosis of CRPS to be established: 1. the presence of an initiating noxious event, or a cause of immobilization; 2. continuing pain, pain with which the pain is disproportionate to the initiating event; 3. confirmation at some time of edema, changes in blood flow, or abnormal sweating activity in the area of the pain such as changes in skin temperature, skin color, or sweating; 4. and the absence of other conditions that would account for the pain and dysfunction. One must rule out the more common conditions that could mimic CRPS such as diabetic or thyroid neuropathies, nerve entrapment syndromes such as the carpal tunnel syndrome, disc disease or the thoracic outlet syndrome. Also, one should consider in the differential diagnosis the following: deep vein thrombosis, cellulitis, vascular insufficiency, lymphedema, and

Clinical Diagnostic Criteria (the "Budapest Criteria") for CRPS: CRPS describes an array of painful conditions that are characterized by a continuing (spontaneous and/or evoked) regional pain that is seemingly disproportionate in time or degree to the usual course of any known trauma or other lesion. The pain is regional (not in a specific nerve territory or dermatome) and usually has a distal predominance of abnormal sensory, motor, sudomotor, vasomotor, and/or trophic findings. The syndrome shows variable progression over time. To make the clinical diagnosis, the following criteria must be met:

1. Continuing pain, which is disproportionate to any inciting event

2. Must report at least one symptom in three of the four following categories: Sensory: Reports of hyperesthesia and/or allodynia. Vasomotor: Reports of temperature asymmetry and/or skin color changes and/or skin color asymmetry. Sudomotor/Edema: Reports of edema and/or sweating changes and/or sweating asymmetry.Motor/Trophic: Reports of

decreased range of motion and/or motor dysfunction (weakness, tremor, dystonia) and/or trophic changes (hair, nail, skin).

3. Must display at least one sign at time of evaluation in two or more of the following categories: Sensory: Evidence of hyperalgesia (to pinprick) and/or allodynia (to light touch and/or temperature sensation and/or deep somatic pressure and/or joint movement), Vasomotor: Evidence of temperature asymmetry (>1 °C) and/or skin color changes and/or asymmetry, Sudomotor/Edema: Evidence of edema and/or sweating changes and/or sweating asymmetry, Motor/Trophic: Evidence of decreased range of motion and/or motor dysfunction (weakness, tremor, dystonia) and/or trophic changes (hair, nail, skin).

4. There is no other diagnosis that better explains the signs and symptoms.

For research purposes, the diagnostic decision rule should be at least one symptom in all four symptom categories and at least one sign (observed at evaluation) in two or more sign categories. The understanding of causation is important in understanding the causes of injuries in individuals. However, a patient need to understand causation as it applies to groups in the population as well. In this case a patient needs to understand a model of causation.

The determination of causation is difficult to ascertain. One needs to initially know what event caused the individual's medical condition. One can use the "but for" theory in the case example presented (a result would not have happened but for the occurrence of a certain event).

One may want to further consider the Bradford Hill model of causation to help establish causation in CRPS cases.[3] Hills Criteria of Causation outlines the minimal conditions needed to establish a causal relationship between two items. These criteria were originally presented by Austin Bradford Hill to determine the causal link between a specific factor (e.g., cigarette smoking) and a disease (lung cancer).

While it is quite easy to claim that smoking causes lung cancer, it is quite difficult when a patient attempt to establish a valid connection between the two events. In many cases of CRPS it is difficult to demonstrate scientifically that such causal relationships exist. Hill's Criteria provide an additional means to evaluate the many theories and hypotheses proposed by the claimants, adjusters, case workers, physicians etc.

Professor Hill and members of the United States Public Health Department developed the following criteria that can help to evaluate criteria to attempt to establish causation when two or more possible causative factors exist. Hill stated however, that cause-effect decisions cannot be based on a set of rules. Hill also stated that both the medical, scientific and legal establishments need to consider costs and benefits when making decisions about health-care interventions.

1.   Temporal Relationship: Exposure always precedes the outcome. If factor "A" is believed to cause a disease, then it is clear that factor "A" must necessarily always precede the occurrence of the disease. This is the only absolutely essential criterion in Hill's first criteria. If the cases presented revealed that each claimant had lumbar degenerative disc disease this makes causation determination more difficult. Degenerative disc disease may cause low back pain but not always. It is a chronic condition. This condition does not have to cause low back pain. However, lifting 40 pound boxes do not always cause low back pain either.

2.   Strength of Association: It is defined by the strength of the association as measured by appropriate statistical tests. The stronger the association, the more likely it is that the relation is causal.

Cigarette smoking can cause lung cancer. An asbestos worker can develop lung cancer. However, if the worker smokes and also works with asbestos the worker has a higher incidence of developing lung cancer. Which factor caused the lung cancer?

3.   Dose-Response Relationship: In some situations an exposure to an activity or exposure can cause significant impairment. If a patient attempts to lift a 500 pound weight he/she may suffer a disc herniation. If a patient keeps attempting this task, the risk of injury increases. An increasing amount of exposure increases the risk. If a dose-response relationship is present, it is strong evidence for a causal relationship. However, the absence of a dose-response relationship does not rule out a causal relationship.

A patient does not have to lift a 40 pound box to develop low back pain. A threshold may exist above which a relationship may develop. At the same time, if a specific factor is the cause of a disease, the incidence of the disease should decline when exposure to the factor is reduced or eliminated. In many instances, a low dose of activity can enable the body to repair simple sprains and strains and enable one's body to repair itself.

4.   Consistency: The association is consistent when results are replicated in different settings using different methods. That is, if a relationship is causal, we would expect to find it consistently in different populations. Sustaining an upper extremity fracture should cause CRPS to

occur in every group of workers to demonstrate consistency among studies if one wanted to establish injury and CRPS causation.

For example, it has taken thousands of highly technical studies of the relationship between cigarette smoking and cancer before a definitive conclusion could be made that cigarette smoking increases the risk of cancer. Similarly, it would require numerous studies of the difference between ages and male and female performance of a specific task by a number of different workers under a variety of different circumstances before a conclusion could be made regarding whether an or gender difference exists in the performance of such behaviors.

If one examines the demographics of the injured workers, their data must be compared to that of the uninjured workers and to workers on other shifts, other departments etc. to attempt to evaluate definite causation.

5. Plausibility: A conclusion can be assumed for which no sound evidence may exist. One may think that a certain virus causes a respiratory infection. However, there may be no conclusive evidence that any certain vector transmits the virus to a patient's body even though a presumptive conclusion is believed to exist between a vector and a disease.

One may correlate that in even years that an overweight president will be elected president. The likelihood that these events are related is minimal and not plausible. On the other hand, the discovery of a correlation between population growth and the use of oil in the United States is logical and plausible.

6. Consideration of Alternate Explanations: In judging whether a factor is the cause of an event then it is necessary to determine the extent to which researchers have taken other possible causes into account and have effectively ruled out alternate explanations.

In other words, it is necessary to consider multiple hypotheses before making conclusions about relationship between any two items under investigation. This is where comparison to placebo groups is important. If factor A causes event B, then event B should not occur. If B occurs without A then other causes of B must be ruled out to state that events A and B are related.

7. Experiment: The condition can be altered by an appropriate experimental regimen. 'smust use caution however, if one tries and extrapolate animal studies with causation in humans. It would be extremely difficult to argue causation of low back pain for example based upon animal studies.

8.Specificity: This is established when a single cause produces a specific event. When a acidic solution contacts litmus paper, the litmus paper turns red. On the other hand, the causes attributed to lung cancer do not meet this criterion. When specificity of an association is found, it provides additional support for a causal relationship.

However, absence of specificity in no way negates a causal relationship. Causality is most often multiple especially when discussing human medical conditions because multiple factors are usually involved. This is the weakest criteria when discussing injury causation or disease causation. Therefore, it is necessary to examine specific causal relationships within a larger systemic perspective to formulate a plausible conclusion.

9. Coherence: This is determined when the cause is consistent with the natural history of the effect. The association should be compatible with existing theory and current medical knowledge. In other words, it is necessary to evaluate claims of causality within the context of the current state of knowledge within a given field.

However, as with the issue of plausibility, research that disagrees with established theory and knowledge are not automatically false. They may in fact, force a reconsideration of accepted beliefs and principles.

A patient should be aware that there is no diagnostic gold standard or an objective test for the diagnosis of CRPS. Abnormal neurohumoral and inflammatory mechanisms have however, been implicated in its causation usually following trivial noxious event in an extremity.4

A variety of other conditions can mimic the signs and symptoms of reflex sympathetic dystrophy and have to be ruled out before a definite diagnosis of RSD can be established. These include: rheumatoid arthritis, gout, lumbar or cervical disk herniation, peripheral neuropathy, diabetic neuropathy, nerve entrapment syndromes, osteomyelitis, septic arthritis, thoracic outlet syndrome, cellulitis, vascular insufficiency, lymphedema, bursitis, tendonitis, patella injuries of the knee, meniscal tears of the knee, femoral/tibial injury or bone fracture.

Some physicians will tell a patient that he/she does not have CRPS because he/she has a normal triple phase bone scan. Insurance companies will deny a patient treatment also because of a normal scan. A normal triple phase bone scan does not rule out CRPS.

In the second phase of CRPS, the bone scan is normal. It is possible that the Herpes Simplex Virus contributes to CRPS as well. Therefore, a virus infection theory is an attractive hypothesis that accounts for many enigmas of CRPS causation.5

Another study indicated that motor nerve injury and female gender are risk factors for CRPS.6 The prevention measures should be focused mainly on females and patients with motor nerve injury in order to reduce the risk of CRPS.

A positive history for allergy/hypersensitivity reactions is a predisposing conditions for CRPS I in orthopedic patients. These hypersensitivity reactions may prove important in gaining a better understanding in the pathophysiology of CRPS I as a regional pain syndrome.7

Significant differences between CRPS patients and healthy persons were found in a family history. The results suggest that headache and a first-degree family history of headache are also risk factors for CRPS.8

Work in a research consortium raised internal validity concerns regarding the IASP criteria for Complex Regional Pain Syndrome, suggesting problems with inadequate sensitivity and specificity. IASP criteria for CRPS have inadequate specificity and are likely to lead to over diagnosis. 9

There is no consensus on the diagnostic or treatment criteria for CRPS. This results in controversies regarding the validity of both the diagnosis and the treatment of this disorder. Physicians must therefore attempt to assign causation of CRPS with attention to relevant evidence based medicine.

Several pathophysiological concepts have been proposed to explain the symptoms of CRPS: 1, facilitated neurogenic inflammation; 2, pathological sympatho-afferent coupling; 3, neuroplastic changes within the CNS; 4. genetic factors may predispose for CRPS.10

Physicians who treat nonspecific disease entities may be asked on occasion to give their expert opinions on causation of a particular pathologic entity. Furthermore, there is no consensus on the diagnostic or treatment criteria for this entity.

This results in controversies regarding the validity of both the diagnosis and the treatment of this disorder. In order to establish CRPS causation, a physician must understand medical and legal causation.

Causation in general, is an event that produces an effect. Causal relevance helps explain if and why one event caused another event. If a patient want to know why an airplane crashed for example, a patient will seek an antecedent event that could have caused the accident such as inclement weather, ice on the wings or runway, engine malfunction etc.

Causation implies that a set of circumstances exists that in their presence, a specific effect occurs and in their absence, the effect does not occur. For example, litmus paper always turns a specific color when placed in an acidic or basic solution.

Medical causation determination is usually not this simple. Medical causation is based on scientific epidemiological studies and on statistical significance ($p < 0.05$). Legal causation on the other hand, is based on probable cause or a "but for principle". The "but for" rule states than an effect would not have occurred but for a specific causative event.based on a probability greater than 50%.

There is no consensus on a single criteria set that can be used to diagnose CRPS. Several criteria sets can be used to diagnose CRPS.11 For example, the diagnosis of CRPS defined by the International Association for the Study of Pain (IASP) clinical criteria for CRPS is as follows: the presence of regional pain and sensory changes following a noxious event, pain is defined as abnormal skin color, temperature change, abnormal sudomotor activity, edema, no distribution of the pain of a single nerve in the extremity and the combination of these findings exceeds their expected magnitude in response to known physical damage during and following the inciting event.1,9 Eisenberg and Melamed on the other hand reported painless CRPS in a group of patients that they studied.12

Thermography however, has been reported to be a useful method to diagnose CRPS.13 Stress infra-red thermography is a sensitive and specific indicator of CRPS-I.14 Infrared thermography (IRT) is a useful tool for assessing skin temperature abnormalities in patients with complex regional pain syndrome and the reliability of IRT for assessing skin temperature abnormalities in CRPS was high when the regions of interest were determined based on patient history and symptoms.15 A temperature difference can be detected via infrared thermography between the affected extremity and the normal extremity.

Concepts of cause and causal inference are largely self-taught from early learning experiences. A model of causation that describes causes in terms of sufficient causes and their component causes illuminates important principles such as multi-causality, the dependence of the strength of component causes on the prevalence of complementary component causes, and interaction between component causes.16

CRPS IASP criteria are reported to have a high sensitivity but a lower specificity.11 If the diagnostic criteria for CRPS I are not used uniformly, the populations in clinical studies may not be uniform either.

Whether different authors are describing the same syndrome and whether their findings can be compared is open to question. It is established that the IASP criteria for CRPS I are poorly used in clinical studies.17

Several pathophysiological concepts have been proposed to explain the symptoms of CRPS: 1, facilitated neurogenic inflammation; 2, pathological sympatho-afferent coupling; 3, neuroplastic changes within the CNS; 4.

Contrary to other authors, sympathetic signs such as hyperhidrosis are reported by Veldman et al to be infrequent and therefore have no diagnostic value.18 It is unlikely that CRPS is a simple exaggeration of post-traumatic inflammation.

CRPS most often follows injury to peripheral nerves or their endings in soft tissue. These neurons undergo central sensitization that lead to a major physiological change of the autonomic, pain and motor systems. The role of the immune system and the sickness response is becoming clearer as microglia are activated following injury and can induce central sensitization while astrocytes may maintain the process.2

Cigarette smoking has also been reported to be been statistically associated with CRPS and may be involved in its pathogenesis by enhancing sympathetic activity or vasoconstriction.19

Because sympathetic hyperactivity is not present in every patient, sympatholytic interventions are only recommended only for patients with sympathetically maintained pain and not for those with sympathetically independent pain.20

There is a consensus that two types of CRPS exist. CRPS I does not involve a partial injury to a nerve or one of its branches but does involve a minor injury following a sprain or fracture. Because there is no consensus on the diagnosis or cause of CRPS, therapy is based on a multidisciplinary approach as well and multiple modalities have been recommended.10,21-24 Non-pharmacological approaches include physiotherapy and occupational therapy.

Accumulating experimental and clinical evidence supports the hypothesis that complex regional pain syndrome type I (CRPS-I) may be a small fiber neuropathy. CRPS-I may be associated with changes in the ultramicroscopic small fiber structure that cannot be visualized with commercially available techniques.25

Alternatively, functional rather than structural alterations of small fibers or pathological changes at a more proximal site such as the spinal cord or brain may be responsible for the syndrome.

Pharmacotherapy is based on individual symptoms and includes steroids, free radical scavengers, treatment of neuropathic pain, and agents interfering with bone metabolism (calcitonin, biphosphonates). Sympathetic blocks may also be beneficial in some patients. Implantation of dorsal column stimulators may benefit some patients as well.

Electro convulsant therapy has also been recommended for the treatment of CRPS.22,26 Therapies to avoid due to lack of efficacy, lack of evidence, or a high likelihood of adverse outcomes are IV regional sympathetic blocks with anything but bretylium, sympathetic ganglion blocks with local anesthetics, systemic IV sympathetic inhibition, acupuncture, and sympathectomy.27

Epidemiologic studies conclude that the incidence of CRPS is low. The estimated overall incidence rate of CRPS reported by de Mos et al was 26.2 per 100,000 person years (95% CI: 23.0-29.7).28 Females were affected at least three times more often than males (ratio: 3.4). The highest incidence occurred in females in the age category of 61-70 years.

The upper extremity was affected more frequently than the lower extremity and a fracture was the most common precipitating event. The severity of nerve damage does not appear to affect the onset of CRPS.

A pseudodystrophy is a disuse dystrophy and must be distinguished from CRPS. They described the signs and symptoms of a pseudodystrophy as severe pain at a joint or part of a limb with major functional disability, cyanosis, coldness and edema or atrophy.

Rothman's concept of causation is another model that may be used to address CRPS causation. In this model the strength of a causal association depends on the relative prevalence of other component causes for the same disease.29 In the Rothman model a single cause is insufficient by itself to cause the disease in question.

Rothman's model of causation describes a cause in terms of sufficient causes and their component causes and illuminates important principles such as multi-causality, the dependence of the strength of component causes on the prevalence of complementary component causes, and the interaction between component causes.16

The Rothman model might be appropriate for CRPS causation determination because a single cause of CRPS has yet to be determined.

Concepts of cause and causal inference are largely self-taught from early learning experiences. A model of causation that describes causes in terms of sufficient causes and their component causes illuminates important principles such as multi-causality, the dependence of the strength of component causes on the prevalence of complementary component causes, and interaction between component causes.16

The determination of CRPS must therefore, be based on sound science. This however, is difficult when one attempts to assign a specific medical diagnosis to a condition that is primarily determined by subjective symptoms and nonspecific physiologic signs and has no valid diagnostic tests to make an accurate diagnosis.

It would furthermore, be unreasonable to attribute CRPS causation to a single factor when clearly other risk factors are present. However, thermography and skin biopsy with small nerve fiber analysis may be helpful as well as reliable is determining a diagnosis of CRPS.

References

1.   Stanton-Hicks M. Reflex sympathetic dystrophy: a sympathetically mediated pain syndrome or not? Curr Rev Pain. 2000;4(4):268-275.

2.   Schwartzman RJ, Alexander GM, Grothusen J. Pathophysiology of complex regional pain syndrome. Expert Rev Neurother. 2006;6(5):669-681.

3.   Hill AB. The Environment and Disease: Association or Causation? Proc R Soc Med. 1965;58:295-300.

4.   Bhattarai B, Shrestha BP, Rahman TR, Sharma SK, Tripathi M. Complex regional pain syndrome (CRPS) type-1 following snake bite: a case report. Nepal Med Coll J. 2008;10(4):278-280.

5.   Muneshige H, Toda K, Kimura H, Asou T. Does a viral infection cause complex regional pain syndrome? Acupunct Electrother Res. 2003;28(3-4):183-192.

6.   Demir SE, Ozaras N, Karamehmetoglu SS, Karacan I, Aytekin E. Risk factors for complex regional pain syndrome in patients with traumatic extremity injury. Ulus Travma Acil Cerrahi Derg. 2010;16(2):144-148.

7.   Li X, Kenter K, Newman A, O'Brien S. Allergy/hypersensitivity reactions as a predisposing factor to complex regional pain syndrome I in orthopedic patients. Orthopedics. 2014;37(3):e286-291.

8.   Toda K, Muneshige H, Maruishi M, Kimura H, Asou T. Headache may be a risk factor for complex regional pain syndrome. Clin Rheumatol. 2006;25(5):728-730.

9.   Bruehl S, Harden RN, Galer BS, et al. External validation of IASP diagnostic criteria for Complex Regional Pain Syndrome and

proposed research diagnostic criteria. International Association for the Study of Pain. Pain. 1999;81(1-2):147-154.

10.   Maihofner C, Birklein F. [Complex regional pain syndromes: new aspects on pathophysiology and therapy]. Fortschr Neurol Psychiatr. 2007;75(6):331-342.

11.   Niehof SP, Beerthuizen A, Huygen FJ, Zijlstra FJ. Using skin surface temperature to differentiate between complex regional pain syndrome type 1 patients after a fracture and control patients with various complaints after a fracture. Anesth Analg. 2008;106(1):270-277, table of contents.

12.   Eisenberg E, Melamed E. Can complex regional pain syndrome be painless? Pain. 2003;106(3):263-267.

13.   Jeong MY, Yu JS, Chung WB. Usefulness of thermography in diagnosis of complex regional pain syndrome type I after transradial coronary intervention. J Invasive Cardiol. 2013;25(9):E183-185.

14.   Gulevich SJ, Conwell TD, Lane J, et al. Stress infrared telethermography is useful in the diagnosis of complex regional pain syndrome, type I (formerly reflex sympathetic dystrophy). Clin J Pain. 1997;13(1):50-59.

15.   Choi E, Lee PB, Nahm FS. Interexaminer reliability of infrared thermography for the diagnosis of complex regional pain syndrome. Skin Res Technol. 2013;19(2):189-193.

16.   Rothman KJ, Greenland S. Causation and causal inference in epidemiology. Am J Public Health. 2005;95 Suppl 1:S144-150.

17.   Reinders MF, Geertzen JH, Dijkstra PU. Complex regional pain syndrome type I: use of the International Association for the Study of Pain diagnostic criteria defined in 1994. Clin J Pain. 2002;18(4):207-215.

18.   Veldman PH, Reynen HM, Arntz IE, Goris RJ. Signs and symptoms of reflex sympathetic dystrophy: prospective study of 829 patients. Lancet. 1993;342(8878):1012-1016.

19.   An HS, Hawthorne KB, Jackson WT. Reflex sympathetic dystrophy and cigarette smoking. J Hand Surg [Am]. 1988;13(3):458-460.

20.   Wilson PR. Complex Regional Pain Syndrome-Reflex Sympathetic Dystrophy. Curr Treat Options Neurol. 1999;1(5):466-472.

21.   Olsson GL, Meyerson BA, Linderoth B. Spinal cord stimulation in adolescents with complex regional pain syndrome type I (CRPS-I). Eur J Pain. 2008;12(1):53-59.

22.   Wolanin MW, Gulevski V, Schwartzman RJ. Treatment of CRPS with ECT. Pain Physician. 2007;10(4):573-578.

23.   Sinis N, Birbaumer N, Gustin S, et al. Memantine treatment of complex regional pain syndrome: a preliminary report of six cases. Clin J Pain. 2007;23(3):237-243.

24.   Ackerman WE, Zhang JM. Efficacy of stellate ganglion blockade for the management of type 1 complex regional pain syndrome. South Med J. 2006;99(10):1084-1088.

25.   Kharkar S, Venkatesh YS, Grothusen JR, Rojas L, Schwartzman RJ. Skin biopsy in complex regional pain syndrome: case series and literature review. Pain Physician. 2012;15(3):255-266.

26.   Fukui S, Shigemori S, Nosaka S. Changes in regional cerebral blood flow in the thalamus after electroconvulsive therapy for patients with complex regional pain syndrome type 1 (preliminary case series). Reg Anesth Pain Med. 2002;27(5):529-532.

27.   Quisel A, Gill JM, Witherell P. Complex regional pain syndrome: which treatments show promise? J Fam Pract. 2005;54(7):599-603.

28.   de Mos M, de Bruijn AG, Huygen FJ, Dieleman JP, Stricker BH, Sturkenboom MC. The incidence of complex regional pain syndrome: a population-based study. Pain. 2007;129(1-2):12-20.

29.   Rothman KJ, Poole C. A strengthening programme for weak associations. Int J Epidemiol. 1988;17(4):955-959.

5. Physiology

In the United States, millions of Americans are affected by chronic pain, which adds heavily to national rates of morbidity, mortality, and disability, with an ever-increasing prevalence. Pain not only exacts its toll on people's lives but also on the economy with an estimated annual economic cost of at least $560 - 635 billion in health care costs and the cost of lost productivity attributed to chronic pain.1

Research into complex regional pain syndrome (CRPS) has made significant progress. Research into the processes that cause pain has resulted in the development of more drugs to block nervous system pathways that transmit pain in the body.

During laboratory experiments and clinical trials, gender differences between men women are well documented with respect to pain responses. Studies of large numbers of people (epidemiological data) clearly show that women are at greater risk for developing certain pain syndromes than men and that this is believed to be a result of hormonal factors and other differences between the sexes.

The Complex regional pain syndrome (CRPS) is a common pain condition with an unknown etiology. Recently added new information enriches our understanding of CRPS pathophysiology. Researches on genetics, biogenic amines, neurotransmitters, and mechanisms of pain modulation, central sensitization, and autonomic functions in CRPS revealed various abnormalities indicating that multiple factors and mechanisms are involved in the pathogenesis of CRPS.

Epigenetics refers to mitotically and meiotically heritable changes in gene expression that do not affect the DNA sequence. As epigenetic modifications potentially play an important role in inflammatory cytokine metabolism, neurotransmitter responsiveness, and analgesic sensitivity, they are likely key factors in the development of chronic pain.2

However, the reason why RSD/CRPS is more prevalent in women is unknown. CRPS patients in an United Kingdom study had chronic disease with a median duration of 29 months; 72.5% were female with a mean age at symptoms onset of 43 years, and were left-handed more than expected Patients reported a delayed diagnosis, with the median time between symptom onset and diagnosis of 6 months.3 In all, 30 patients

(12.5%) had multiple limb involvement and (83.3%) had a contiguous spread of CRPS.

Pain is the body's way of telling a patient that something is harming the body. For example, chest pain tells a patient that a patient may be having a heart attack. Pain will cause the body to become restricted or immobile so that healing can occur.

When the pain becomes severe, it tells a patient to seek medical attention. The problem exists when the body's pain alarm system fails to quit working and the pain continues. When pain becomes uncontrolled, depression, anxiety, and loss of sleep can result, making the perception of the pain worse.

The onset of depression or anxiety happens when the pain reduces certain levels of chemicals in the brain and spinal cord. Pain is an individual experience that is difficult to study. The International Association for the Study of Pain defines pain as an unpleasant emotional and sensory experience that results from tissue injury or the threat of tissue injury.

The sensation of pain in different places on the body usually begins with the peripheral nervous system. The peripheral nervous system includes all nerves located outside of the spinal cord and brain, such as in the arms and legs. The spinal cord and brain together are called the central nervous system. Nerve fibers in the peripheral nervous system send painful impulses from nerve endings in the body directly to the spinal cord and brain.

Two main classes of nerve fibers exist that transmit pain in the body to the brain. The first class of pain fibers is called Alpha delta fibers. These fibers are able to send sharp pain and transmit pain impulses rapidly. The second class of pain fibers is called C fibers. These are smaller fibers and send burning types of pain more slowly than the Alpha delta fibers.

If a patient were to hit the finger with a hammer, a patient would experience two components of pain. First, a patient would feel a fast, sharp pain (Alpha delta fiber), followed by a second slow, throbbing or burning (C fiber) pain.

The throbbing or burning types pain last longer than sharp pain. Specific pathways exist that transmit pain information from the damaged part, or "tissue," through the spinal cord to a center of pain perception in the brain cortex called the post central gyrus.

When a patient is hurt, chemicals called neurotransmitters are released by the injured tissue that stimulates the nerve endings to feel pain. As a result, the pain a patient feel comes from the place of the tissue injury. The effects of several of these neurotransmitters have been well studied. Some of these chemical substances make the nerve endings more sensitive to pain. This process is called transduction.

The body does have neurochemicals in the spinal cord that can decrease the pain intensity. Remember that pain is the body's protective mechanism to tell a patient that something is wrong with an area of the body. A patient will then protect that particular area of the body that is injured.

In a rate study, injury and immobilization cause peripheral changes in neuropeptide signaling and inflammatory mediator production acutely, but central spinal changes may be more important for the persistent nociceptive changes in this CRPS model.4

If a type of neurotransmitter called prostaglandin is in the painful area of the tissue, the size of the blood vessels will grow and increase the blood circulation to that area. This will cause a patient to have swelling, redness and warmth in the injured area. The pain impulse travels along the length of the nerve to a junction where the nerve enters the spinal cord. This junction between the nerve and the spinal cord is the command center for many pain syndromes.

Transmission occurs when the pain impulse from the injured tissue flows to the junction at the spinal cord. From this area, the sensation of pain is transmitted to the back of the spinal cord. When the pain impulse reaches the spinal cord, it can lessen the sensation of pain. This process is called modulation.

The patients with CRPS in another study did have a moderate to serious disease activity and impairment. In plasma, no changes of mediators of inflammation were observed. In blister fluid, however, significantly higher levels of IL-6 (interleukin) and TNF-(alpha tumor necrosis factor-alpha) in the involved extremity were observed in comparison with the uninvolved extremity.5

Nerves "talk" with each another when neurotransmitter chemicals are released, causing other nerves around the injured area to transmit painful impulses. Another chemical released from injured tissue is bradykinin. Bradykinin causes C fibers to transmit pain, and also causes another type of neurotransmitter called prostaglandins to be produced. Prostaglandins decrease the level of pain tolerance that C fibers can withstand, which causes an increased sensitivity to feelings of pain.

There are some medications available that can block these prostaglandins from casing pain. A common prostaglandin blocker is Ibuprofen. When the pain fibers enter the spinal cord, they terminate in different parts of the spinal cord.

Ultimately these fibers will terminate in the cortex where a patient will experience painful sensations. CRPS is associated with the presence of a proinflammatory state in the blood, blister fluid, and CSF.6 Different inflammatory profiles were found for acute and chronic cases.

Prostaglandins fulfil many conversion functions and are involved in vasoactive processes, pain, and inflammation. They play an intermediating role between the activity of the autonomic nervous system and local occurrences. The insufficiently explored conversion function of prostaglandins as a cofactor may be related to the development of CRPS at sites which have had minor injuries in the past.7

Nerve cells in the spinal cord receive and respond to pain impulses from both the large and small fibers. Activation of receptors by the continual bombardment by pain impulses can result in a significant increase in the pain.

The spinal cord is "upregulated" to magnify pain impulses and result in excruciating disabling pain. Dendrites carry pain toward the neuron. Axons carry pain fibers away from the neuron and direct them to the dendrites of the next neuron until they terminate in the brain or spinal cord.

The axons and dendrites do not touch. They form synapses or clefts between the axon and dendrite. The synapse has chemicals in the axon nerve ending. These chemicals allow communication between the neurons. Drugs are chemicals that can interrupt the communication between the neurons at the synapses.

Another type of pain fiber exists that transmits impulses from the peripheral nervous system to the spinal cord. The third fiber that is important in understanding the transmission of pain is large nerve fibers called A beta fibers. These fibers respond to non-pain-producing stimuli such as touch, pressure or movement of joints.

These fibers also end at the spinal cord. They are important because these nerves can either activate or inhibit pain impulses. The convergence of different types of nerves on the spinal cord including pain-producing nerves as well as touch and pressure producing nerves can be a source of an unusual experience referred to as referred pain.

Referred pain occurs when an individual feels pain, for example, in the shoulder when the actual pain producing tissue is the heart as is noted when an individual suffers a heart attack. This referred pain from the heart travels to the shoulder because some of the receptors in the spinal cord also receive nervous impulses from both the peripheral nervous system and arms and legs as well as within the organs within the body. In this case, the brain misinterprets the location of the injured tissue stimulus.

Referred pain is pain felt at a site other than where the cause is situated. An example is the pain from the pancreas, which is felt in the back. When a hammer strikes the finger, rubbing the injured finger can result in considerable pain relief. This phenomenon was explained in 1965 by two pain researchers who published the gate-control theory of pain.

Their studies revealed that only a limited amount of sensory information can be processed by the brain and spinal cord at any given moment. When pain fibers from the periphery such as the arms or legs, activate pain transmission cells in the spinal cord, signals from the non-pain-producing large fibers can inhibit or increase activation of these the pain impulses from these pain transmitting nerves.

As a result, pain impulses appear to be dependent on a balance of activity in both the large and small fibers. This is the basis of the gate-control theory of pain. When the balance of nerve activity is directed toward the pain transmission fibers, the gate is open which allows transmission of painful signals to go from the spinal cord to the brain.

On the other hand, when the large non-pain fibers are the dominant electrical impulses, the gate is closed and the pain signals are decreased. In some instances they may be completely blocked.

Once the pain impulses have reached the spinal cord, the pathways for pain become crossed. Pain originating from peripheral nerves on the left side of the body is transmitted to the spinal cord on the left side of the body and across the spinal cord on the right side of the body.

Pain transmission then reaches the brain by two main pathways, called tracts. Chronic pain can make pain nerve endings more sensitive which results in more pain that continues to worsen over time.

After a while the pain from the pain transmitting fibers can "cross wires" with the large nerves that transmit touch and movement sensation so that even a slight change in movement or light touch can cause severe agony to a patient. This is probably how CRPS patients complain of severe pain to light touch. This is called allodynia which is present in patients suffering from CRPS. Allodynia must be present for one to make a diagnosis of CRPS.

The brain and spinal cord develop when a patient are in the mother's womb. In other words, gender differences in body structure and brain function develop when a fetus is still in the mother's womb. These differences show themselves in childhood. These factors combine with family lifestyles and school and socio-cultural sex roles to act uniquely on the individual.

All of these events factor into gender-specific patterns of pain perception. During adolescence, gender differences in pain syndromes emerge, such as dysmenorrhea in women and cluster headaches in men. Smoking and other dangerous activities can influence the onset of these chronic pain syndromes in both men and women.

When acute pain becomes chronic, a self-perpetuating cycle of maladies can occur, resulting in changes in the body as well as behavior that make the pain worse. For example, after an injury, changes can occur in the regrowth of damaged nerve endings and where pain nerves connect with other nerves. This can result in muscle tension, making muscles extra sensitive because they are tense rather than relaxed.

The increased stress from chronic pain can increase the release of a naturally occurring chemical in the brain called norepinepherine, eventually leading to its depletion and resulting depression and exhaustion. The depression can magnify the physical pain, which in turn depletes serotonin in both the spinal cord and brain. Persistent pain can decrease the sleep. This sleep deprivation depletes the body's supply of endorphins, which are chemicals that decrease pain.

Endorphins work on pain fibers essentially like morphine. With the depletion of endorphins in the brain and spinal cord, the pain can become worse and a patient may become depressed.. As a result of the increase in pain, people often place themselves into guarded positions to avoid pain.

However, these unnatural positions can strain other muscles, which in turn spread more pain to other parts of the body. Other, unused muscles shrink, or atrophy, with a resulting loss of strength causing more discomfort. The goal and purpose of pain medicine is to interrupt this vicious cycle.

Endorphins, mentioned previously, can shut the gate to pain. Endorphins are natural morphine like drugs (chemically related to opium) that switch off the pain alarm. Several types have been identified that modulate pain at the spinal cord and the brain. Because pain can affect breathing, blood flow, heart rate, and digestion, the body naturally releases endorphins to deal with pain.

Moreover, pain can affect the limbic system, which is a complex area of nerve pathways in the brain that controls emotions such as mood, self-preservation, rage, fear, and pleasure. Certain areas of the spinal cord contain high concentrations of endorphin receptors. The body also produces enkephalins and dynorphins, two neurochemicals also involved in pain modulation.

Another important neurochemical in CRPS pain modulation is gamma aminobutyric acid (GABA), an inhibitory pain mediator (baclofen). GABA inhibits pain transmission in the spinal cord when neurons are stimulated. The nerves that conduct pain go to the spinal cord that allows pain signals to ultimately reach the brain. Areas of the body that have many pain receptors include the skin, the outer aspect of bone called the periosteum, ligaments, joints, teeth and gums and the cornea of the eye.

Muscle also contains pain fibers but not as many per square meter (a measure of area) as the previously mentioned structures. Where the nerves from the body enter the spinal cord, aspartic and glutamic acid are produced. These acids increase pain impulse generation. NMDA may also be produced.

GABA (gamma-aminobutyric acid) in the spinal cord on the other hand, decreases the number of pain impulses that reach the brain. GABA inhibits pain impulse transmission   Norepinepherine and serotonin are two more chemicals in the spinal cord which attenuate the number of pain impulses which reach the brain.

The brain and spinal cord regulate pain by the production of naturally occurring narcotic-like substances that decrease pain transmission in specific areas of the brain. These narcotic-like drugs are called enkephalins, dynorphins and beta-endorphins. Some of these substances also decrease pain transmission in the spinal cord. Enkephalins are located in areas of the brain related to pain modulation.

Enkephalins inhibit pain at the spinal cord level. Enkephalins bind to narcotic receptors. When the narcotic receptors are activated, they inhibit pain signals. Dynorphins exist in both the brain and spinal cord but are more prevalent in the brain. Like enkephalins these substances bind to narcotic receptors in the brain and spinal cord. Pain impulses that enter the spinal cord cross over to the other side and then progress upward to the brain.

Autoantibodies may be associated with the pathophysiology of CRPS, at least in a subset of patients. Further research is needed into defining this subset and into the role of autoantibodies in the pathogenesis of CRPS.[8] The natural beta-endorphins in the body exhibit morphine-like activity. They work like morphine to decrease the pain. Following injury or stress these endorphins are released into the blood stream.

The effects of beta-endorphins are similar to morphine. Beta-endorphins like narcotics can cause respiratory depression, constipation, euphoria, tolerance and physical dependence. The exact biochemical actions of all of the substances mentioned are complex.

Stress can influence an animal's response to pain. There is a difference in stress-induced analgesia between male and female rodents, with the females having a greater pain response to stress. The reason for this observation is unknown and is believed not to be a result of the effect of hormones.

On the other hand, estrogen, a female hormone, regulates the formation of the pain transmitter chemical substance P as well as some of the other chemicals in the nervous system that do cause pain

This may be a reason why RSD/CRPS occurs more in females than in males. Women go through a 5- to 10-year period of menopause. During this time, changes occur in hormones, most notably a decrease in the hormones in the female bloodstream.

Collectively, data suggests that miR-939 may regulate multiple proinflammatory genes and that downregulation of miR-939 in CRPS patients may increase expression of these genes, resulting in amplification of the inflammatory pain signal transduction cascade.[9]

In men hormone changes occur over approximately 20 years. Body structure changes occur in both males and females. Lifestyle changes also occur during this time. Increases in the incidence of disease occur during this time in both men and women.

There also is an alteration of drug metabolism in both men and women. It is interesting that the incidence of CRPS in women following menopause is the same as men.

Nicotine can have an effect on pain intensity as well in patients with CRPS. It has been shown that nicotine increases the amount of stimulus needed to cause pain in men but not in women. However nicotine can enhance a patient's sympathetic nervous system which can intensify the pain associated with CRPS.

In human patients, the overall effects of pain-relieving drugs are greater in men than in women. However, men report greater pain relief than women when morphine or morphine like drugs are used for pain control.

In contrast, drugs that stimulate other receptors than the morphine receptors, such as butorphanol (Stadol), provide greater pain relief in women than men in a clinical setting. These differences in opioid medications are discussed in a later chapter.

According to physiologic cardiovascular parameters in a laboratory setting, male rodents exhibit greater levels of analgesia following stressful laboratory manipulations than female rodents. This may be a result of the effects of stress on the pain systems in these animals.

It is known that significant differences exist between men and women as to sensitivity to painful stimuli. Laboratory studies show that sex hormones do affect pain perception. When sex hormones are at their peak in the female, pain sensitivity is decreased.

Epidemiological studies done in 1996 and repeated in 1997 indicated that women report more severe pain intensity and more frequent pain as well as pain in multiple areas of the body and pain of a longer duration than do males.

Reflex sympathetic dystrophy (CRPS) is a chronic condition that usually affects the arms or legs and causes intense aching and burning pain along with swelling, skin discoloration and temperature changes) is more prevalent in females as is a piriformis muscle syndrome (a spasm of the gluteal [buttocks] muscles).

The pain stimulus differs among the sexes. Pressure and electrical pain stimuli result in larger gender specific responses than do heat or cold stimuli. However, if heat stimuli are administered repeatedly, the gender-specific difference increases.

In a laboratory setting, males demonstrate greater sensitivity than females to painful stimuli applied to areas near the genitals. A high sugar and fat intake can increase the pain in both males and females.

Phantom pain is another aspect of pain that is hard to define and note in the research lab. Phantom pain occurs after an arm, tooth or a leg is amputated. Phantom limb pain can mimic RSD. Many patients who have had a foot amputated still complain of pain in the "foot" for many months or even years. This is due to changes within the brain and spinal cord.

A patient may believe that the pain is in the foot even though the foot is not there, but the actual pain is experienced in areas of the brain that correspond to the foot. Right now it is not known whether women or men have a higher incidence of phantom pain. It also is not known whether hormones affect the incidence of phantom pain.

Cutaneous sympathetic pathophysiology in complex regional pain syndrome type 1 (CRPS-1) is not yet completely understood. It may reflect underlying damage to the sympathetic postganglionic fibers.10

COX-2 inhibitors have been reported to be effective for CRPS management. COX-2 might however be less important than previously assumed for the treatment of CRPS.11

The sympathetic nervous system and its release of pain neuro-stimulating chemicals can increase a woman's susceptibility to reflex sympathetic dystrophy (RSD) or causalgia. Reflex sympathetic dystrophy and causalgia are usually caused by trauma to a nerve. These entities are more common in women.

Patients with longstanding CRPS have serum antibodies to alpha-1a receptors, and that measurement of these antibodies may be useful in the diagnosis and management of the patients.12

In patients with complex regional pain syndrome (CRPS), the temperature of the affected side often differs from that of the contralateral side. In the acute phase, the affected side is usually warmer than the contralateral side, the so-called 'warm' CRPS.

This thermal asymmetry can develop into a colder affected side, the so-called 'cold' CRPS.13 The complex regional pain syndrome is thought to have an auto-immune component.

One such target recently proposed from the effects of auto-immune IgGs on $Ca(2+)$ transients in cardiac myocytes and cell lines is the alpha1-adrenoceptor.14

Reflex sympathetic dystrophy is a pain syndrome caused by a bruise or compression of the nerve, whereas causalgia is defined as direct trauma to the nerve (where the nerve is not completely severed). The hormonal status at the time of a nerve injury may be important for the development of reflex sympathetic dystrophy (now called complex regional pain syndrome).

After trauma, some inflammation is physiological; in acute CRPS, this inflammation persists for months. There is an abundance of inflammatory and a lack of anti-inflammatory mediators. This proinflammatory network (cytokines and probably also other mediators) sensitizes the peripheral and spinal nociceptive system; it facilitates the release of neuropeptides from nociceptors inducing the signs of inflammation.

Trauma may also expose nervous system structures to the immune system and triggers autoantibodies binding to adreno- and acetylcholine receptors. In an individual time frame, the pain in this inflammatory phase pushes the transition into "centralized" CRPS, which is dominated by neuronal plasticity and reorganization.

Birklein and Schlereth have postulated that sensory-motor integration becomes disturbed, leading to a loss of motor function; the body representation is distorted leading to numbness and autonomic disturbances.15

CRPS usually develops after a noxious event, but spontaneous onsets have been described in 3-11% of the cases. CRPS may develop both with and without a precipitating noxious event.16 However, there are no other published references that support CRPS spontaneous onset.

Spontaneous-onset CRPS patients generally develop the syndrome at a younger age, possibly indicating a susceptibility to develop the condition.

The longer disease duration in spontaneous-onset cases may reflect a more gradual disease onset, poorer prognosis, or a delay in diagnosis, possibly as a result of reluctance to make this diagnosis in the absence of a clear initiating event.

Differences in the mechanisms of pain inhibition in the brain and spinal cord are presently being studied. This is important because preliminary studies have noted that equivalent doses of pain-relieving drugs differ for males and females. The quality and intensity of pain differs for men and women.

The differences in body structure and physiology of men and women needs to be studied as well and further addressed, especially when developing new physical modalities as well as new drugs for the management of pain.

Previous studies essentially used a majority of male subjects. No one took into consideration the differences of the effects of medications on men and women. Further studies and research into gender differences with respect to pain management may eliminate misleading information regarding the best way to manage a male's or female's pain.

It is obvious that men and women differ with respect to pain. This is also true with regard to the treatment of pain. Doctors are beginning to realize that men and women respond differently to different pain therapies. As stated earlier, the effects of the absorption and metabolism of drugs differ in men and women. It also has been mentioned that different types of drugs such as opioids and antidepressants may work differently in men and women.

The menstrual cycle results in women being affected more than men with respect to the absorption of drugs through their stomach and intestine. Women experience a decreased absorption of drugs in the mid cycle of the menstrual period.

When women are using hormones, there is a decreased attachment of drugs to proteins in their bloodstream after the drug has been absorbed through the intestine. Removal of drugs from the bloodstream by the kidneys appears to be equal in males and females, and this "clearance" appears to decrease as both men and women age.

The treatment of RSD may involve utilization of occupational therapy or physical therapy and sometimes chiropractor therapy. Little information is available that addresses the gender differences in the efficacy of physical therapy and chiropractic therapy. However, women are more likely to use effective forms of pain relief such as relaxation, massage, and manipulation.

Studies in healthy women have demonstrated that their sensitivity to massage therapy and heat therapy can change during the menstrual cycle. Women need to consider this factor when considering the effects of heat packs or cold packs as well as massage for pain treatment.

References

1.	Kosharskyy B, Almonte W, Shaparin N, Pappagallo M, Smith H. Intravenous infusions in chronic pain management. Pain Physician. 2013;16(3):231-249.

2.	Wang F, Stefano GB, Kream RM. Epigenetic modification of DRG neuronal gene expression subsequent to nerve injury: etiological contribution to complex regional pain syndromes (Part I). Med Sci Monit. 2014;20:1067-1077.

3.	Shenker N, Goebel A, Rockett M, et al. Establishing the characteristics for patients with chronic Complex Regional Pain Syndrome: the value of the CRPS-UK Registry. Br J Pain. 2015;9(2):122-128.

4.   Wei T, Guo TZ, Li WW, Kingery WS, Clark JD. Acute versus chronic phase mechanisms in a rat model of CRPS. J Neuroinflammation. 2016;13(1):14.

5.   Huygen FJ, De Bruijn AG, De Bruin MT, Groeneweg JG, Klein J, Zijlstra FJ. Evidence for local inflammation in complex regional pain syndrome type 1. Mediators Inflamm. 2002;11(1):47-51.

6.   Parkitny L, McAuley JH, Di Pietro F, et al. Inflammation in complex regional pain syndrome: a systematic review and meta-analysis. Neurology. 2013;80(1):106-117.

7.   van der Veen P. CRPS: A contingent hypothesis with prostaglandins as crucial conversion factor. Med Hypotheses. 2015;85(5):568-575.

8.   Dirckx M, Schreurs MW, de Mos M, Stronks DL, Huygen FJ. The prevalence of autoantibodies in complex regional pain syndrome type I. Mediators Inflamm. 2015;2015:718201.

9.   McDonald MK, Ramanathan S, Touati A, et al. Regulation of proinflammatory genes by the circulating microRNA hsa-miR-939. Sci Rep. 2016;6:30976.

10.   Poudel A, Asahina M, Fujinuma Y, et al. Skin sympathetic function in complex regional pain syndrome type 1. Clin Auton Res. 2015;25(6):367-371.

11.   Breuer AJ, Mainka T, Hansel N, Maier C, Krumova EK. Short-term treatment with parecoxib for complex regional pain syndrome: a randomized, placebo-controlled double-blind trial. Pain Physician. 2014;17(2):127-137.

12.   Dubuis E, Thompson V, Leite MI, et al. Longstanding complex regional pain syndrome is associated with activating autoantibodies against alpha-1a adrenoceptors. Pain. 2014;155(11):2408-2417.

13.   Dirckx M, Stronks DL, van Bodegraven-Hof EA, Wesseldijk F, Groeneweg JG, Huygen FJ. Inflammation in cold complex regional pain syndrome. Acta Anaesthesiol Scand. 2015;59(6):733-739.

14.   Reilly JM, Dharmalingam B, Marsh SJ, Thompson V, Goebel A, Brown DA. Effects of serum immunoglobulins from patients with complex regional pain syndrome (CRPS) on depolarisation-induced calcium transients in isolated dorsal root ganglion (DRG) neurons. Exp Neurol. 2016;277:96-102.

15.   Birklein F, Schlereth T. Complex regional pain syndrome-significant progress in understanding. Pain. 2015;156 Suppl 1:S94-103.

16.   de Rooij AM, Perez RS, Huygen FJ, et al. Spontaneous onset of complex regional pain syndrome. Eur J Pain. 2010;14(5):510-513.

6. Epidemiology

The nervous system consists of two key parts: the central nervous system and the peripheral nervous system: The central nervous system is made up of the brain and spinal cord. The peripheral nervous system is made up of the nerve fibers that branch off from the spinal cord and extend to all parts of the body, including the neck and arms, torso, legs, skeletal muscles and internal organs cells of the sensory nervous system send information to the CNS from internal organs. The Autonomic Nervous System controls involuntary muscles, such as smooth and cardiac muscle.

It is not clear why complex regional pain syndrome (CRPS) develops in some patients but not in others, despite similar initiating events. One study indicated that motor nerve injury and female gender are risk factors for CRPS. The prevention measures should be focused mainly on females and patients with motor nerve injury in order to reduce the risk of CRPS.[1]

A study showed that although CRPS is a progressive disease, after 1 year, the majority of the signs and symptoms were well developed and although many variables worsen over the course of the illness, the majority demonstrated only moderate increases with disease duration.[2] Complex regional pain syndrome has an incidence of 8.3% after CTR surgery without association with the anesthetic techniques investigated.[3]

Anxiety, pain-related fear, and disability are associated with poorer outcomes in CRPS and could be considered as target variables for early treatment. The findings support the theory that CRPS represents an aberrant protective response to perceived threat of tissue injury.[4]

The autonomic nervous system is divided into the sympathetic nervous system and the parasympathetic nervous system. An A delta fiber is a type of sensory nerve fiber. "A" delta fibers carry cold, pressure and some pain signals. These nerve fibers are associated with acute sharp pain. Slowly conducting, unmyelinated C fibers, by contrast, carry slow, burning pain.

A-delta nerve fibers are insulated with myelin. C-nerve fibers are unmyelinated. The thickness of the nerve fiber is correlated to the speed with which information travels in it. Seventy per cent of pain nerve fibers are C fibers. A pain score of 5 or greater in the first week after fracture should be considered a "red flag" for probable CRPS.

The term Complex Regional Pain Syndrome (CRPS) was adopted as from 1994 by the International Association for Study of Pain (IASP) Consensus. In an epidemiologic study patients had chronic CRPS disease (median duration: 29 months) 72.5% were female, with a mean age at symptoms onset of 43 years, and were left-handed. Patients reported a delayed diagnosis, with the median time between symptom onset and diagnosis of 6 months. In all, 12.5% had multiple limb involvement and 83.3%) had a spread of CRPS.

Another study found that CRPS patients had seen on average 4.8 different physicians before referral to a pain center and had received an average of five different kinds of treatments both prior to and during pain clinic treatment. The mean duration of CRPS symptoms prior to a pain center evaluation was 30 months. The estimated overall incidence rate of CRPS was 26.2 per 100,000 person years (95% CI: 23.0-29.7).

Females were affected at least three times more often than males (ratio: 3.4). The highest incidence occurred in females in the age category of 61-70 years. The upper extremity was affected more frequently than the lower extremity and a fracture was the most common precipitating event (44%).5 CRPS can be familial and hence may have a genetic basis in some families as well.6

A study previously published suggested that anxiety, pain-related fear, and disability are associated with poorer outcomes in CRPS and could be considered as target variables for early treatment. The findings support the theory that CRPS represents an aberrant protective response to perceived threat of tissue injury.4

Glial activation contributes to the maintenance of central nociceptive sensitization in CRPS. Treatments inhibiting glial activation and spinal inflammation may be therapeutic for CRPS.7 Twenty seven (33%) of the 82 CRPS patients of whom serum was available showed a positive ANA test.8 This prevalence is significantly higher than in the general population.

Six patients (7.3%) showed a positive result for typical antineuronal antibodies. This proportion, however, does not deviate from that in the general population. These findings suggest that autoantibodies may be associated with the pathophysiology of CRPS, at least in a subset of patients. Further research is needed into defining this subset and into the role of autoantibodies in the pathogenesis of CRPS.8

Fibromyalgia and CRPS also seem to share many pathophysiological mechanisms, among which the most important are those involving central effects. Nonetheless, peripheral effects, such as neurogenic neuroinflammation, are also important contributors to the clinical features of each of these disorders.9 The alpha1-adrenoceptor as a target for CRPS auto-immunity.10

The diagnosis is clinical and the pathophysiology involves combinations of small-fiber axonopathy, microvasculopathy, inflammation, and brain plasticity/sensitization.11 Females have a much higher risk and workplace accidents are a well-recognized cause. Inflammation and dysimmunity, perhaps facilitated by injury to the blood-nerve barrier, may contribute.

Collectively, it has been shown that CD20-positive B cells produce antibodies that ultimately support the CRPS-like changes in the murine fracture/cast model.12 Therapies directed at reducing B-cell activity may be of use in treating patients with CRPS.

Postmenopausal woman appeared to be at the highest risk for the development of CRPS. It has been postulated that CRPS-1 is not an illness but rather a 'disuse syndrome' as a result of immobilization, or there may be a missed underlying diagnosis. Patients with familial CRPS however, develop the disease at a younger age and have a more severe phenotype than sporadic cases, suggesting a genetic predisposition to develop CRPS.

It is not clear why complex regional pain syndrome (CRPS) develops in some patients but not in others, despite similar initiating events. CRPS was diagnosed in 84 patientsin a study.1 Female/male ratio was higher in patients with CRPS versus those without. The mean age was higher in patients with CRPS. The affected forearm/hand was the dominant side in 62.9% of patients without CRPS and in 64.2% of patients with CRPS.

The CRPS incidence was higher in patients with motor nerve injury and in patients with sensory nerve injury. A logistic regression showed that risk for CRPS was higher in patients with motor nerve injury and in females. This study indicates that motor nerve injury and female gender are risk factors for CRPS.

The basic working unit of the nervous system is a cell called a neuron. Neurons communicate with each other using axons and dendrites. When a neuron receives a message from another neuron, it sends an electrical signal down the length of its axon. At the end of the axon, the electrical signal is converted into a chemical signal, and the axon releases chemical messengers called neurotransmitters. The neurotransmitters are released into the space between the end of an axon and the tip of a dendrite from another neuron. This space is called a synapse.

Complex regional pain syndrome usually occurs following an injury. However, a heart attack or stroke can cause you to have complex regional pain syndrome. It can also be seen in the knee as well as in the shoulder. In complex regional pain syndrome, 40 percent of the cases followed an injury to a muscle or a nerve. Simple bruises or sprains can trigger complex regional pain syndrome. Fractures account for 25 percent of complex regional pain syndrome cases.

In animal pain models spinal glial cell activation results in nociceptive sensitization. Data support the hypothesis that C-fiber afferent substance P signaling chronically supports spinal neuroglial activation after limb fracture and that glial activation contributes to the maintenance of central nociceptive sensitization in CRPS.7 Treatments inhibiting glial activation and spinal inflammation may be therapeutic for CRPS.

Twenty percent of the CRPS patients were postoperative on an arm or leg, whereas 12 percent occurred after a heart attack. Three percent occurred after a stroke. Approximately 37 percent of patients have emotional disturbances at the time of the onset of the complex regional pain syndrome. There is evidence that inflammatory processes are involved in at least the early phase of complex regional pain syndrome.

It was once thought that complex regional pain syndrome was a result of an emotional problem. However, many people do not suffer from emotional problems at the time of onset of complex regional pain syndrome. To prevent you from having permanent disability, treatment needs to be started immediately. Treatment usually consists of oral medications as well as injection therapy by an anesthesiologist using local anesthetics. Steroids may also be used effectively to treat CRPS.

Recent evidence, however, suggests that an autoimmune attack on self-antigens found in the peripheral and central nervous system may underlie a number of CRPS symptoms. From both animal and human studies, evidence is accumulating that neuroinflammation can spread, either anterograde or retrograde, via axonal projections in the CNS, thereby establishing neuroinflammatory tracks and secondary neuroinflammatory foci within the neuraxis.

A previous definition of causalgia was referred to the syndrome associated with known nerve injury, whereas complex regional pain syndrome included those patients whose pain and associated symptoms were followed by a variety of causes. Injury associated with causalgia was more severe, whereas that associated with CRPS was relatively minor. Now complex regional pain syndrome is referred to as complex regional pain syndrome I, whereas causalgia is referred as complex regional pain syndrome II.

Chemical substances in the tissues activate the pain fibers. These chemicals cause the blood vessels to increase their diameter. As the blood vessels enlarge in diameter, a patient may also have swelling in the tissue. Chemicals such as acetylcholine, potassium, and serotonin can stimulate pain in the tissues. However, when these chemicals are in the brain or spinal cord they do not cause pain.

Histamine in the tissues can also be a chemical that can cause a patient to have pain. However, histamine is being used in creams to decrease the pain in the skin and muscles. Further studies have shown that the release of histamine into the spinal cord can decrease the pain as well. The mechanisms by which histamine either cause pain or help relieve pain remain to be studied and elucidated.

Prostaglandins are also released. As mentioned previously, prostaglandins themselves do not produce pain; when they are around pain nerves, however, they sensitize these nerves to pain. Prostaglandins can intensify any inflammation that a patient may have and increase the action of bradykinin on the nerve endings. Substance P in the tissues can be a cause of significant pain. It is important for a patient to realize that there are many pain producing chemicals especially in complex regional pain syndrome.

Over time the treatment of complex regional pain syndrome included repetitive sympathetic blocks or removal of the sympathetic nerves, either surgically or by chemicals such as phenol. Sympathetic blocks involve placing a local anesthetic about the bundles of nerves which exist outside of the central nervous system.

These nerve bundles which are called ganglia are in the neck as well as the lower back. The ganglion in the neck influences the arm pain while the ganglion in the lower back influences CRPS pain in the leg. These procedures for many years have been the standard treatment for the treatment of complex regional pain syndrome.

Finally, doctors who regularly treat complex regional pain syndrome critically evaluated the effectiveness of early description of complex regional pain syndrome included injuries without obvious nerve damage. Causalgia, on the other hand, was the description given to symptoms of complex regional pain syndrome where a nerve had been actually injured, such as in a gunshot wound that was described by Dr. Mitchell during the Civil War. Sprains and strains can also be a cause of these syndromes as well as bursitis and tendonitis. Arthritis can also cause either complex regional pain syndrome or causalgia.

As the CRPS progresses, the blood vessels to the extremity will decrease in diameter. They go from the enlarged diameter to a normal appearing diameter. This is phase II. A three-phase bone scan will, therefore, appear normal at this time. You will have some swelling as well at this time and global pain about the extremity and sweating of the extremity as the sympathetic nervous system becomes overactive. This phase can progress on to phase III. In this systematic assessment of the incidence of widespread pain in a large cohort of patients with CRPS, important widespread pain affected > 10% of patients13

During this phase, the blood vessels become extremely small and a patient has decreased blood flow to the hand, foot, or the affected extremity. This will cause the skin to become cold. By this time, you will notice that the skin has become shiny and that the sweating in the hand or foot may have increased. A three-phase bone scan at this time can detect a significant decrease in the blood flow to the extremity.

After a patient has reached phase three of complex regional pain syndrome, the disease is irreversible. The success rate for phase I is extremely high, which does decrease as a patient progresses to phase II. Be aware that on rare occasions CRPS can spread into more than one extremity.

This observation suggests that an individual may have a predisposition to develop CRPS. Even though some investigators have questioned the existence of the sympathetic nervous system's influence on the pain associated with complex regional pain syndrome, there is clinical evidence that this influence does actually exist.

This led investigators to describe two types of pain. One is sympathetically maintained pain and is pain associated with chemicals released by the sympathetic nervous system. Sympathetically maintained pain is frequently diagnosed clinically by assessing the analgesic effect of an appropriate sympathetic block.

In patients with CRPS in multiple limbs, spontaneous spread of symptoms generally follows a contralateral or ipsilateral pattern whereas diagonal spread is rare and generally preceded by a new trauma. Spread is associated with a younger age at onset and a more severely affected phenotype.14

Acute CRPS patients also had increased mast cell accumulation in the affected skin, but there was no increase in mast cell numbers in chronic CRPS.15 Autoimmunity has been suggested as one of the pathophysiologic mechanisms that may underlie complex regional pain syndrome (CRPS).8,16 Screening for antinuclear antibodies (ANA) is one of the diagnostic tests, which is usually performed if a person is suspected to have a systemic autoimmune disease. Antineuronal antibodies are autoantibodies directed against antigens in the central and/or peripheral nervous system.

There is a report that decreased cortical thickness in the prefrontal cortex and neurocognitive dysfunctions is present in patients with CRPS.17 These findings may contribute to the understanding of pain-related impairments in cognitive function and could help explain the symptoms or progression of CRPS.

There are numerous etiological pathophysiological events that have been incriminated in development of CRPS, including inflammation, autoimmune responses, abnormal cytokine production, sympathetic-sensory disorders, altered blood flow and central cortical reorganization.

However, the number of studies that have included appropriate controls and have sufficient numbers of patients to allow statistical analysis with appropriate power calculations is vanishingly small. This has led to over-diagnosis and often excessive pharmacotherapy and even unnecessary surgical interventions.18

The other type of pain is sympathetically independent pain, which is not associated with the chemicals liberated by the sympathetic nervous system into the bloodstream. In early stages the pain is sympathetically maintained, but with time becomes sympathetically independent. Sympathetically maintained pain usually has a decrease in the pain component following a sympathetic block.

The disturbances in the sympathetic nervous system in CRPS I patients are systemic and not limited to the affected limb. Sympathetically maintained pain can be seen in other entities besides complex regional pain syndrome. It may be seen in neuropathies, phantom limb pain, and shingles as well as neuralgias.

More recent studies have determined that the COX-2 enzyme may be responsible for the pain associated with complex regional pain syndrome. Furthermore, there may be an interaction between COX-2 enzyme and stimulation of the sympathetic nervous system. Central spinal changes on the other hand may be more important for the persistent nociceptive changes in a CRPS model.19 The most important other factor for diagnosing CRPS is the exclusion of a neuropathic, musculoskeletal, or non-biomedical condition accounting for the presentation.20

The treatment of CRPS is multidisciplinary and aims to educate patients about the condition, sustain or restore limb function, reduce pain and provide psychological intervention.21 Among the types of apparatus used for diagnostics, triple phase bone scintigraphy and temperature measurement have a certain importance. A multimodal therapy started as early as possible is the most promising approach for successful treatment. As part of a multimodal rehabilitation the main focus of therapy lies on pain relief and functional aspects.22

References

1.   Demir SE, Ozaras N, Karamehmetoglu SS, Karacan I, Aytekin E. Risk factors for complex regional pain syndrome in patients with traumatic extremity injury. Ulus Travma Acil Cerrahi Derg. 2010;16(2):144-148.

2.   Schwartzman RJ, Erwin KL, Alexander GM. The natural history of complex regional pain syndrome. Clin J Pain. 2009;25(4):273-280.

3.   da Costa VV, de Oliveira SB, Fernandes Mdo C, Saraiva RA. Incidence of regional pain syndrome after carpal tunnel release. Is there a correlation with the anesthetic technique? Rev Bras Anestesiol. 2011;61(4):425-433.

4.   Bean DJ, Johnson MH, Heiss-Dunlop W, Lee AC, Kydd RR. Do psychological factors influence recovery from complex regional pain syndrome type 1? A prospective study. Pain. 2015;156(11):2310-2318.

5.   de Mos M, de Bruijn AG, Huygen FJ, Dieleman JP, Stricker BH, Sturkenboom MC. The incidence of complex regional pain syndrome: a population-based study. Pain. 2007;129(1-2):12-20.

6.   Shirani P, Jawaid A, Moretti P, et al. Familial occurrence of complex regional pain syndrome. Can J Neurol Sci. 2010;37(3):389-394.

7.   Li WW, Guo TZ, Shi X, et al. Substance P spinal signaling induces glial activation and nociceptive sensitization after fracture. Neuroscience. 2015;310:73-90.

8.   Dirckx M, Schreurs MW, de Mos M, Stronks DL, Huygen FJ. The prevalence of autoantibodies in complex regional pain syndrome type I. Mediators Inflamm. 2015;2015:718201.

9.   Littlejohn G. Neurogenic neuroinflammation in fibromyalgia and complex regional pain syndrome. Nat Rev Rheumatol. 2015;11(11):639-648.

10.   Reilly JM, Dharmalingam B, Marsh SJ, Thompson V, Goebel A, Brown DA. Effects of serum immunoglobulins from patients with complex regional pain syndrome (CRPS) on depolarisation-induced calcium transients in isolated dorsal root ganglion (DRG) neurons. Exp Neurol. 2016;277:96-102.

11.   Oaklander AL, Horowitz SH. The complex regional pain syndrome. Handb Clin Neurol. 2015;131:481-503.

12.   Li WW, Guo TZ, Shi X, et al. Autoimmunity contributes to nociceptive sensitization in a mouse model of complex regional pain syndrome. Pain. 2014;155(11):2377-2389.

13.   Birley T, Goebel A. Widespread pain in patients with complex regional pain syndrome. Pain Pract. 2014;14(6):526-531.

14.   van Rijn MA, Marinus J, Putter H, Bosselaar SR, Moseley GL, van Hilten JJ. Spreading of complex regional pain syndrome: not a random process. J Neural Transm (Vienna). 2011;118(9):1301-1309.

15.   Birklein F, Drummond PD, Li W, et al. Activation of cutaneous immune responses in complex regional pain syndrome. J Pain. 2014;15(5):485-495.

16.   Tajerian M, Sahbaie P, Sun Y, et al. Sex differences in a Murine Model of Complex Regional Pain Syndrome. Neurobiol Learn Mem. 2015;123:100-109.

17.   Lee DH, Lee KJ, Cho KI, et al. Brain alterations and neurocognitive dysfunction in patients with complex regional pain syndrome. J Pain. 2015;16(6):580-586.

18.   Borchers AT, Gershwin ME. Complex regional pain syndrome: a comprehensive and critical review. Autoimmun Rev. 2014;13(3):242-265.

19.   Wei T, Guo TZ, Li WW, Kingery WS, Clark JD. Acute versus chronic phase mechanisms in a rat model of CRPS. J Neuroinflammation. 2016;13:14.

20.   Mailis-Gagnon A, Lakha SF, Allen MD, Deshpande A, Harden RN. Characteristics of complex regional pain syndrome in patients referred to a tertiary pain clinic by community physicians, assessed by the Budapest clinical diagnostic criteria. Pain Med. 2014;15(11):1965-1974.

21.   Goebel A. Complex regional pain syndrome in adults. Rheumatology (Oxford). 2011;50(10):1739-1750.

22.   Harhaus L, Neubrech F, Hirche C, et al. [Complex regional pain syndrome following distal fractures of the radius : Epidemiology, pathophysiological models, diagnostics and therapy]. Unfallchirurg. 2016;119(9):732-741.

7. Patient Assessment

There is controversy regarding the importance of psychological/psychiatric factors in the development of the Complex Regional Pain Syndrome (CRPS).1 Anxiety, pain-related fear, and disability are associated with poorer outcomes in CRPS and could be considered as target variables for early treatment.2 Most pain assessments are done with in the form of a scale. The scale is explained to the patient and they give a score. A rating is taken before administering any medication and after the specified time frame to rate the efficacy of a treatment. RSD/CRPS can be very painful. Several different techniques are available for patient's doctor to use in determining patient's level of pain. Commonly used techniques include verbal, visual, and psychological tests.

Psychological and behavioral factors can exacerbate the pain and dysfunction associated with complex regional pain syndrome (CRPS) and could help maintain the condition in some patients. Effective management of CRPS requires that these psychosocial and behavioral aspects be addressed as part of an integrated multidisciplinary treatment approach.3

Both a patient and his/her doctor are responsible for documenting and recording trends in the intensity and frequency of patient's pain. This information tells each of the patients whether a patient's pain has really improved or whether it has worsened. Charting patient's pain levels will help patient's doctor see patient's long-range pain trends, which are ultimately more important than patient's day-to-day pain trends.

A patient may wonder why a patient needs to measure patient's pain. A pain-experience measurement is extremely valuable to both the patient and patient's doctor. It provides a baseline for patient's doctor to assess any therapy or medications patient are currently taking, and it also helps patient's doctor to prescribe future therapy methods. Patient's doctor also needs to be able to determine how much disability patient have in order to prescribe the appropriate types of therapy for patient.

The spread of complex regional pain syndrome (CRPS) has been well documented. A study was done to assess pain that spread within a patient's body. Twenty patients with CRPS were studied.4 Each patient stated that they suffered from total body pain. Five patients with CRPS had signs of CRPS over 100% of their body (20%). One patient had pain over 87% and another had pain over 90% of their body area. The average percentage of body involvement was 62% (range 37% - 100%). All patients with CRPS had at least one sensory parameter abnormality in all body regions.

All patients with CRPS had lower pain thresholds for static allodynia in all body areas, while 50% demonstrated a lower threshold for dynamic allodynia in all body regions compared to the healthy participants. Cold allodynia had a higher median pain rating on the Likert pain scale in all body areas versus healthy participants except for the chest, abdomen, and back.

Eighty-five percent of the patients with CRPS had a significantly lower pain threshold for mechanical hyperalgesia in all body areas compared to the healthy participants. The results of this study implied that not only extremity pain should be assessed but also total body pain should be assessed.

Many of the test instruments that mentioned in this chapter enable doctors to diagnose a specific pain condition. They also help doctors determine whether the patient is truly in pain or just making it up. Patient should be able to easily understand the test patient is being given so that it is as accurate as possible at measuring patient's level of pain.

After reading this chapter a patient will be able to see that patient and patient's doctor can use several different pain-assessment forms to monitor patient's pain-medicine therapy. Which form is best for patient? There is no definite answer to this question. The assessment form that patient feel most comfortable with and the one that patient will use is the best pain assessment for both patient and patient's doctor.

These assessment scales help patient and patient's doctor plan an individualized pain-management program. Look over patient's pain-assessment evaluations carefully. If patient are not decreasing patient's pain, or if patient's pain is becoming worse, patient and patient's physician must evaluate other treatments for patient's pain. Patient and patient's doctor must develop a partnership in the control of patient's pain.

A patient's doctor will depend on a patient for accurate and reliable answers to questions about the pain patient feel. Because pain involves many aspects such as sensory, emotional, and behavioral factors, it is difficult to measure the amount of pain patient feel based on one thing. Patient's doctor will carefully instruct patient as to how to report patient's pain when going through a pain-assessment test.

The choice of a pain-assessment test depends on the needs of both patient and patient's doctor. Two common tests are a Number Scale and a Faces Scale. Using a Number Scale, patients rate pain on a scale from 0-10, 0 being no pain and 10 being the worst pain ever imaginable. The Faces Scale is a scale with corresponding faces depicting various levels of pain is shown to the patient and they select one.

A functional evaluation, such as reports of patient's daily activities, must be included in patient's assessment. If patient's doctor does not ask about patient's daily activities, voluntarily tell him patient's further limitations with respect to work, recreation, dressing, fixing meals, and any other daily activities. Use a daily pain diary and tell patient's doctor whether patient's pain is becoming worse or is getting better.

This will enable patient's doctor to assess patient's medication and therapy needs. Positive effects of therapy are best assessed when patient's doctor keeps a database of patient's pain progression. This type of data is easily stored on a computer. This type of database is even more valuable because patient's doctor can graph important data from each of patient's visits.

The assessment and measurement of pain has received considerable attention in the past two decades. Progress continues to be made in developing pain-assessment tools. Patient or patient's doctor should not oversimplify patient's pain assessment. The objective reports patient are able to give, as well the observations patient's doctor is able to make about patient's behavior, are important to accurate pain management decisions.

Because pain is subjective and can be observed only by patient, it is important that the reports of patient's pain levels come from patient. This will give the patient's doctor a more accurate measurement of the type of pain patients are experiencing.

For example, if patient just complains of a toothache, patient's doctor will have almost no way of knowing how severe patient's pain is. On occasion, patient's doctor will need to rate patient's level of pain if patient are not able for some reason to identify patient's level of pain.

In general, patient should be able to accurately describe patient's level of pain. If a patient is not able to rate the pain it should be done only by a patient's doctor or other type of health-care provider.

Each doctor's approach to managing pain may differ. Therefore, it is important that patient and patient's doctor have a healthy doctor-patient relationship and that patient's doctor understands patient's situation. The situations and causes of each person's pain differ, and therefore patient's doctor may suggest different combinations of methods to help relieve patient's pain.

The current methods doctors have available to measure patient's pain are imperfect. The perception of pain is based on many things that affect patient, and can range from memories of a previous painful event to psychological influences.

Pain is not necessarily just a sensory experience, but it is also a result of processes that occur at a higher level in the brain, making pain a psychological experience. There is no general consensus among pain medicine doctors as to the best test for the measurement of pain.

An ideal test for the assessment of pain must bring together experimental as well as clinical knowledge. Right now, there are no adequate tests that can differentiate gender with respect to the assessment of pain. In order to provide adequate pain management, a doctor must combine all of the data given by patient concerning patient's pain complaints.

Hopefully a universally accepted pain assessment test will become available in the near future. In the meantime, patient and patient's doctor must talk not only about pain complaints, but also about patient's feelings of depression and anxiety during each office visit. Patient and patient's doctor must develop a healthy relationship so that the appropriate pain modalities can be rationally prescribed specifically for patient.

Pain is subjective and does not allow itself to be measured accurately. In other words, it is impossible to visualize "pain." When patient's doctor interviews patient about patient's pain complaints, he or she will begin by asking the following questions: the time of the onset of patient's pain, the location of the pain on patient's body, how long it lasts, and how often it occurs during the day.

The patient's doctor also will ask patient whether patient's pain is sharp, dull, or cramping. Patient should tell patient's doctor whether patient's pain is mild, moderate, or severe. Women in general are more able to express their pain experiences than men. Patient must provide patient's doctor with enough information so that he or she can come up with a reasonable and accurate diagnosis for patient.

What follows is an initial pain-assessment form. This assessment addresses a patient's pain and psychosocial issues and leaves room for patient's doctor's evaluation of patient's condition. Patient's doctor will give patient a copy of this assessment form. Patient will be asked questions such as when the pain began, how long it lasts, what makes it worse, what makes it better, what medications patient are taking, what effects medications are having on patient's pain, and what patient's emotional status is during episodes of pain.

One way of assessing patient's pain is to use a numeric scale. This is the simplest method for attempting to measure patient's pain. During this test, patient are asked to rate patient's pain on a scale of 0 to 5 or to use words such as "none," "slight," "moderate," or "severe." This assessment is also a quick, simple, and reliable way to evaluate the effectiveness of any medications patient are taking to manage patient's pain.

On the numeric scale, 0 equals no pain, 1 equals mild pain, 2 equals moderate pain, 3 equals distressing pain, 4 equals horrible pain, and 5 equals excruciating pain confining patient to bed rest. This method is easily understood and may be helpful in guiding the treatment plans patient's doctor creates for patient.

Another type of verbal scale asks patient to rate patient's pain on a scale of 1 to 10, with 1 being equivalent to pain that is barely noticeable and 10 relating to excruciating pain. A verbal numeric scale is easily understood. All patient have to do is choose a number to represent patient's level of pain.

The following numeric pain-intensity scale is the most popular test used by pain-medicine specialists. Patient circle a number on the scale that corresponds to how much pain patient feel. It only uses numbers from 0 through 10 along the length of the horizontal scale. A score of 0 indicates no pain, whereas a score of 10 means that patient feel the worst pain ever imagined. Another method used by some doctors is a pain diary.

This is a descriptive report patient keep to assess patient's pain. The pain diary shows a written account of patient's day-to-day experiences. It can be used to help diagnose the cause of patient's pain.

The value of the pain diary is that patient and patient's doctor can monitor patient's day-to-day variation of painful states and patient's response to therapy. Patient need to keep a diary of patient's pain patterns when patient are sitting, standing, and lying down. Patient should also record sleep patterns and sexual activity.

A patient also must note the amount of pain medication patient is taking and whether it lessens patient's pain. Because pain can interfere with eating patterns, keep a diary of the amount of food patient eat and at what time patient ate. Be sure to include any types of recreational activities and whether patient's pain felt better or worse afterward. Patients have to be diligent in patient's record keeping. This form enables patient to record an entire month of pain-intensity scores, patient's activities, the location of patient's pain, and a medication log. Patient's physician will find this diary extremely helpful in working with patient to plan patient's pain therapy.

Pain drawings offer a visual way to evaluate patient's pain. Patient will be asked to shade in areas on a human figure outline that correspond to the areas of patient's pain. The drawing will help patient's doctor determine where patient's pain is coming from and how widespread it is on patient's body. Over time, patient's pain drawings can be compared to show the changes of patient's pain and how patient are responding to therapy.

The following is a sample pain-assessment tool that includes diagrams for patient to shade to tell patient's doctor whether patient's pain is confined to one area of patient's body or whether patient's pain is widespread throughout patient's body. This form allows patient to shade the areas of patient's body where patient are feeling patient's pain.

A common method of determining the behavioral component of patient's pain is for patient to be directly observed by patient's doctor. Patient must be observed while sitting, walking to and from the office, and getting in and out of vehicles. Patient's doctor will focus his or her attention on the area of patient's major pain complaint.

Behavioral influences affecting patient's perception of pain include the amount of medications patient use and the number of doctor visits required. Limping and facial grimacing also are appropriate behavioral evaluations of pain.

Depression and anxiety are emotional factors that can be measured by tests. Because the experience of pain is impossible to measure directly, patient's doctor must observe patient's displays of appropriate or inappropriate physical behavior.

After observing patient's behavior, a patient's doctor may classify patient using the following four-class system: Class 1 consists of patients with low physical injury but high levels of abnormal behavior patterns related to their pain. Class 2 consists of patients with lower physical injury and low behavior pattern abnormalities. Class 3 consists of patients with significant tissue injury in addition to high behavioral pattern abnormalities. Class 4 consists of patients with a high tissue injury and normal behavioral patterns.

A visual analog scale is another method of assessment that attempts to measure patient's level of pain. Instead of choosing a number, patient are asked to mark a point on a horizontal line that is labeled with "no pain" at one end and "the worst possible pain" at the opposite end.

The line is divided into 10 equal spaces, and patient chooses number from 1 to 10 based on patient's level of pain. It is slightly more difficult to administer than the numeric method, but some doctors and researchers think that the visual analog scale is more accurate than the numeric scale for pain measurements.

A patient will circle a point on the line that indicates how much pain patient feel. Descriptive words are placed along the horizontal scale, which enables patient to describe the severity of patient's pain. Another visual scale that is easy to use, especially for children, is the face scale. It shows pictures of happy to grimacing faces and patients are asked to circle the face that shows what kind of pain they feel. Using descriptive words is one method of describing patient's pain.

Self-reports have been used by doctors since 1939. A pain-rating index consists of groups of words associated with pain. This index has been incorporated into the McGill pain questionnaire, a type of verbal assessment that uses word

For the following pain assessment form patient will circle the words that best describe patient's pain. Since they are in no particular order, there is no obvious progression of pain shown.

A McGill pain questionnaire is a method for assessing pain psychologically. A McGill pain questionnaire gives a multidimensional pain score. Patient are given 20 word sets that describe a different dimension of patient's pain. Patients are asked to select words relevant to patient's pain from each of these 20 sets.

For example, one set includes the words "jumping," "flashing," and "shooting." Another set includes the words "tingling," "itching," "smarting," and "stinging." Patient circle the word that relates closest to the pain patient feel throughout the 20 word sets.

This questionnaire is difficult to administer as well as to interpret. However, it has characteristic response patterns for different pain syndromes such as back pain, arthritis, and cancer. The validity of this questionnaire continues to be studied. The McGill pain questionnaire consists of four different parts. The first part consists of a human figure drawing on which patient are instructed to mark the location of patient's pain. The second part is the pain-rating index that contains 78 words divided into 20 groups.

Each set contains up to six words. Five of these groups describe tension or fear. Each word is assigned a value according to its position within a subclass. The third part of this test asks additional questions about prior pain experiences, as well as the location of the pain and current usage of pain medications.

The fourth part consists of a present pain intensity index. This aspect of the test requests a pain score from 0 to 5 with word descriptors such as no pain, mild pain, discomforting pain, distressing pain, or horrible and excruciating pain. These words also are assigned different values.

All the values are added to obtain a total score. All the scores are then evaluated to attempt to assess patient's total pain experience. The problem with this test is that there is no specific mechanism within the test itself to determine which component truly reflects patient's pain experience.

The value of this test, however, is that it treats pain as a multidimensional experience. There also is a short form of the McGill pain questionnaire that has been developed. This questionnaire contains fewer words and categories than the long form. This test is sensitive to evaluations of reduction in pain experiences. This test is more useful for rapid evaluation of data following procedures or surgery.

Some simple tests have been developed that patient's physician can administer in his or her office. These tests are not as comprehensive as the McGill Questionnaire but do give a quick estimate of how patient's pain compares with other pain patients. Certain psychological tests exist, including the P-3® and the BBHITM that assist healthcare practitioners in the assessment of biopsychosocial factors that can affect the effective diagnosis and treatment of patient's pain.

A patient must realize that if patient's physician requires patient to take a psychological test that he or she does not think that patient are imagining patient's pain. The goal is to determine how much suffering patient are experiencing as a result of patient's pain syndrome. This information is helpful in planning an overall treatment plan for patient.

Clinicians can consider a rating of greater than 5/10 to the question "What is patient's average pain over the last 2 days?" to be a "red flag" for CRPS.5

The following is a pain diary that may be of some help to patient and patient's physician. Patient should fill the form out daily; when patient awaken, at noon and in the evening. Patient are instructed to rate patient's pain on a score from 0 to 10 with 0 being no pain and 10 the worst imaginable. Patient can create patient's own pain diary using a computer spreadsheet program or a word processing program. Some patients like to use a notebook.

Some patients prefer to graph their pain scores to watch their pain trends. No matter which pain diary that patient use, patient need some data to give to patient's physician, therapist and/or chiropractor so that any further treatment can be assessed. Patient can create patient's own pain diary as below.

Pain-related fear might be a promising concept in the understanding of pain disability in patients with neuropathic pain.6   Chronic pain due to CRPS has a profound impact on many aspects of the lives of both patients and their spouses.7

Despite the variety of outcome measurement tools reported for CRPS rehabilitation, large gaps in both comprehensiveness and supporting psychometric evidence remain. Comprehensive, relevant and psychometrically sound tools for monitoring treatment outcomes are needed to address the pain and functional limitations experienced by this population.8

A sample daily patient pain assessment diary is presented. Any form can be utilized. It is important to know when the patient's pain was the worst so that appropriate medication dosing can be established. It is important to know what activity worsens the pain. Furthermore, do the medications decrease the pain an hour after taking the medicine? It is important to know if the patient does therapy or exercise and the effect on his/her. Any side effects and/or new problems must be addressed as well.

Date_____   **Daily Pain Assessment**

Time	Where is the pain? Rate the pain (0-10), or list the word from the scale that describes your pain.	What were you doing when the pain started or increased?	Did you take medicine? What did you take? How much?	What other treatments did you use?	After an hour, what is your pain rating?	Other problems or side effects? Comments.
morning						
noon						
evening						

A paper was published which is intended to provide assistance to physicians asked to evaluate impairment- and disability-related issues and is not primarily geared to guide treatment of the CRPS I patient.9 Evaluators should perform a comprehensive assessment of patients with CRPS I to make an accurate diagnosis and exclude other conditions that could explain the symptoms and signs of the condition.

While radiological, laboratory, and other diagnostic studies may be of assistance in making the diagnosis, in the final analysis, this is a clinical diagnosis. Impairment is based on objectively validated limitation in activities of daily living.

Litigation may be involved in some CRPS cases. Forensic activity in a practice has been reviewed with reference to the differing roles of the pain clinician and the independent expert. Ethical guidelines and recommendations for assessment, documentation, record review, and court testimony are discussed.

Specific issues include the assessment of disability and impairment, malingering, and application of the Daubert standard in forensic pain practice. Examples of case law are reviewed for civil liability and CRPS, malpractice with opioid prescribing, and practice issues in a correctional setting.10

References

1.   Monti DA, Herring CL, Schwartzman RJ, Marchese M. Personality assessment of patients with complex regional pain syndrome type I. Clin J Pain. 1998;14(4):295-302.

2.   Bean DJ, Johnson MH, Heiss-Dunlop W, Lee AC, Kydd RR. Do psychological factors influence recovery from complex regional pain syndrome type 1? A prospective study. Pain. 2015;156(11):2310-2318.

3.   Bruehl S, Chung OY. Psychological and behavioral aspects of complex regional pain syndrome management. Clin J Pain. 2006;22(5):430-437.

4.   Edinger L, Schwartzman RJ, Ahmad A, Erwin K, Alexander GM. Objective sensory evaluation of the spread of complex regional pain syndrome. Pain Physician. 2013;16(6):581-591.

5.   Moseley GL, Herbert RD, Parsons T, Lucas S, Van Hilten JJ, Marinus J. Intense pain soon after wrist fracture strongly predicts who

will develop complex regional pain syndrome: prospective cohort study. J Pain. 2014;15(1):16-23.

6.   de Jong JR, Vlaeyen JW, de Gelder JM, Patijn J. Pain-related fear, perceived harmfulness of activities, and functional limitations in complex regional pain syndrome type I. J Pain. 2011;12(12):1209-1218.

7.   Kemler MA, Furnee CA. The impact of chronic pain on life in the household. J Pain Symptom Manage. 2002;23(5):433-441.

8.   Packham T, MacDermid JC, Henry J, Bain J. A systematic review of psychometric evaluations of outcome assessments for complex regional pain syndrome. Disabil Rehabil. 2012;34(13):1059-1069.

9.   Aronoff GM, Harden N, Stanton-Hicks M, et al. American Academy of Disability Evaluating Physicians (AADEP) position paper: complex regional pain syndrome I (RSD): impairment and disability issues. Pain Med. 2002;3(3):274-288.

10.   Kulich RJ, Kreis PG, Fishman SM, et al. Forensic issues in pain: review of current practice. Pain Pract. 2001;1(2):119-135.

8. Psychological Factors

Psychological and behavioral factors can exacerbate the pain and dysfunction associated with the complex regional pain syndrome (CRPS) and could help maintain the condition in some patients. Effective management of CRPS requires that these psychosocial and behavioral aspects be addressed as part of an integrated multidisciplinary treatment approach. The risk of CRPS type I was significantly increased in patients with high trait anxiety scores.[1]

Because of the uncertain origins of the condition, professionals have considered the role of psychological factors, either in the development of the condition or in its continuance. However, research does not reveal support for specific personality or psychopathology predictors of the condition.

Cognitive and sensory changes observed in chronic pain patients are derived from observations regarding cortical representation and reorganization, and thus these domains are complementary to each other, reinforcing the idea that the brain abnormalities do result in very specific changes in information processing.[2]

Anxiety, pain-related fear, and disability are associated with poorer outcomes in CRPS and could be considered as target variables for early treatment. The findings support the theory that CRPS represents an aberrant protective response to perceived threat of tissue injury. Even in the early stages of CRPS, a cycle of pain, disability, depression, and work absence can emerge.

Anxiety, pain-related fear, and disability are associated with poorer outcomes in CRPS and could be considered as target variables for early treatment. [3] CRPS represents an aberrant protective response to perceived threat of tissue injury. Management of CRPS is challenging, partly because of a lack of clinical data regarding the efficacy of the various therapies, and partly because successful treatment of CRPS requires a multidisciplinary, patient-tailored approach.

In CRPS, disability and pain severity were more strongly associated with psychological factors than they were in low back pain. In CRPS, disability and pain severity were more strongly associated with psychological factors than they were in low back pain.[4]

The risk of CRPS type I was significantly increased in patients with high trait anxiety scores. Early traumatic experiences were reported in 87% of the CRPS-I patients and were found to be moderately related to somatoform dissociative experiences, indicating that early traumatic experiences might be a predisposing, although not a necessary factor for the development of CRPS-I-related dystonia.

All patients with chronic CRPS should receive a thorough psychological evaluation, followed by cognitive-behavioral pain management treatment, including relaxation training with biofeedback. Patients making insufficient overall treatment progress or in whom comorbid psychiatric disorders/major ongoing life stressors are identified should additionally receive general cognitive-behavioral therapy to address these issues.[5] It is interesting to note that psychological factors are not associated with CRPS onset.[6]

CRPS patients with allodynia manifest clinical signs of special psychological distress. The high incidence of personality pathology in CRPS patients may represent an exaggeration of maladaptive personality traits and coping styles as a result of a chronic, intense, state of pain. Stressful life events are more common in the CRPS group, which indicates that there may be a multiconditional model of CRPS.

CRPS is comorbid with depression, anxiety, and insomnia, but this relationship is not psychopathological. Medical and health professionals should not dismiss symptoms related to CRPS as caused by emotional distress.[7] When CRPS sufferers are grouped as mentally ill, serious consequences follow. Primarily, CRPS patients will not have access to treatment interventions such as pharmacotherapy and physical rehabilitation that could improve quality of life, daily functioning, and thwart disease progression.

There may be decreased cortical thickness in the prefrontal cortex and neurocognitive dysfunctions in patients with CRPS.[8] These findings may contribute to the understanding of pain-related impairments in cognitive function and could help explain the symptoms or progression of CRPS.

Patients who have an anxious personality have a higher risk of developing CRPS type I.[1] Following these patients closely for the development of CRPS type I is important so that a rapid diagnosis and treatment can be instituted in a timely fashion. Based on recent research into the neurobiology of CRPS a supraspinal mechanism has been proposed as an etiological element which could explain how emotional stress can produce both symptoms and signs of CRPS.9

There is controversy regarding the importance of psychological/psychiatric factors in the development of the Complex Regional Pain Syndrome.10 The high incidence of personality pathology in CRPS patients may represent an exaggeration of maladaptive personality traits and coping styles as a result of a chronic, intense, state of pain.

Investigations are typically normal, but many patients fulfil strict criteria for a somatoform disorder/psychogenic dystonia. In a proportion of patients, however, no conclusive features of somatoform disorder or psychogenic disorder can be found and, in these patients, whether this disorder is primarily neurological or psychiatric remains an open question.11 Whilst the prognosis is overall poor, remissions do occur, particularly in those patients who are willing and able to undergo multidisciplinary treatment including physiotherapy and psychotherapy.

A significantly large number of cases of CRPS are being missed by their health care providers, most of them being attributed to psychogenic issues rather than pain from CRPS. Suspecting that psychological factors are entirely responsible for influencing CRPS carries the implication that pain is all in the patient's head, and ultimately blames the patient for their pain.7

When an injury elicits a pain response, guarding the affected site is an innate response to prevent further injury; if the pain is unrelenting, than this guarding behavior of the arm or leg immobilizes the limb in question. A higher pain score was predictive of higher depression, anxiety, and anger scores in CRPS patients.12 Only life events seemed to be associated with CRPS1: patients who experienced more life events appeared to have a greater chance of developing CRPS 1.

A Somatoform disorder is characterized by physical symptoms that mimic physical disease or injury for which there is no identifiable organic cause. If there is an identifiable cause for physical symptoms, such as pain or neurological deficits, the symptoms cannot be fully explained by the nature of the injury and are thought to be psychologically maintained.

Symptoms resulting from a Somatoform disorder are said to be due to the manifestation of mental distress or have a psychogenic origin. Symptoms of body and sensory disturbances common in CRPS pathology are often mistaken for somatoform disorders, particularly conversion disorder or pain disorder. The main CRPS criterion is that the pain must be out of proportion to the trauma and this unfortunately is also the same criterion for pain disorder; a type of somatoform disorder.

There is compelling evidence against the psychogenic model of CRPS onset. Psychiatrists do not have expertise in the clinical diagnosis of CRPS, but they are able to assess the presence of co-morbid psychiatric conditions.13 They can assist the court as experts in the underlying neurophysiological and psychological processes which may explain some of the important features of CRPS and an individual's psychological vulnerability to CRPS.

It has been suggested that anxiety, pain-related fear, and disability are associated with poorer outcomes in CRPS and could be considered as target variables for early treatment.3 The findings support the theory that CRPS represents an aberrant protective response to perceived threat of tissue injury.

Because psychosocial factors play an important role, it is recommended to provide psychological evaluation and cognitive behavioral treatment as soon as possible.14 Their expertise in psychological and psycho-pharmacological interventions should be considered for any multidisciplinary treatment program for CRPS along with the likely contribution of these interventions to the overall prognosis.

The psychogenic model cannot account for the neurological and neuroanatomical deficits related to CRPS pathology.15 Psychological factors play a role in CRPS, but the exact relationship is unknown. CRPS onset is not likely due to psychogenic factors.

Although many patients with CRPS have been stigmatized as being psychologically different, a relationship between this disease and several psychological factors cannot be derived. The search for a predisposing psychologic personality structure are obsolete and useless.16 Management of pain and pain-related impairments, however, are based on the personality of the affected persons.

When pain treatment fails, CRPS is associated with negative outcomes, both psychological and psychosocial in nature.17 However, research does not reveal support for specific personality or psychopathology predictors of the condition. What is proven however, is that psychiatrists because of their expertise in psychological and psycho-pharmacological interventions should be considered for any multidisciplinary treatment program for CRPS patients along with the likely contribution of these interventions to the overall prognosis.

The controversy surrounding the disorder of CRPS centers around the nature of the problem and whether it is a primary organic disorder or a primary psychogenic disorder associated with the accomplishment of some secondary gain. If it is the former, then clearly research should continue to determine the nature and etiology of the malfunctioning organ.

If, on the other hand, RSD is a psychogenic disorder, then the medical community does well to focus mainly on the peripheral manifestations of the problem. In that instance, therapy should be primarily psychological and cognitive with regard to the secondary gain, and persistent organic treatments are unlikely to improve the condition in general and worsen individual cases.18

A biopsychosocial hypothesis which considers the possible role of psychophysiological and behavioral aspects of helplessness in the precipitation, maintenance, and/or enhancement of RSD may be considered.19 Another study concluded that there is no particular psychological or personality pattern predisposing one to develop RSD.20 Most experts believe that a multidisciplinary approach including pharmacotherapy, physiotherapy, and psychotherapy is warranted.

Stressful life events are more common in the CRPS group, which indicates that there may be a multiconditional model of CRPS. The experience of stressful life events besides trauma or surgery are risk factors, not causes, in such a model.21

Psychological and behavioral factors can exacerbate the pain and dysfunction associated with complex regional pain syndrome (CRPS) and could help maintain the condition in some patients.5 Anxiety, pain-related fear, and disability are associated with poorer outcomes in CRPS and could be considered as target variables for early treatment.

Complex regional pain syndrome is a disabling pain condition poorly understood by medical professionals. Because CRPS is particularly enigmatic, and has significant impact on patient function, researchers have examined psychological processes present among patients with this diagnosis. Research does not reveal support for specific personality or psychopathology predictors of the condition.17

Although the psychological profile of the patients with CRPS-I-related dystonia shows some elevations, there does not seem to be a unique disturbed psychological profile on a group level.22   CRPS patients with allodynia manifest clinical signs of special psychological distress. In chronic CRPS depressive syndrome frequently develops and psychological treatment can be recommended.23

Anxiety, pain-related fear, and disability are associated with poorer outcomes in CRPS management and could be considered as target variables for early treatment. The findings support the theory that CRPS represents an aberrant protective response to perceived threat of tissue injury.3

As stated in the first paragraph of this chapter, patients who have an anxious personality have a higher risk of developing CRPS type I. Following these patients closely for the development of CRPS type I may be advantageous for early preventative and therapeutic interventions.1

The findings support the theory that CRPS represents an aberrant protective response to perceived threat of tissue injury.3   Furthermore, evidence indicates that chronic pain is associated with a specific cognitive deficit, which may impact everyday behavior especially in risky, emotionally laden, situations.24

In summary one can conclude that in most instances that patients who eventually develop CRPS have neither a unique psychological pattern nor displayed more symptoms of depression than those who recovered uneventfully in a previous published study on CRPS.25

References

1.   Dilek B, Yemez B, Kizil R, et al. Anxious personality is a risk factor for developing complex regional pain syndrome type I. Rheumatol Int. 2012;32(4):915-920.

2.   Apkarian AV. Human Brain Imaging Studies of Chronic Pain: Translational Opportunities. In: Kruger L, Light AR, eds. Translational Pain Research: From Mouse to Man. Boca Raton, FL2010.

3.   Bean DJ, Johnson MH, Heiss-Dunlop W, Lee AC, Kydd RR. Do psychological factors influence recovery from complex regional pain syndrome type 1? A prospective study. Pain. 2015;156(11):2310-2318.

4.   Bean DJ, Johnson MH, Kydd RR. Relationships between psychological factors, pain, and disability in complex regional pain syndrome and low back pain. Clin J Pain. 2014;30(8):647-653.

5.   Bruehl S, Chung OY. Psychological and behavioral aspects of complex regional pain syndrome management. Clin J Pain. 2006;22(5):430-437.

6.   de Mos M, Huygen FJ, Dieleman JP, Koopman JS, Stricker BH, Sturkenboom MC. Medical history and the onset of complex regional pain syndrome (CRPS). Pain. 2008;139(2):458-466.

7.   Hill RJ, Chopra P, Richardi T. Rethinking the psychogenic model of complex regional pain syndrome: somatoform disorders and complex regional pain syndrome. Anesth Pain Med. 2012;2(2):54-59.

8.   Lee DH, Lee KJ, Cho KI, et al. Brain alterations and neurocognitive dysfunction in patients with complex regional pain syndrome. J Pain. 2015;16(6):580-586.

9.   Grande LA, Loeser JD, Ozuna J, Ashleigh A, Samii A. Complex regional pain syndrome as a stress response. Pain. 2004;110(1-2):495-498.

10.   Monti DA, Herring CL, Schwartzman RJ, Marchese M. Personality assessment of patients with complex regional pain syndrome type I. Clin J Pain. 1998;14(4):295-302.

11.   Schrag A, Trimble M, Quinn N, Bhatia K. The syndrome of fixed dystonia: an evaluation of 103 patients. Brain. 2004;127(Pt 10):2360-2372.

12.   Beerthuizen A, van 't Spijker A, Huygen FJ, Klein J, de Wit R. Is there an association between psychological factors and the Complex Regional Pain Syndrome type 1 (CRPS1) in adults? A systematic review. Pain. 2009;145(1-2):52-59.

13.   Neal LA. Complex regional pain syndrome: the role of the psychiatrist as an expert witness. Med Sci Law. 2009;49(4):241-246.

14.   Kachko L, Efrat R, Ben Ami S, Mukamel M, Katz J. Complex regional pain syndromes in children and adolescents. Pediatr Int. 2008;50(4):523-527.

15.   Schwartzman RJ, Alexander GM, Grothusen JR, Paylor T, Reichenberger E, Perreault M. Outpatient intravenous ketamine for the treatment of complex regional pain syndrome: a double-blind placebo controlled study. Pain. 2009;147(1-3):107-115.

16.   Lesky J. [Sudeck syndrome (CRPS) caused by unique personality traits: myth and fiction]. Z Orthop Unfall. 2010;148(6):716-722.

17.   Lohnberg JA, Altmaier EM. A review of psychosocial factors in complex regional pain syndrome. J Clin Psychol Med Settings. 2013;20(2):247-254.

18.   Pawl RP. Controversies surrounding reflex sympathetic dystrophy: a review article. Curr Rev Pain. 2000;4(4):259-267.

19. Van Houdenhove B, Vasquez G. Is there a relationship between reflex sympathetic dystrophy and helplessness? Case reports and a hypothesis. Gen Hosp Psychiatry. 1993;15(5):325-329.

20. Zyluk A. [Are mental disorders the cause of reflex sympathetic dystrophy: a review]. Wiad Lek. 1999;52(9-10):500-507.

21. Geertzen JH, de Bruijn-Kofman AT, de Bruijn HP, van de Wiel HB, Dijkstra PU. Stressful life events and psychological dysfunction in Complex Regional Pain Syndrome type I. Clin J Pain. 1998;14(2):143-147.

22. Reedijk WB, van Rijn MA, Roelofs K, Tuijl JP, Marinus J, van Hilten JJ. Psychological features of patients with complex regional pain syndrome type I related dystonia. Mov Disord. 2008;23(11):1551-1559.

23. Rommel O, Willweber-Strumpf A, Wagner P, Surall D, Malin JP, Zenz M. [Psychological abnormalities in patients with complex regional pain syndrome (CRPS)]. Schmerz. 2005;19(4):272-284.

24. Apkarian AV, Sosa Y, Krauss BR, et al. Chronic pain patients are impaired on an emotional decision-making task. Pain. 2004;108(1-2):129-136.

25. Puchalski P, Zyluk A. Complex regional pain syndrome type 1 after fractures of the distal radius: a prospective study of the role of psychological factors. J Hand Surg Br. 2005;30(6):574-580.

9. Diagnosis

It is important to remember that there is no test validated for CRPS diagnosis. A gold standard in diagnosing CRPS has not been found yet, diagnostics are based on the patient's medical history and correlating clinical signs. The various tests that might be suggested and their relation to CRPS causation and diagnosis are presented.

Dr. John J. Bonica proposed a staging of CRPS. In a consensus conference held in Budapest in 2003, it was proposed a new classification system that included the presence of at least two clinical signs included in the four categories and at least three symptoms in its four categories.

Complex regional pain syndrome is a neuropathic pain disorder with significant autonomic features. Few treatments have proven effective, in part, because of a historically poor understanding of the mechanisms underlying the disorder

Relative contributions of the mechanisms underlying CRPS may differ across patients and even within a patient over time, particularly in the transition from "warm CRPS" (acute) to "cold CRPS" (chronic). Enhanced knowledge regarding the pathophysiology of CRPS increases the possibility of eventually achieving the goal of mechanism-based CRPS diagnosis and treatment.[1]

The complex regional pain syndrome is a neurologic disorder that often results in debilitating chronic pain, but the diagnosis may elude providers as it is one of exclusion. The incidence and disease course of the complex regional pain syndrome has been unclear until recently. This was due to inconsistent diagnostic criteria used in previous studies and a lack of large-scale prospective datasets.

Multiple mechanisms of CRPS have been suggested, and recent research has begun to explain how inflammation, the immune system and the autonomic nervous system may interact with aberrant central neuroplasticity to produce the clinical picture.[2]

The final step will be to assess large cohorts and to analyze these data together with data from public resources using a bioinformatics approach. Clinicians could then develop diagnostic toolboxes for individual pathophysiology and select focused treatments or develop new ones.

Because of a lack of a simple objective diagnostic test, diagnosis is reliant on clinical assessment. Prospective studies have repeatedly demonstrated a higher incidence than retrospective studies, an observation that has been challenged owing to the lack of uniformity of diagnostic criteria across specialties and workers researching the condition.3

There have been other classification systems proposed for the diagnosis of CRPS, such as Veldman's diagnostic criteria based on the presence of at least 4 signs and symptoms of the disease associated with a worsening of the same following the use of the limb and their location in the same area distal to the one that suffered the injury.

On the other hand, the Atkins diagnostic criteria are much more objective than those proposed by IASP and are specifically applicable to an orthopedic context. However, current classification systems and related criteria proposed to make a diagnosis of CRPS, do not include instrumental evaluations and imaging, but rely solely on clinical findings.4

It has been reported that there is a significant reduction of bone mineral density in patients with CRPS after a stroke. The reduction in bone mineral density correlates with the severity of shoulder hand syndrome score, degree of weakness, duration of hemiplegia, and the severity of stroke.5

A three-phase bone scan, before conventional radiography shows morphological changes in CRPS 1, represents a valuable diagnostic tool thanks to the depiction of pathognomonic findings and the localization ability in all 3 phases.6

In late or subsequent stages the lack of scintigraphic uptake seems to represent the end of the active disease process. The role of three-phase bone scintigraphy in CRPS I is to support or even confirm the diagnosis, given its various presentations.

Furthermore, it enables exclusion of other diagnoses such as arthritis, benign or malignant bony lesions, or even metabolic bone diseases such as Paget's disease, particularly if an integrated SPECT/CT is added. Moreover, the earlier the diagnosis is finally established and treatment of CRPS I is initiated, the better the prognosis.

Therefore, bone scintigraphy potentially has a major impact on patient management of this disorder. Conventional MRI may be helpful, when repeated for monitoring the treatment response in patients with CRPS.7

Reasonable tests for the diagnosis of CRPS are conventional X-ray examination comparing sides, magnetic resonance imaging and a 3-phase bone scintigraphy. Moreover, electrophysiological examinations can prove a nerve lesion and differentiate between CRPS type I and II.

A temperature difference can be detected via infrared thermography. Furthermore, quantitative sensory testing can verify the magnitude of the sensory disturbance and can be beneficial to objectify therapeutic effects.

Use of these diagnostic tools, even after achievement of normal findings, cannot exclude a CRPS and the decision for therapeutic initiation should not be influenced thereby.8

X rays are useful because this method is less invasive than some of the other diagnostic tests mentioned, it is often used as a preliminary test to view bone mineralization status and track it through the disease process.

The three-phase bone scan, which uses immediate and delayed images to study blood flow, is especially useful to CRPS study. This modality emphases the role of scintigraphy in the management of this multisystem disorder.9

The measured pain, temperature, volume and range of motion can be used as diagnostic indicators for establishing presence or absence of CRPS I. Infrared thermometry records the distribution of skin temperature. In CRPS testing, each area of the skin is then compared with the identical contralateral area with a goal of determining temperature between the side with CRPS and the normal side.

Vascular abnormalities are dynamic. The maximal skin temperature difference that occurs during the thermoregulatory cycle distinguishes CRPS I from other extremity pain syndromes with high sensitivity and specificity.10

It is suggested that, in CRPS I, unilateral inhibition of sympathetic vasoconstrictor neurons leads to a warmer affected limb in the acute stage. Secondary changes in neurovascular transmission may lead to vasoconstriction and cold skin in chronic CRPS I, whereas sympathetic activity is still depressed.

The maximal skin temperature difference that occurs during the thermoregulatory cycle distinguishes CRPS I from other extremity pain syndromes with high sensitivity and specificity.

Skin temperature measurement results using infra-red thermometers support reliability. This equipment demonstrated excellent reliability for the diagnosis of CRPS, with little difference in the reliability of measurement sites.11

Laser doppler flowmetry measures the skin's blood flow to local thermal stimulation.12 When a peripheral vascular disease is suspected, the blood flow deviates from the normal pattern, which also affects the skin temperature. Unlike thermography, which can measure a specific area, laser doppler flowmetry is more effective over a larger area.

Laser Doppler flux metric perfusion studies were performed by Ackerman et. al on the normal and CRPS I hands pre- and post-stellate ganglion block therapy which was useful in ascertain blood flow in the CRPS extremity as well as the normal extremity.13

Infrared thermography uses an electronic thermographic apparatus to create computer-generated images that display changes in temperature. A temperature difference can be detected via infrared thermography. Furthermore, quantitative sensory testing can verify the magnitude of the sensory disturbance and can be beneficial to objectify therapeutic effects. Use of these diagnostic tools, even after achievement of normal findings, cannot exclude a CRPS and the decision for therapeutic initiation should not be influenced thereby.8

Excessive sweating of the affected limb is an important feature of CRPS I.14 The quantitative sudomotor axon reflex test (QSART) is used for sweating abnormalities as increased sweating of an affected extremity may be associated with CRPS.15

EMG/NCV testing suggests that Subtype 2 may reflect CRPS-Type 2 (causalgia) if nerve damage is evident by nerve conduction tests.16 Nerve conduction velocity tests define the health of peripheral nerves by testing the speed of the signals through the nerve.

In a group of patients with short- and long-term (chronic) duration of complex regional pain syndrome type I (CRPS I) motor cortical representation was determined, using a transcranial magnetic stimulation (TMS) mapping method. This was done, starting with suprathreshold intensities at the location of the largest amplitude, mapping systematically in all directions.

Patients were compared to a group of healthy subjects. In both patient groups it was found that there was significantly larger motor cortical representation for the unaffected hand muscles compared to the affected side. This asymmetry was absent in healthy subjects. Such motor cortical representation asymmetry can be considered an effect of altered sensomotor cortical representation which can be useful in the diagnosis of CRPS.17

Cortical reorganization occurs in chronic neuropathic pain patients even without peripheral nerve damage. It is possible that cortical reorganization is related to chronic pain, regardless of its etiology.18

Some experts advocate serial measurement of skin temperatures, based upon evidence from one small study that a 2°C difference for the affected versus unaffected side was supportive of the diagnosis of CRPS.

However, this method requires monitoring for five to eight hours with recording of skin temperature at one minute intervals using temperature sensors applied to the index fingers. Thus, it is not practical as a routine clinical test.

Chronic CRPS patients have a normal vasodilatory response to external heating and that skin temperature differences between the affected and unaffected lower limbs, which were highly variable during daytime, disappeared during sleep. 19

Quantitative sensory testing (QST) is another diagnostic test and with this modality it has been conclude that hemisensory impairment in patients with CRPS Type I is probably related to functional disturbances in processing of noxious events in the thalamus and may be a clinical correlate of subcortical brain plasticity in chronic pain.20 QST uses a computer testing system to measure how the nerves involved react to vibration and changes in temperature. These test results are then compared to unaffected patients and the patient's unaffected side.

The development of surgical and percutaneous neurodestructive methods have been developed in order to target and destroy various components of afferent nociceptive pathways. Sympathetic nerve blocks are not neurodestructive and essentially injections of a local anesthetic at various places in the body, which in turn block the sympathetic nerves of each area which can relieve pain associated with CRPS.

Sympathetic blocks are applied for the treatment of various vascular diseases including critical limb ischemia. Other indications for thoracic and lumbar sympathectomy include complex regional pain syndrome (CRPS), chronic tumor associated pain and hyperhidrosis. Neurolysis of the celiac plexus is an effective palliative pain treatment particularly in patients suffering from pancreatic cancer. Percutaneous dorsal root ganglion rhizotomy can be performed in selected patients with radicular pain that is resistant to conventional pharmacological and interventional treatment.21

Sympathetic blocks may also relieve CRPS pain. Systemic alpha-adrenergic blockade with phentolamine is a diagnostic test for sympathetically maintained pain. Raja et al pointed out that only some patients with CRPS respond to a sympathetic nerve blockade, and they proposed that patients' pain be defined as "sympathetically-maintained" or "sympathetically-independent" according to their response to temporary sympathetic nerve blocks.22

The use of intravenous regional blocks or diagnostic intravenous infusions remains questionable for the diagnosis of CRPS.23   While sympathetic blocks can be helpful in the reduction of mechanical allo-dynia, and thus the facilitation of physical and occupational therapy, ultimate response to a regime that includes medications is not predicted by sympathetic block alone.24

Accumulating experimental and clinical evidence supports the hy-pothesis that complex regional pain syndrome type I (CRPS-I) may be a small fiber neuropathy.25   CRPS-I may be associated with changes in the ultramicroscopic small fiber structure that cannot be visualized with commercially available techniques.

Alternatively, functional rather than structural alterations of small fibers or pathological changes at a more proximal site such as the spinal cord or brain may be responsible for the syndrome. As a result, a skin biopsy may be of benefit in the diagnosis of CRPS where the affected extremity is compared to the normal extremity. CRPS-I is specifically associated with post-trauma in many instances affecting nociceptive small-fibers. This type of nerve injury will remain undetected in most clinical settings.26

Phentolamine mesylate (Regitine) is a short-acting alpha-adrenergic blocking agent that acts at both alpha-1 and alpha-2 adrenergic receptor sites. As a test to diagnose RSD, patients are usually given an intravenous infusion of 25 to 75 mg phentolamine for 20 mins. Pain relief following phentolamine administration is then taken as a confirmation of RSD. However, the value of the phentolamine test in diagnosing RSD has been challenged by many investigators.27

No specific laboratory diagnostic tests confirm the presence of CRPS. However, the differential diagnosis includes other neuropathic conditions, as well metabolic, systemic, vascular, and rheumatological disorders. Blood work for inflammatory arthropathy and vasculitis is indicated, which includes a complete blood count (CBC), erythrocyte sedimentation rate, C-reactive protein, antinuclear antibody, and a rheu-matoid factor.

A study was previously done to assess the relation between the subjectively assessed and objectively measured diagnostic signs and symptoms in the complex regional pain syndrome type I and to quantify their severity. The bedside evaluation of CRPS I criteria was shown to be in good accord with psychometric or laboratory testing of the criteria recommended for the diagnosis of CRPS.28

In some cases damage to the peripheral nervous system can be objectively assessed using electromyoneurography. New diagnostic methods, such as quantitative sensory testing (CST), challenge this division because the CST findings in patients with CRPS I can suggest damage to A delta peripheral nerve fibers. Except for distinguishing type I and type II disease, it is important to bear in mind the diversity of clinical presentation of CRPS in acute and chronic phase of the disease.

This regional pain syndrome typically includes the autonomic and motor signs and thus differs from other peripheral neuropathic pain syndromes. The complexity of the clinical presentation indicates the likely presence of different pathophysiological mechanisms underlying this disease.29

There is no gold standard in diagnosis of this entity, and a multidisciplinary approach is necessary for proper diagnosis.30   Raising awareness of CRPS may help physicians make the correct diagnosis early, as well as initiate a collaborative effort between neurology, anesthesiology, and dermatology to provide the patient the most favorable outcome.31

References
1.   Bruehl S. An update on the pathophysiology of complex regional pain syndrome. Anesthesiology. 2010;113(3):713-725.
2.   Rockett M. Diagnosis, mechanisms and treatment of complex regional pain syndrome. Curr Opin Anaesthesiol. 2014;27(5):494-500.
3.   Thomson McBride AR, Barnett AJ, Livingstone JA, Atkins RM. Complex regional pain syndrome (type 1): a comparison of 2 diagnostic criteria methods. Clin J Pain. 2008;24(7):637-640.
4.   Iolascon G, de Sire A, Moretti A, Gimigliano F. Complex regional pain syndrome (CRPS) type I: historical perspective and critical issues. Clin Cases Miner Bone Metab. 2015;12(Suppl 1):4-10.
5.   Kumar V, Kalita J, Gujral RB, Sharma VP, Misra UK. A study of bone densitometry in patients with complex regional pain syndrome after stroke. Postgrad Med J. 2001;77(910):519-522.
6.   Nitzsche EU. [Nuclear medicine imaging for diagnosis of CRPS I]. Handchir Mikrochir Plast Chir. 2011;43(1):20-24.
7.   Poll LW, Weber P, Bohm HJ, Ghassem-Zadeh N, Chantelau EA. Sudeck's disease stage 1, or diabetic Charcot's foot stage 0? Case

report and assessment of the diagnostic value of MRI. Diabetol Metab Syndr. 2010;2:60.

8.   Peltz E, Seifert F, Maihofner C, Internationale Gesellschaft zum Studium des S. [Diagnostic guidelines for complex regional pain syndrome]. Handchir Mikrochir Plast Chir. 2012;44(3):135-141.

9.   Intenzo CM, Kim SM, Capuzzi DM. The role of nuclear medicine in the evaluation of complex regional pain syndrome type I. Clin Nucl Med. 2005;30(6):400-407.

10.   Wasner G, Schattschneider J, Heckmann K, Maier C, Baron R. Vascular abnormalities in reflex sympathetic dystrophy (CRPS I): mechanisms and diagnostic value. Brain. 2001;124(Pt 3):587-599.

11.   Packham TL, Fok D, Frederiksen K, Thabane L, Buckley N. Reliability of infrared thermometric measurements of skin temperature in the hand. J Hand Ther. 2012;25(4):358-361; quiz 362.

12.   Schurmann M, Gradl G, Zaspel J, Kayser M, Lohr P, Andress HJ. Peripheral sympathetic function as a predictor of complex regional pain syndrome type I (CRPS I) in patients with radial fracture. Auton Neurosci. 2000;86(1-2):127-134.

13.   Ackerman WE, Zhang JM. Efficacy of stellate ganglion blockade for the management of type 1 complex regional pain syndrome. South Med J. 2006;99(10):1084-1088.

14.   Chemali KR, Gorodeski R, Chelimsky TC. Alpha-adrenergic supersensitivity of the sudomotor nerve in complex regional pain syndrome. Ann Neurol. 2001;49(4):453-459.

15.   Stanton-Hicks M. Complex regional pain syndrome. Anesthesiol Clin North America. 2003;21(4):733-744.

16.   Bruehl S, Harden RN, Galer BS, Saltz S, Backonja M, Stanton-Hicks M. Complex regional pain syndrome: are there distinct subtypes and sequential stages of the syndrome? Pain. 2002;95(1-2):119-124.

17.   Krause P, Forderreuther S, Straube A. [Motor cortical representation in patients with complex regional pain syndrome: a TMS study]. Schmerz. 2006;20(3):181-184, 186-188.

18.   Vartiainen N, Kirveskari E, Kallio-Laine K, Kalso E, Forss N. Cortical reorganization in primary somatosensory cortex in patients with unilateral chronic pain. J Pain. 2009;10(8):854-859.

19.   Schilder JC, Niehof SP, Marinus J, van Hilten JJ. Diurnal and nocturnal skin temperature regulation in chronic complex regional pain syndrome. J Pain. 2015;16(3):207-213.

20.   Rommel O, Malin JP, Zenz M, Janig W. Quantitative sensory testing, neurophysiological and psychological examination in patients with complex regional pain syndrome and hemisensory deficits. Pain. 2001;93(3):279-293.

21.   Bale R. [Ganglion block. When and how?]. Radiologe. 2015;55(10):886-895.

22.   Raja SN, Treede RD, Davis KD, Campbell JN. Systemic alpha-adrenergic blockade with phentolamine: a diagnostic test for sympathetically maintained pain. Anesthesiology. 1991;74(4):691-698.

23.   Boas RA. Sympathetic nerve blocks: in search of a role. Reg Anesth Pain Med. 1998;23(3):292-305.

24.   Hartrick CT, Kovan JP, Naismith P. Outcome prediction following sympathetic block for complex regional pain syndrome. Pain Pract. 2004;4(3):222-228.

25.   Kharkar S, Venkatesh YS, Grothusen JR, Rojas L, Schwartzman RJ. Skin biopsy in complex regional pain syndrome: case series and literature review. Pain Physician. 2012;15(3):255-266.

26.   Oaklander AL, Rissmiller JG, Gelman LB, Zheng L, Chang Y, Gott R. Evidence of focal small-fiber axonal degeneration in complex regional pain syndrome-I (reflex sympathetic dystrophy). Pain. 2006;120(3):235-243.

27.   Kingery WS. A critical review of controlled clinical trials for peripheral neuropathic pain and complex regional pain syndromes. Pain. 1997;73(2):123-139.

28.   Oerlemans HM, Oostendorp RA, de Boo T, Perez RS, Goris RJ. Signs and symptoms in complex regional pain syndrome type I/reflex sympathetic dystrophy: judgment of the physician versus objective measurement. Clin J Pain. 1999;15(3):224-232.

29.   Blazekovic I, Bilic E, Zagar M, Anic B. [Complex Regional Pain Syndrome]. Lijec Vjesn. 2015;137(9-10):297-306.

30.   Ersoy H, Pomeranz SJ. Complex Regional Pain Syndrome. J Surg Orthop Adv. 2016;25(2):117-120.

31.   Carr ES, De La Cerda A, Fiala K. Complex regional pain syndrome. Proc (Bayl Univ Med Cent). 2016;29(3):333-334.

Studies focusing on children with CRPS are on the rise. Once considered rare among children, it is now thought that this may have been caused by under-recognition of the disorder. The complex regional pain syndrome (CRPS in children and adolescents) is characterized by a painful mottled appearing, swollen limb with allodynia and hyperalgesia.1

While complex regional pain syndrome (CRPS) is a well-established entity in adults, its occurrence in children was doubted for a long time. However, in the last few years several case reports and some comparative studies have described CRPS in children and adolescents.

The complex regional pain syndrome is therefore, a relatively new diagnostic entity in pediatrics. Among physicians it is not common knowledge that CRPS also affects children. Chronic pain is an important clinical problem affecting significant numbers of children and their families. While the complex regional pain syndrome (CRPS) can happen at any age, CRPS in children is less common than in adults. Few studies on RSD have been done that included children.

The estimated incidence of CRPS is 1.2/100 000 children 5-15 years old. The diagnosis of CRPS is often delayed. CRPS has a significant impact on children and their families.2 Children often respond more quickly and positively to CRPS treatment than adults. An early diagnosis and active treatment may reduce the duration of the condition considerably.

The complex regional pain syndrome is a chronic, intensified localized pain condition that can affect children and adolescents as well as adults, but is more common among adolescent girls.3 Because psychosocial factors play an important role, it is recommended to provide psychological evaluation and cognitive behavioral treatment as soon as possible. Symptoms include limb pain; allodynia; hyperalgesia; swelling and/or changes in skin color of the affected limb; dry, mottled skin; hyperhidrosis and trophic changes of the nails and hair.

Complex regional pain syndrome I is defined by the International Association for the Study of Pain (IASP) criteria to include pain that is disproportionate to the inciting event, sensory disturbances such as allodynia/ hyperalgesia, autonomic dysfunction, and motor dysfunction that usually occurs after trauma that is frequently trivial and generally expressed in an extremity. These symptoms are well described in the adult population, but there are relatively few data or reports of its prevalence in the pediatric population.

Recent studies have demonstrated that unlike the adult population, about 90% of the cases reported are females in a range of 8 to 16 years, the youngest being 3 years old. There tends to be delay in recognizing the diagnosis, which may be as long as 4 months. In contrast to adults, the response to treatment, particularly exercise therapy with behavioral management will achieve almost 97% remission.[4]

The exact mechanism of CRPS is unknown, although several different mechanisms have been suggested. The child population differs from adults in that the skin temperature of the involved extremity at onset was more often cooler, the lower extremity was involved more frequently and neurological and sympathetic symptoms were less pronounced.[5]

Many children with amplified extremity pain have CRPS. It can occur in more than one body area. Some children with CRPS have spreading pain that includes areas without overt autonomic dysfunction but still with extreme amplified pain. Pediatric CRPS is under-recognized by clinicians, resulting in diagnostic delays, but has a favorable outcome to noninvasive treatment in that complete resolution of symptoms and signs occur in most patients.

Although it has been widely held that CRPS in children is intrinsically different from adults, there appear to be relatively few differences. However, there is a marked preponderance of lower extremity cases in children.[6] Clinical judgment dictates the extent of medication or interventional therapy added to the treatment to facilitate rehabilitation. In many ways, the approach to the treatment of children mirrors that of adults, with perhaps greater restraint in the use of medications and invasive procedures.

The diagnosis is clinical, with the aid of the adult criteria for CRPS. Standard care consists of a multidisciplinary approach with the implementation of intensive physical therapy in conjunction with psychological counseling. Pharmacological treatments may aid in reducing pain in order to allow the patient to participate fully in intensive physiotherapy. The prognosis in pediatric CRPS is favorable.

The estimated incidence of CRPS is 1.2/100 000 children 5-15 years old. The diagnosis of CRPS is often delayed. CRPS has a significant impact on children and their families. CRPS requires a coordinated, multidisciplinary approach. Physical rehabilitation is an important component of long-term treatment. Unfortunately, patients with significant allodynia or hyperalgesia characteristic of CRPS-1 often have difficulty progressing through a physical therapy (PT) regimen.

CRPS in children is more common, and more debilitating, than is commonly known. Although there have been no large-scale studies on the incidence of RSD in children, some generalizations can be made about the children who get this condition. CRPS I in children has a different presentation than in adults.5

The incidence of RSD/CRPS increases dramatically between 9 and 11 years old, and it is found predominantly in young girls. The estimated incidence of CRPS is 1.2/100 000 children 5-15 years old.7 The diagnosis of CRPS is often delayed. CRPS has a significant impact on children and their families. In contrast to adults most of the involved children are female, suffering from CRPS after an initial event that is typically a minor trauma.8

Furthermore, CRPS occurs more frequently in the lower extremity than in the upper extremity when compared to adults. Since neither radiological findings nor laboratory parameters are able to confirm CRPS, the diagnosis is made from a detailed description of the clinical signs and symptoms characterized by a remarkable intra- and inter-individual variability. Genetic factors are suggested to play a role in complex regional pain syndrome (CRPS), but familial occurrence has not been extensively studied.9

Children do not develop the severe, disabling pain or the patchy osteoporosis (Sudeck's atrophy) which are considered essential features of reflex sympathetic dystrophy in adults. CRPS in children and adolescents is characterized by a painful, mottled appearing, swollen limb with allodynia and hyperalgesia. For most patients, pain is severe, resulting in significant functional disability. More recent evidence suggests that a rehabilitative program results in improvement in both pain and functional measures.1

In contrast to the adult variety, reflex sympathetic dystrophy in children is a self-limiting condition which usually responds well to mild analgesics and physical therapy.10 Symptoms of CRPS vary, but the most common symptom is prolonged pain in one area. A child's pain may be constant, and can range from mildly uncomfortable to severe.

A child may complain of a burning, squeezing, or "pins and needles" sensation, and pain can spread throughout an entire arm or leg. The child's limb may also be sensitive to touch. In many ways, the approach to the treatment of children mirrors that of adults, with perhaps greater restraint in the use of medications and invasive procedures.6

Children will fall into several diagnostic groups. First are those who are permanently cured by treatment. The second is a group of children whose conditions are improved, but then show a high recurrence of RSD/CRPS. Fortunately each subsequence occurrence of RSD/CRPS seems less severe.

A third and relatively small group of children with RSD/CRPS get progressively worse despite treatment and require aggressive intervention, even sympathectomy. A high percentage of children will improve with active mobilization of the affected extremity and psychosocial conditioning alone.

As a group, clinic-referred children with CRPS may be more functionally impaired and experience more somatic symptoms compared with children with other pain conditions.11 However, overall psychological functioning as assessed by self-report appears to be similar to that of children with other chronic pain diagnoses. Comprehensive assessment using a biopsychosocial framework is essential to understanding and appropriately treating children with symptoms of CRPS.

Studies have shown that physical therapy alone may be effective in many cases of children with CRPS. In one study, 90 percent of participants effectively alleviated CRPS symptoms after undergoing physical therapy for up to six hours a day with no medication.

Reflex sympathetic dystrophy in children differs in presentation and clinical course from the syndrome in adults. It is best treated in a multidisciplinary fashion.12 In spite of a sometimes long and variable clinical course the prognosis in most cases is excellent and usually results in complete functional restoration.8

Physicians need to remain vigilant for a recurrence of RSD/CRPS when a child goes into remission following a bout with RSD/CRPS. Recurrent episodes of RSD/CRPS in children can occur in up to 40% of patients; however, most of these recurrent episodes were milder than the initial episode.

CRPS-1 may occur following immunization with rubella and hepatitis B vaccines.13 CRPS-1 may also follow immunization with rubella and hepatitis B vaccines. CRPS can occur in younger than expected age ranges of children who experience the unique emotional stressor of a deployed military family member.14

The prognosis of RSD/CRPS in the children is excellent. This is due to the surge of growth hormone, endorphins, sex hormones, and other hormones during adolescence which afford the body with excellent control of healing with respect to the sympathetic system. In this age group it is rare to see a child progress to stage III.

Even sympathectomy, which practically universally fails in adults with RSD/CRPS, is helpful in young patients. Early treatment with continuous epidural anesthesia may be a promising option for the management of complex regional pain syndrome during childhood.15

Not all patients with RSD/CRPS move from stage to stage in an orderly progression, especially not children. Stage one is called the acute stage. The child's onset of CRPS may occur immediately after the initial injury or may not occur until several weeks after the event. Either way, the child experiences pain that is out of proportion to the injury.

A child may have swelling (i.e., edema), redness or inflammation of the skin (i.e., erythema) and increased warmth; however, some children initially may have a cool extremity. Stage two is called the dystrophic stage and typically occurs three to six months after symptoms begin. RSD/CRPS can markedly disable a child and depress activities of daily living.

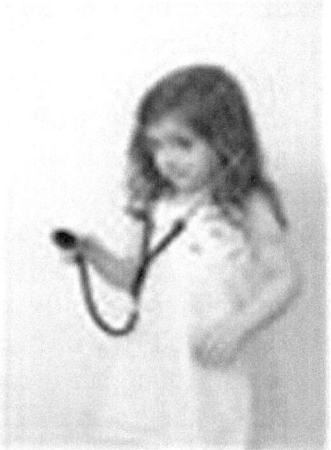

Figure 1. It is important to diagnose pediatric RSD/CRPS in a timely fashion. This disease entity can be overlooked in children.

You may notice skin and nail bed changes in your child during this stage and your child's physician may find bony demineralization by taking radiographic images. The third stage of CRPS is called the atrophic stage where a progressive decline of skin and muscle and osteopenia (i.e., a condition in which bones are not mineralized normally) can occur.

Children seldom progress to the atrophic stage although stage three is not unheard of in children. Children who have CRPS type I more frequently are affected in one of their lower extremities. Children's lower extremities are affected about five times more often than upper extremities. Adults, on the other hand, are twice as likely to be affected in an upper extremity.

Most children with CRPS type I are from upper middle class families and are athletic. A typical pediatric patient with CRPS type I is a female who participates in ballet, soccer or gymnastics. Researchers have hypothesized that there may be a genetic predisposition to CRPS type I. Most children who have the syndrome are Caucasian.

Standard care consists of a multidisciplinary approach with the implementation of intensive physical therapy in conjunction with psychological counseling. Pharmacological treatments may aid in reducing pain in order to allow the patient to participate fully in intensive physiotherapy. The prognosis in pediatric CRPS is favorable.3

Recent studies have demonstrated that unlike the adult population, about 90% of the pediatric RSD cases reported are females in a range of 8 to 16 years, the youngest being 3 years old.4 There tends to be delays in recognizing the diagnosis, which may be as long as 4 months.

In contrast to adults, the response to treatment, particularly exercise therapy with behavioral management will achieve almost 97% remission. While the pathophysiology is poorly understood, many features, particularly the neurologic abnormalities, suggest both peripheral and central nervous system involvement.

Treating RSD/CRPS in children typically requires a combination of anti-inflammatory medications coupled with neuropathic medications that are typically used for the treatment of pain associated with childhood diabetes. In addition, your child's pediatrician may recommend the use of physical therapy in an effort to improve the mobility and use of the arm that is affected.

Children with CRPS experienced more stressful life events than children with chronic headaches or abdominal pain. Prospective long-term studies are needed to further explore the potential role of stressful life events in the etiology of CRPS.16

Detailed psychological and psychiatric evaluation is recommended in individuals with CRPS because psychiatric support and improvement of associated psychosocial concerns in addition to pregabalin seems to facilitate RSD treatments in some patients.17

When not effectively treated, RSD/CRPS can continue into adulthood and become a debilitating health condition, affecting quality of life and even causing work related disability. The key to a child's optimal health, however, will lie in early diagnosis and aggressive treatment of RSD/CRPS from not only a physical standpoint but also a mental health standpoint.

CRPS should be considered as a differential diagnosis of unexplained persistent limb pain even in childhood for early and appropriate management.18   Reflex sympathetic dystrophy in children differs in presentation and clinical course from the syndrome in adults. It is best treated in a multidisciplinary fashion.

Like many chronic pain conditions, it is often associated with significant disability and a detrimental effect on quality of life. It has a complex pathophysiology that remains poorly understood but provides many potential targets for treatments. Management involves a biopsychosocial formulation that encompasses physical and psychological interventions alongside pharmacological strategies.

The prognosis of childhood-onset CRPS I seems less favorable than usually reported, and is comparable to the prognosis of the adult-onset CRPS I in view of a decreased quality of life and a large relapse percentage (33%) at long-term follow-up.19

Childhood onset CRPS I affects predominantly preadolescent girls at the ankle.20 For a minority of patients who prove to be resistant to such therapies, spinal cord stimulation (SCS) may be tried.21 The favorable outcome in all seven cases with no or minor remaining symptoms and without severe recurrences illustrates that SCS may also be an efficient treatment in pediatric cases with exceptionally therapy resistant forms of CRPS I.

No high-quality clinical research studies into the etiology and pathogenesis and treatment of CRPS-I in children and adolescents are available to date.22   Consequently, the management of CRPS in the pediatric population presents an even greater challenge than in adults, partly because there is a lack of clinical data concerning the efficacy of the diverse treatment methods available, and partly because successful treatment of CRPS involves a multidisciplinary approach.

There is debate as to what constitutes the most effective treatment for pediatric CRPS. Treatment that has been reported to be successful in adults may not necessarily apply to children. Invasive techniques have been used to treat CRPS over the last few decades but the evidence for their use is still very weak. Invasive management should be contemplated only when high-standard conservative management has failed to work.23

CRPS is frequently unrecognized in children, leading to family anxiety and unnecessary para-clinical costs. Pediatricians and pediatric neurologists should be aware of this syndrome in order to avoid delay in diagnosis, unnecessary studies, and multiple visits to specialists, with a view to providing effective treatment.24

References

1.   Borucki AN, Greco CD. An update on complex regional pain syndromes in children and adolescents. Curr Opin Pediatr. 2015;27(4):448-452.

2.   Abu-Arafeh H, Abu-Arafeh I. Complex regional pain syndrome in children: incidence and clinical characteristics. Arch Dis Child. 2016;101(8):719-723.

3.   Weissmann R, Uziel Y. Pediatric complex regional pain syndrome: a review. Pediatr Rheumatol Online J. 2016;14(1):29.

4.   Stanton-Hicks M. Plasticity of complex regional pain syndrome (CRPS) in children. Pain Med. 2010;11(8):1216-1223.

5.   Tan EC, Zijlstra B, Essink ML, Goris RJ, Severijnen RS. Complex regional pain syndrome type I in children. Acta Paediatr. 2008;97(7):875-879.

6.   Wilder RT. Management of pediatric patients with complex regional pain syndrome. Clin J Pain. 2006;22(5):443-448.

7.   Abu-Arafeh H, Abu-Arafeh I. Complex regional pain syndrome in children: incidence and clinical characteristics. Arch Dis Child. 2016.

8.   Fitze G. [Complex regional pain syndrome in children]. Unfallchirurg. 2011;114(5):411-416.

9.   de Rooij AM, de Mos M, Sturkenboom MC, Marinus J, van den Maagdenberg AM, van Hilten JJ. Familial occurrence of complex regional pain syndrome. Eur J Pain. 2009;13(2):171-177.

10.   Ruggeri SB, Athreya BH, Doughty R, Gregg JR, Das MM. Reflex sympathetic dystrophy in children. Clin Orthop Relat Res. 1982(163):225-230.

11.   Logan DE, Williams SE, Carullo VP, Claar RL, Bruehl S, Berde CB. Children and adolescents with complex regional pain syndrome: more psychologically distressed than other children in pain? Pain Res Manag. 2013;18(2):87-93.

12.   Wilder RT, Berde CB, Wolohan M, Vieyra MA, Masek BJ, Micheli LJ. Reflex sympathetic dystrophy in children. Clinical characteristics and follow-up of seventy patients. J Bone Joint Surg Am. 1992;74(6):910-919.

13.   Richards S, Chalkiadis G, Lakshman R, Buttery JP, Crawford NW. Complex regional pain syndrome following immunisation. Arch Dis Child. 2012;97(10):913-915.

14.   Pearson RD, Bailey J. Complex regional pain syndrome in an 8-year-old female with emotional stress during deployment of a family member. Mil Med. 2011;176(8):876-878.

15.   Saito Y, Baba S, Takahashi A, et al. Complex regional pain syndrome in a 15-year-old girl successfully treated with continuous epidural anesthesia. Brain Dev. 2015;37(1):175-178.

16.   Wager J, Brehmer H, Hirschfeld G, Zernikow B. Psychological distress and stressful life events in pediatric complex regional pain syndrome. Pain Res Manag. 2015;20(4):189-194.

17.   Saltik S, Sozen HG, Basgul S, Karatoprak EY, Icagasioglu A. Pregabalin Treatment of a Patient With Complex Regional Pain Syndrome. Pediatr Neurol. 2016;54:88-90.

18.   Matsui M, Ito M, Tomoda A, Miike T. Complex regional pain syndrome in childhood: report of three cases. Brain Dev. 2000;22(7):445-448.

19.   Tan EC, van de Sandt-Renkema N, Krabbe PF, Aronson DC, Severijnen RS. Quality of life in adults with childhood-onset of Complex Regional Pain Syndrome type I. Injury. 2009;40(8):901-904.

20.   Bayle-Iniguez X, Audouin-Pajot C, Sales de Gauzy J, Munzer C, Murgier J, Accadbled F. Complex regional pain syndrome type I in children. Clinical description and quality of life. Orthop Traumatol Surg Res. 2015;101(6):745-748.

21.   Olsson GL, Meyerson BA, Linderoth B. Spinal cord stimulation in adolescents with complex regional pain syndrome type I (CRPS-I). Eur J Pain. 2008;12(1):53-59.

22.   Lascombes P, Mamie C. Complex regional pain syndrome type I in children: What is new? Orthop Traumatol Surg Res. 2016.

23.   Rodriguez MJ, Fernandez-Baena M, Barroso A, Yanez JA. Invasive Management for Pediatric Complex Regional Pain Syndrome: Literature Review of Evidence. Pain Physician. 2015;18(6):621-630.

24.   Pedemonte Stalla V, Medici Olaso C, Kanopa Almada V, Gonzalez Rabelino G. Complex regional pain syndrome type i. An analysis of 7 cases in children. Neurologia. 2015;30(6):347-351.

11. Elderly

Medication nonadherence is a frequent problem in the treatment of chronic conditions. Physicians should monitor older patients with chronic nonmalignant pain more closely and pay more attention to patients' beliefs regarding analgesics to ensure better adherence to pharmacological therapy.1

Adherence to pharmacological therapy prescribed for chronic nonmalignant pain in patients aged 65 and older, 57% of patients indicated that they did not take prescribed analgesics exactly as the physician prescribed. Elderly patients however rarely have a severe acute pain as younger patients may complain of.

Many nursing home residents are often unable to communicate with nursing home staff members because of disease or mental illness. The facility staff might notice the resident crying out in pain for no apparent reason, but this pain, especially if constant and severe, can be an indicator of RSDS. Many nursing homes have large resident populations, which increases the likelihood of a resident's pain being ignored or concern over constant pain being minimized.

Elderly nursing home residents have an increased risk for dangerous slips and falls. These falls can result in bone fractures, and other injuries. These injuries, which often affect the limbs, can be a source of trauma that puts them at increased risk to develop RSD. CRPS is rare in the elderly.

If the nursing home facility does not properly monitor the resident's pain and recovery following an injury, the resident might not be properly diagnosed with CRPS. Delirium in older ED patients has negative consequences and is an independent predictor of prolonged hospitalizations.2

Disorders of the skeleton are one of the most common causes of chronic pain and long-term physical disability in the world.3 In addition to CRPS, chronic skeletal pain is caused by a remarkably diverse group of conditions including trauma-induced fracture, osteoarthritis, osteoporosis, low back pain, orthopedic procedures, celiac disease, sickle cell disease and bone cancer.

In patients with CRPS in multiple limbs, spontaneous spread of symptoms generally follows a contralateral or ipsilateral pattern whereas diagonal spread is rare and generally preceded by a new trauma. Spread is associated with a younger age at onset and a more severely affected phenotype and is not common in elderly patients.4

While these disorders are diverse, what they share in common is that when chronic skeletal pain occurs in these disorders. New therapeutic options for treating and/or preventing chronic pain in the injured, diseased and aged skeleton must be found. The mean age in one study was higher in patients with CRPS. The affected forearm/hand was the dominant side in 62.9% of patients without CRPS and in 64.2% of patients with CRPS.

CRPS incidence was higher in patients with motor nerve injury and in patients with sensory nerve injury. A logistic regression showed that risk for CRPS was higher in patients with motor nerve injury and in females.5

CRPS is not uncommon in elderly patients (65 years and over). It may occur following a stroke, heart attack, bone fractures etc. Elderly patients react differently to treatments than younger patients. Pain management in general in elderly patients can be a challenge. Elderly patients can be taking many different medications. Some of these drugs can adversely interact with some pain medications.

Postmenopausal woman appeared to be at the highest risk for the development of CRPS. The highest incidence occurred in females in the age category of 61-70 years. The upper extremity was affected more frequently than the lower extremity and a fracture was the most common precipitating event (44%).6

Senile patients may forget to take their medications as prescribed. Their kidneys do not function as well as in younger patients. The kidneys are responsible for eliminating drugs. As a result, drugs like morphine can accumulate within an elderly patient's body which could cause an overdose.

The liver metabolizes drugs. Liver function decreases with age. An elderly patient's body mass may be decreased as well. As a result, there is less body volume where a drug can go. A dose of drug will be distributed through various body tissues. If a patient is emaciated, a dose of drug will remain in the blood stream instead of being distributed throughout the body. As a result, the concentration of drug in the blood stream may be higher than expected.

Because older adults often experience chronic health conditions that require treatment with multiple medications, there is a greater likelihood of experiencing unwanted drug side effects. Older people can also be more sensitive to certain medications. A study concluded that loss of quality of life in CRPS patients is due mainly to reduced physical health.

A comparison with data available from the literature shows that CRPS patients generally report poorer quality of life than patients with other chronic pain conditions, particularly in the physical domains. Pain correlated moderately with quality of life and therefore deserves ongoing attention by physicians.

To help one make better informed decisions about the medications, and to lower the chances of overmedication and serious drug reactions, the American Geriatrics Society Foundation for Health in Aging recommends that older people be cautious about using some types of medications like opioids or sedatives, including some that can be purchased without a prescription.

With respect to pain management, older patients handle pain medications differently than younger patients. The kidneys become smaller with age. As a result, there is decreased blood flow to the kidney and less effective filtration with removal of a drug from the kidney. As one ages, the liver undergoes a decrease in mass and blood flow.

Decreased saliva noted in some older patients may interfere with swallowing. Drugs prescribed by mouth may be absorbed differently because of changes in stomach acid levels in older patients. The changes in physiology with aging may alter the side effect profile of many drugs.

Depression is common in older patients. Inactivity can lead to deconditioning. Many elderly patients take pain for granted and do not mention it unless they are asked. The assessment of patients with impaired cognition may be challenging. Patients with dementia may be able to describe their current symptoms but unable to reliably report their previous symptoms. Depression, secondary gain, personality disorders, and psychologic stress should be evaluated in all elderly patients.

Chronic nonmalignant neuropathic pain is difficult to manage. Chronic neuropathic pain subsequent to a thoracotomy syndrome and a resultant reflex sympathetic dystrophy syndrome must be diagnosed in a timely fashion.[7]

The patient's physical examination should focus on the musculoskeletal system and include palpation for trigger points, evaluation for joint swelling and inflammation, and evaluation for pain with passive range of motion. Pain is suggested by facial grimacing, frowning, or repetitive eye blinking. In the elderly, pain often has multiple causes, and no single predominant cause can be identified.

Poor pain management decreases the patient's quality of life and may contribute to suicide. The elderly are more likely than younger patients to experience adverse effects of analgesics. Drug dosing starting low and going upward slowly. Oral analgesic administration is usually preferred because it is convenient and results in relatively steady blood levels.

Home care nursing isn't just changing dressings, checking blood pressure, or even giving i.v. therapy. It's providing a critical interface between the patient, the health system, and the patient's family.8

RSD and myofascial pain patients appear comparable with respect to a wide range of demographic, clinical, and psychological functioning indices. A specific psychological profile, uniquely neurotic or otherwise, has yet to be demonstrated in terms of any etiologic or maintenance factors in RSD.9

Other studies have reported that female patients developed CRPS I more frequently, and the patients who developed CRPS I were older and more likely to sustain a high energy injury or have a comminuted fracture.

Acetaminophen is the analgesic of choice for most elderly people with mild to moderate pain. Despite its relative lack of anti-inflammatory activity, acetaminophen is usually the best drug for initial treatment of osteoarthritis. NSAIDs are indicated when inflammation contributes significantly to pain. Adverse effects vary, and a patient may tolerate one NSAID better than another. NSAIDs tend to have a ceiling analgesic dose which means that more medicine will not result in greater pain relief.

The most common adverse effect of all NSAIDs is gastrointestinal upset, which may require stopping the drug. Ulceration and GI bleeding can occur. Ulceration with or without bleeding can occur simultaneously or independently of each other.

The risk of ulcers and GI bleeding for people 65 years or over is 3 to 4 times higher than that for middle-aged people. NSAIDs can impair renal function and cause sodium and water retention; they should be used cautiously in the elderly, particularly in those who have a renal disorder. Nonacetylated salicylates may have less renal toxicity and fewer antiplatelet effects than other NSAIDs.

Opioids are the most potent analgesics. Opioids act by blocking receptors in the brain and spinal cord. In the elderly, opioids have an increased half-life and possibly a greater analgesic effect than in younger patients. Nonetheless, the most common error in prescribing these drugs is to give them too infrequently, allowing breakthrough pain. A few opioids have specific advantages and disadvantages in elderly patients.

Fentanyl in a patch form causes less histamine release and thus less vasodilation and hypotension. Meperidine should be avoided in elderly patients. Meperidine is less effective when given orally and can cause confusion; also, it is metabolized to an active form that tends to accumulate and thus may lead to central nervous system excitement and seizures.

Opioid agonist-antagonists, which have both agonist and antagonist effects on opiate receptors, often have psychotomimetic effects in the elderly. For this reason, pentazocine (Talwin) and butorphanol (Stadol) are rarely appropriate for the elderly patient. The analgesic effect of propoxyphene (Darvon is similar to that of aspirin or acetaminophen, but dependency and renal impairment may occur.

As a result, propoxyphene (has been removed from pharmacies) should not be used in the elderly. In patients with renal insufficiency, excretion of morphine and codeine may be delayed, resulting in undesirably long therapeutic or adverse effects, particularly with sustained-release formulations. In these patients, hydromorphone or oxycodone is less likely to accumulate and may be preferred.

Unlike NSAIDS, opioids have no ceiling analgesic effect as dosage is increased. The maximum dose is whatever is needed to relieve pain. However, adverse effects may limit the maximum dose that is used. Opioids cause dose-related sedation and respiratory depression. Most elderly patients taking opioids should not drive and should take precautions to prevent falls.

Opioids may cause confusion. If confusion is due to an opioid, pupils are usually very constricted. Sometimes decreasing the dose may relieve confusion without significantly decreasing analgesia. If this approach is ineffective, a different analgesic may be necessary. Opioids almost always cause constipation or urinary retention. Patients do not develop tolerance to these adverse effects.

When an opioid is started, the patient's intake of fluid and fiber should be increased to try to prevent constipation. If a laxative is needed, a fiber laxative may be used. Gabapentin (Neurontin) is frequently prescribed in elderly patients. Dose reductions of gabapentin are recommended in patients with renal insufficiency. Dizziness and drowsiness are common adverse effects. Pregabilin (Lyrica) is frequently used in elderly patients with post herpetic neuralgia.

Antidepressant medications are also prescribed as adjunct medications for elderly patients who suffer from pain. The analgesic mechanism of antidepressants involves interruption of brain mechanisms mediated by norepinephrine and serotonin. For tricyclic antidepressants, there is little evidence that one is better than another; however, amitriptyline which is highly sedating and anticholinergic, should be avoided in the elderly.

Physical therapy can reduce pain due to musculoskeletal disorders in elderly patients. Aquatic therapy can help muscle and joint pain. Pain due to muscle spasm may be reduced by stretching, muscle massages, cold therapy or heat therapy.

Ultrasound therapy may relieve musculoskeletal pain originating in the deep tissues. Transcutaneous electrical nerve stimulation (TENS) can relieve many types of pain as well. Alternative therapies are also used by many patients to control their pain. Occupational therapy can be helpful as well as this modality can teach patients energy saving techniques to be used around their residences.

Elderly patients can have a pronounced effect to sympathetic blocks. In other words, a patient's blood pressure can significantly drop and stellate ganglion blocks can not only decrease an elderly patient's blood pressure but can also dangerously decrease the heart rate. In summary, RSD/CRPS pain management can be challenging in elderly patients.

Elderly patients can be difficult to treat. Many elderly patients do not like taking medications, doing therapy or having injections.

References
1.   Markotic F, Cerni Obrdalj E, Zalihic A, et al. Adherence to pharmacological treatment of chronic nonmalignant pain in individuals aged 65 and older. Pain Med. 2013;14(2):247-256.
2.   Han JH, Eden S, Shintani A, et al. Delirium in older emergency department patients is an independent predictor of hospital length of stay. Acad Emerg Med. 2011;18(5):451-457.
3.   Mantyh PW. The neurobiology of skeletal pain. Eur J Neurosci. 2014;39(3):508-519.
4.   van Rijn MA, Marinus J, Putter H, Bosselaar SR, Moseley GL, van Hilten JJ. Spreading of complex regional pain syndrome: not a random process. J Neural Transm (Vienna). 2011;118(9):1301-1309.
5.   Demir SE, Ozaras N, Karamehmetoglu SS, Karacan I, Aytekin E. Risk factors for complex regional pain syndrome in patients with

traumatic extremity injury. Ulus Travma Acil Cerrahi Derg. 2010;16(2):144-148.

6.   de Mos M, de Bruijn AG, Huygen FJ, Dieleman JP, Stricker BH, Sturkenboom MC. The incidence of complex regional pain syndrome: a population-based study. Pain. 2007;129(1-2):12-20.

7.   Pullen RL, Jr. Pain management of chronic nonmalignant neuropathic pain. Home Healthc Nurse. 2002;20(6):387-392.

8.   Kennison M. A case study in care. RN. 1999;62(1):46-48.

9.   Nelson DV, Novy DM. Psychological characteristics of reflex sympathetic dystrophy versus myofascial pain syndromes. Reg Anesth. 1996;21(3):202-208.

Whether a patient is a man or a woman affects every aspect of a patient's life. A patient may not realize it, but there is a difference between how and why men and women feel pain differently. For example, most women have a lower tolerance for pain than men do, but they are more sensitive and likely to express their feelings of pain than men.

This means that, on average, women are more likely to recognize their long-term pain and admit to it than men. The causes and treatment of pain are different for men and women. The study of the differences between how men and women feel pain and are treated for it is a relatively new branch of medicine.

A patient's age, physical design, hormones, psychological issues, and social issues all play a part in why a patient feel pain. These things also determine how a patient's doctor will treat a patient's pain. In the future, doctors will be able to design treatments that are specific to men and women. Simply stated, sex (male or female) is determined by chromosomes (XX for women, XY for men) and a patient body's particular anatomy. A patient's gender (man or woman) is determined by a patient's body's anatomical features and social issues.

Concerning social issues, in most cases men have been programmed since they were children to be macho when dealing with pain. When playing athletic events, boys are often told to "tough it out" when they are hurt. On the other hand, women since childhood have been allowed to express their pain freely. It is socially acceptable for a girl to cry, but it is not so for a boy. These distinct differences are important when a doctor tries to figure out how to treat pain and other medical problems.

Pain is a very individual and personal experience. Things that cause pain in a patient may not cause pain in someone else. Without a psychological component to a type of pain, the repeated experience of the same type of pain would not be considered to be as painful as the first episode. This is the reason why a professional football player continues to play in a big game in spite of a broken bone.

The estimated overall incidence rate of CRPS was 26.2 per 100,000 person years. Females are affected at least three times more often than males (ratio: 3.4). The highest incidence occurred in females in the age category of 61-70 years. The upper extremity was affected more frequently than the lower extremity and a fracture was the most common precipitating event (44%).1

Since complex regional pain syndrome (CRPS) shows a clear female predominance, researchers investigated the association between the cumulative as well as current exposure to estrogens, and CRPS. This study did not find an association between CRPS onset and cumulative endogenous estrogen exposure.2 Postmenopausal woman however, appeared to be at the highest risk for the development of CRPS.1

The psychology of the game distracts the broken-bone pain. Pain perception varies between person to person based on gender and age. When a patient feels pain, a response is to stay away from everything that would cause a patient to feel more pain. This is the response that aids a body in tissue healing. Sex differences affect the absorption, metabolism (breakdown of drugs), and excretion (elimination of drugs) of many medications.

Women respond more favorably to a class of antidepressant medications called serotonin-specific reuptake inhibitors, or SSRIs (for instance, Prozac), than to other antidepressants known as tricyclics (for instance, Elavil). Sexual differences between men and women are important with respect to drug action, especially because the menstrual cycle can affect the amount of medication in the blood (blood levels).

If a female retains fluid, the excess fluid will dilute the action of the drug. Oral contraceptives (for instance, "the pill") can decrease the blood levels of some anticonvulsant medications such as Dilantin. On the other hand, oral contraceptives can increase the blood level of some medications such as Valium. Hormone replacement in women does enhance the effects of antidepressant medications.

Approximately two thirds of antidepressant medications in the United States are used by women. Women have more side effects with antidepressant-type medications than men. They suffer more fatigue, gastrointestinal affects, and other adverse effects than men. Gonadal hormonal changes in women that occur monthly (before, during and after the menstrual cycle) alter the metabolism (breakdown of drugs in the liver) of certain drugs and can affect their removal from the body.

One of the reasons why men and women differ in the perception of pain results from the effects of the female hormones estrogen and progesterone on the brain and spinal cord (the nervous system). The effects of the menstrual cycle on the nervous system vary before, during, and after menses. In the future, sexual and/or gender differences may allow a doctor to individualize treatments that are specific for each sex. It has also been found that low testosterone in males can also lower the pain threshold.

The wiring of the central nervous system is influenced by differences in sex. Male and female brains have approximately the same number of receptors for estrogen and androgen. Estrogen is primarily a female hormone, whereas androgen is primarily a male hormone. A receptor is an area on the outer covering, or membrane, of a cell where hormones or drugs attach and start to take action. The way receptors respond to drugs and hormones effects the body's response to both drugs and hormones.

For example, giving estrogen to a man does not affect his brain like it does a woman. In the same way, giving androgens (male hormones) to a female brain does not cause the same response as in a male. Researchers have therefore concluded that hormone and hormonal receptor differences between men and women also influence the regulation and transmission of the nervous impulses that transmit pain. Studies that suggest that the pathogenesis of CRPS is due in part to central neuroimmune activation in both men and women.3

Estrogen (the female hormone) affects the central nervous system levels of dopamine and serotonin, which are involved with mood disorders. Women experience more depression than males. Men may have more serotonin receptors, which may be a reason why they suffer from a lower incidence of depression.

As a result, a woman's greater sensitivity to pain may be dependent on the fact that she has less serotonin in the brain and spinal cord. Studies show that sex hormones modulate neural function and affect the central nervous system with respect to the perception of pain. Recent studies in rats have shown that hormone receptors for male and female hormones are also present and modulate the function of the peripheral nerves (nerves outside the brain and spinal cord).

Exaggerated inflammation and oxidative stress are possibly involved in the pathogenesis of Complex Regional Pain Syndrome. A study in 2013 showed no elevation of systemic markers of oxidative stress in CRPS patients compared to matched healthy volunteers.4

Patients are encouraged to stay informed of the new developments in gender-specific pain medicine. This will require some effort on a patient's part. A patient must keep a pain diary that a patient can bring with a patient when a patient visits a doctor. If a patient has any concerns about a pain management, he/she should discuss it with the doctor.

Take control of a patients pain by becoming better informed as to why a patient are suffering from pain and the methods available for the treatment of a patients pain. This can include not only conventional medicine, but also methods that could be offered by complementary and alternative medicine health-care providers.

A patient should be aware that women and men really are different. Ultimately, a better understanding of these differences will enhance a doctor's ability to diagnose and treat all types of pain. Further research should shed more light on the influence of disease on the perception of pain by men and women (and its treatment). For example, diabetes or thyroid abnormalities are diseases that ultimately can cause pain.

Social issues also play a part in how pain will affect a patient. Pain may begin as damage to a patient's body, but a patient's final experience of pain will be at the brain level with a patients emotional feelings. The patient's social and cultural surroundings also can affect the emotions a patient have about a patient's level of pain.

Studies into how and why men and women feel pain differently have begun in the past few years. These studies are important and must cross the life cycle of men and women, because age can also affect hormones and physical characteristics. Researchers at the University of California at San Francisco have found that men and women respond differently to different kinds of pain-relieving medicines. Depending on the kind of medicine given, both the duration of effect and the degree to which pain was relieved differed in men and women. Pain perception will vary from person to person.

While, men and women report the same number of negative (or adverse) reactions during and following treatment with therapeutic medications, negative effects of medicines are higher and more serious in women than in men. This disparity may be influenced by the fact that women use medications more often than men and in different doses, and also because the different ways the drugs are absorbed, metabolized (broken down), and removed from the body by men and women.

Women often report more migraine headaches and arthritic pain than men. Women also have a greater discomfort for the same type of pain than men and are more likely to develop long-term pain after an injury. Women also use more over-the-counter pain medications and have more doctor visits than men.

Because of these differences, research (called "clinical trials" or "clinical drug research") is being done on why women are more likely to suffer from painful conditions such as RSD/CRPS than men and which medications work better for men and women. Media advertising often recommends a certain medication for a specific condition, but none of the advertisements discuss doses with respect to the body size of a man or woman. Body size determines the amount of a medicine needed to treat a painful condition.

Take a look at an aspirin bottle label. Does it tell a patient the dosage for a man or woman? The answer is no. Reviews of major medical journals show clinical drug studies rarely test to determine how medication will affect men and women differently. Women are excluded from many clinical drug study trials.

Because of the potential for pregnancy and the potential harmful effects of a new drug on a developing baby, most researchers have been hesitant to include women in their studies. Early studies mainly consisted of male prisoners. High energy injuries, severe fractures, and the female gender contribute to the development of CRPS I in a reported study.5

In 1977, the U.S. Food and Drug Administration (FDA) prohibited women of child-bearing age from being involved in clinical trials. As a result, many drug studies were done only on men until recently. In 1985, a U.S. public health service task force addressed the Department of Health and Human Services and expressed the need to establish a policy that included women in clinical drug studies.

In 1990, the Government Accounting Office issued a report and concluded that there was a lack of compliance in including women in clinical drug trials. So in 1993, Congress made it mandatory that women, as well as minorities, be included in clinical drug trials.

Also in 1993, the FDA began allowing women of child-bearing age to take part in clinical drug trials. In 1994, the National Institutes of Health issued guidelines to grant applications to confirm that researchers complied with the inclusion of women of child-bearing age in their studies. Recent studies in 1997 showed that women exceeded 50 percent of the study participants. (U.S. Food and Drug Administration website, www.fda.gov)

Published clinical trial results today often include data analyzing how the studied drug affected men and women. Data submitted to the FDA for drug approval must include the gender, age, height, and weight of each participant. It also has been recommended that the data include whether any participating women are pre- or postmenopausal, because levels of hormones can affect how pain much pain is felt.

The anatomic differences between men and women also influence their reactions to medications. In general, women have lower body weights and organ sizes and a higher percentage of body fat, factors that need to be taken into account when discussing the way the body handles drugs and their use in men and women. For example, the muscle relaxant Valium (diazepam) causes more impairment of voluntary muscle control in women than in men, probably because of lower body weight of women as compared to men.

Differences in drug reactions are caused by differences in the way men and women process drugs. The transport of drugs within the bloodstream and the chemicals that break down drugs differ in men and women. Enzymes in the patient's liver help to metabolize drugs. One of these enzymes is the CYP 3A4 liver enzyme. This enzyme breaks down more than 50 percent of all therapeutic drugs. In women, drugs that have been metabolized in the liver are delivered more slowly to the bloodstream, where they are then sent to the kidneys for excretion from the body.

Because more of the pain medications are not taken out of the liver, a higher concentration of these drugs in the liver requires processing. The liver enzymes in women have to process higher concentrations of the drugs than males. Liver enzymes in women may also not metabolize the antidepressants of the selective serotonin-specific reuptake inhibitor class.

Women have a lower stomach acid secretion than men. This can increase the absorption of drugs such as Elavil or Valium, and decrease the absorption of acidic drugs such as Dilantin and barbiturates. Women weigh less than men and have a lower total blood value than men. Body fat is 11 percent higher in women between the ages of 25 and 35. After a drug is absorbed from either the stomach or the small intestine, the drug is distributed throughout the tissues in the body.

Drugs that have a high affinity for fat and are called fat-soluble drugs. If an individual has a high body fat content, some drugs may rapidly enter the fatty tissue. This action will decrease the level of medication in the blood and make it less effective.

However, if repetitive administration of a drug causes a high concentration of that drug in body fat, it will eventually be released back into the bloodstream, which can cause a significantly higher blood level of the drug at that time.

The liver breaks down and eliminates most drugs. Biologic systems, including the liver, may be more efficient in men than in women. Drugs may be eliminated from the body more effectively by the kidneys in men when compared to women. As a result, equal doses of medication could result in a higher blood level of that particular drug in a woman than in a man. This in turn could cause serious side effects in the woman but not in the man.

Alcohol is sometimes used by individuals for pain relief, too. When women smoke and consume alcohol, the effect of the tobacco enhances the effects of the alcohol, whereas in men the opposite is true. Women absorb alcohol differently than men. They also metabolize the alcohol differently than men. Women have less total body water than men at a similar body weight. Therefore, women achieve a higher concentration of the alcohol in their bloodstream after drinking an equal amount of the same alcohol.

If a patient has less body water, the concentration of the drug in a patient's bloodstream is higher. In other words, it is not diluted out. Males who have an increase in body water will dilute out the drug that they take. On the other hand, women eliminate alcohol from their bloodstreams faster than males.

Women experience more severe withdrawal symptoms than men when they stop smoking. Women who smoke have an increased risk of heart attack as compared to male smokers. Smoking also increases the levels of the bad cholesterol (LDL) in women more than men. Some people take illicit drugs to attempt to control their pain.

Sex hormones can have an effect on illicit drugs. Women who take amphetamines say that the effects of the amphetamines differ depending on which phase of the menstrual cycle they are experiencing. Women experience fewer side effects than men when smoking cocaine. The phase of the menstrual cycle will affect whether women get high from the ingestion of cocaine. After smoking cocaine, women have a higher blood level of the drug than men. It is believed that all the effects are hormonal related. Biochemical data shows differences in the spinal cord levels of the glutamate receptor NR2b, suggesting sex differences in mechanisms of central sensitization that could account for differences in duration and severity of CRPS symptoms between the male and female groups.[6]

Men and women differ with respect to their response to medications. Note, therefore, that the dosage for men and women must differ. However, many doctors are unaware of the gender specific differences between men and women with respect to their responses to medications, as well as the differences between men and women with respect to body weight. An obese woman may require more medication to achieve the same pain relief than a thin woman.

Before men and women with painful conditions can be treated properly, many research questions need to be answered with respect to the different effects of drugs on men and women. As a patient can see, attention to gender is important not only in the specialty of pain management but also in other medical specialties.

Sex hormones influence the effects of analgesics and many other drugs. The menstrual cycle, pregnancy, and menopause affect how drugs react in women's bodies, such that the same drug will have a different effect depending on the stage of the menstrual cycle and whether the woman is pre- or postmenopausal.

When a patient take a pill, the amount of medication that a patient is taking may not be appropriate for a patient depending on the previously mentioned factors. This may be the reason why a drug "just stops working." In some instances, if a patient mentions this to a patient's doctor, the doctor may think a patient is just seeking more drugs.

The way in which antidepressant medications are absorbed, distributed in the bloodstream, and eliminated by the kidneys differs in men and women. Monthly hormone cycles in women can influence the effects of some antidepressants. Further, oral contraceptives and hormones can alter drug interactions in women.

For example, acetaminophen (Tylenol) is made inactive in women taking oral contraceptives when compared to women who are not taking oral contraceptives. High blood levels of estradiol (a female hormone) sensitize a female to thermal (heat) pain.

Premenopausal women take longer to empty stomach content such as food and medication. In essence, this means that medications in the stomach are slower to leave the stomach to go into the small intestine. The small intestine has a greater absorptive capacity than the stomach. If a medication is delayed in passage from the stomach to the small intestine, medicine will be absorbed more slowly into the blood. Consequently, the blood level of the drug may be decreased. The effects of hormones on neurotransmitters in the brain during the premenstrual cycle can affect the sensitivity of neurotransmitters or nervous system receptors.

A doctor may have to increase the total dosage of a specific medication throughout the entire menstrual cycle and may have to decrease the medication two to three days after the cycle has been completed. Oral contraceptives used by some women can decrease the effect of anti-anxiety drugs such as the Valium. Studies are currently investigating whether estrogen can be effective in treating depression in women.

The effects of estrogen on certain drugs in postmenopausal women is also currently under study. Men and women respond differently to antidepressant medications. In women, pre- and postmenopausal effects must be taken into account when prescribing an antidepressant medication.

Age also influences the effects of drugs. Because older people break down drugs more slowly, older individuals typically need a smaller dose of a drug. However, age effects are less prevalent in women than in men. Older men have a decreased ability to excrete drugs than women. Age can also influence how sensitive a patient may be to pain. The intensity of pain felt by children lessens as they grow older.

As puberty approaches, girls will notice and report more pain than boys do. Osteoarthritis, which affects 40 percent of middle-age patients and approximately 70 percent of geriatric patients, essentially will have the same degree of input into the central nervous system of men and women. However, patient responses to the degree of pain differ. Women appear to cope better with pain related to osteoarthritis than men.

Stressful life events are more common in the CRPS group, which indicates that there may be a multiconditional model of CRPS.7 The experience of stressful life events besides trauma or surgery are risk factors, not causes, in such a model.

Gender can bias can occur in a doctor's management of pain. Men and women may be treated differently by some doctors because of a gender-stereotyped attitude. Both men and women doctors contributed to the gender-disparate treatment. Male doctors frequently emphasize the importance of patient compliance to female patients, whereas female doctors emphasize the importance of patient compliance to male patients.

Current estrogen exposure at CRPS onset was retrieved from the electronic medical records and determined by current pregnancy or by the use of oral contraceptive (OC) drugs or hormonal replacement therapy. Researchers did not find an association between CRPS onset and cumulative endogenous estrogen exposure.2

It is concluded that gender differences should be taught in medical school to promote awareness of this problem. CRPS I occurs frequently during the third and fourth week after cast removal, especially in women who report severe pain and impairment of physical quality of life.8

Early traumatic experiences were reported in 87% of the CRPS-I patients and were found to be moderately related to somatoform dissociative experiences, indicating that early traumatic experiences might be a predisposing, although not a necessary factor for the development of CRPS-I-related dystonia.9 Although the psychological profile of the patients with CRPS-I-related dystonia shows some elevations, there does not seem to be a unique disturbed psychological profile on a group level.

Complex Regional Pain Syndrome (CRPS) Types I and II showed no correlation with the patient's gender or weight in a previous study.3 These results are consistent with studies that suggest that the pathogenesis of CRPS is due in part to central neuroimmune activation. Further studies demonstrated no association between CRPS onset and cumulative endogenous estrogen exposure as mention previously.2

Pain medicine is still in its infancy, as is gender-specific medicine. Treatment methods are constantly changing. It is unknown why females have a higher incidence of RSD/CRPS than males. A patient with CRPS should do as much research as a patient can to learn about the different methods available for a patient to treat a patient's RSD/CRPS pain.

A patient must feel free to methods of treatment with a patient's doctor and ask any questions that a patient may have. Understanding a patient's condition will help a patient to take charge of the patient's own treatment and help make that treatment as successful as possible. Motor nerve injury and female gender are risk factors for CRPS.

References
1.   de Mos M, de Bruijn AG, Huygen FJ, Dieleman JP, Stricker BH, Sturkenboom MC. The incidence of complex regional pain syndrome: a population-based study. Pain. 2007;129(1-2):12-20.
2.   de Mos M, Huygen FJ, Stricker BH, Dieleman JP, Sturkenboom MC. Estrogens and the risk of complex regional pain syndrome (CRPS). Pharmacoepidemiol Drug Saf. 2009;18(1):44-52.
3.   Alexander GM, van Rijn MA, van Hilten JJ, Perreault MJ, Schwartzman RJ. Changes in cerebrospinal fluid levels of pro-inflammatory cytokines in CRPS. Pain. 2005;116(3):213-219.
4.   Fischer SG, Perez RS, Nouta J, Zuurmond WW, Scheffer PG. Oxidative stress in Complex Regional Pain Syndrome (CRPS): no systemically elevated levels of malondialdehyde, F2-isoprostanes and

8OHdG in a selected sample of patients. Int J Mol Sci. 2013;14(4):7784-7794.

5.   Roh YH, Lee BK, Noh JH, et al. Factors associated with complex regional pain syndrome type I in patients with surgically treated distal radius fracture. Arch Orthop Trauma Surg. 2014;134(12):1775-1781.

6.   Tajerian M, Sahbaie P, Sun Y, et al. Sex differences in a Murine Model of Complex Regional Pain Syndrome. Neurobiol Learn Mem. 2015;123:100-109.

7.   Geertzen JH, de Bruijn-Kofman AT, de Bruijn HP, van de Wiel HB, Dijkstra PU. Stressful life events and psychological dysfunction in Complex Regional Pain Syndrome type I. Clin J Pain. 1998;14(2):143-147.

8.   Jellad A, Salah S, Ben Salah Frih Z. Complex regional pain syndrome type I: incidence and risk factors in patients with fracture of the distal radius. Arch Phys Med Rehabil. 2014;95(3):487-492.

9.   Reedijk WB, van Rijn MA, Roelofs K, Tuijl JP, Marinus J, van Hilten JJ. Psychological features of patients with complex regional pain syndrome type I related dystonia. Mov Disord. 2008;23(11):1551-1559.

13. Neuropathy

The word "pain" is derived from the Latin word poena that means punishment. St. Augustine wrote in the 5th century that all diseases afflicting Christians were derived from demons. Ancient tribal concepts of pain were based on beliefs that evil spirits were sent as punishment from their gods to invade one's body and cause severe pain. In the book of Genesis, Eve was condemned to pain during childbirth as a result of her encounter with the devil in the Garden of Eden.

It has been reported that a shaman could suck an evil spirit from a wound to decrease one's pain. The ancient Greeks such as Aristotle were the first individuals who believed that pain was derived from various nerves in the body. The exact cause of pain was unknown to them. Unfortunately, not unlike ancient times, the diagnosis and treatment of many chronic painful conditions today remains mostly guesswork.

Pain medicine is for the most part subjectively based, because pain is a subjective symptom while other medical specialties are based upon objective medical evidence. Pain in general is not bad. Pain is a protective mechanism that warns a patient that the body has something wrong at some location. The sensation of pain tells a patient to stop activity or to at least slow down the activity. For example if a patient sprains the ankle, the pain is a warning for a patient not to put weight on that leg.

The International Association for the Study of Pain defines pain as" an unpleasant sensory and emotional experience associated with tissue injury as a result of trauma (eg. bone fracture) or disease (eg. cancer, shingles). The efferent sympathetic nervous system is organized into subsystems that innervate and regulate via separate peripheral sympathetic pathways the different autonomic target organ.1

Pain has psychological effects in some instances especially when pain is severe. Pain may cause anxiety and depression. Acute pain is associated with injury, bone fractures, surgery or sprains and strains. Once these entities have healed sometimes, the pain continues. Arthritis is another example of chronic pain. Arthritic pain is caused by continuous joint destruction. However, once the pain becomes chronic, the pain it becomes a problem.

Not only does pain become a personal problem but pain can become a social problem with creation of family problems, loss of self-esteem and lost wages. Fibromyalgia patients have alterations in CNS anatomy, physiology, and chemistry that potentially contribute to the symptoms experienced by these patients

Pain impulses are in essence, electrical signals that travel from various areas of the body such as the extremities, heart, appendix etc. to the spinal cord and eventually reach the brain where the pain signals are processed like data in a computer. The brain is like a computer hard drive, which stores painful experiences that ultimately results in the suffering associated with chronic pain. Pain is produced by unpleasant stimuli to nerve endings throughout the body which include chemical, extreme heat cold and mechanical injury. These nerve endings are silent until mechanical, heat or cold injures tissue. In order to experience pain we need these pain receptors and the nerve fibers that transmit pain to the spinal cord and then to the brain.

Nerves, which conduct pain impulses to the spinal cord, are composed of neurons (nerve cells) that make up nerve fibers that form neurons. Two common pain fibers are the C fibers and the A-delta fibers. A-delta fibers conduct fast onset sharp pain impulses. The C fibers conduct slow onset dull, aching or burning pain. If a patient hit the finger with a hammer, a patient will experience a sudden pain response followed by a dull pain response.

Other types of fibers that transmit touch and vibration exist do not cause pain in most instances. However, these fibers can become hypersensitive and may contribute to the total pain experience. A neuron is an electrically excitable cell in the nervous system that processes and transmits information. Neurons are the significant core components of the brain and spinal cord as well as the peripheral nerves.

Neurons are typically composed of a cell body, a dendrite and an axon. Neurons receive input from dendrites and transmit output via the axon. Neurons are the building blocks of nerves. In other words, multitudes of neurons are necessary to form a nerve. Nerves that exist outside of the central nervous system are called a ganglion. The stellate ganglion in the neck is an example.

An injection into this ganglion may relieve pain associated with Reflex Sympathetic Dystrophy (now called Complex Regional Pain Syndrome). Various ganglia may form a plexus. An example of a plexus is the celiac plexus. Sometimes this plexus is blocked with numbing medicine or phenol or alcohol to relieve severe abdominal pain.

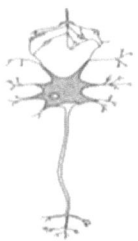

Figure 1. A nerve is composed of neurons. A neuron has one axon that takes nerve signals away from the neuron. The long end of the axon communicates with multiple dendrites.

Action potentials generated by the neuron initiate pain signals. If the skin is pinched a mechanical pain receptor begins and action potential. An action potential begins after a depolarization (a change in the electrical activity within the neuron) such that it could cause a membrane transitory modification, turning prevalently permeable to sodium ions more than to potassium ions. Sodium permeability can cause an action potential.

Neuropathy generates a local accumulation of sodium channels, with a consequent increase of density. This remodel seems to be the basis of neuro hyperexecitably. Males and those with lower levels of baseline pain and disability experienced the lowest CRPS severity scores over 12 months.[2]

Those with lower baseline anxiety and disability had the lowest pain intensity over the study period, and those with lower baseline pain and pain-related fear experienced the least disability over the 12 months. This suggests that anxiety, pain-related fear, and disability are associated with poorer outcomes in CRPS and could be considered as target variables for early treatment. The findings support the theory that CRPS represents an aberrant protective response to perceived threat of tissue injury.

Only life events seemed to be associated with CRPS1: patients who experienced more life events appeared to have a greater chance of developing CRPS1.[3] More studies with greater methodological quality and more participants should be performed on the association between psychological factors and the development and course of CRPS 1.

Excessive baseline pain in the week after an extremity injury greatly elevates the risk of developing CRPS.[4] Clinicians can consider a rating of greater than 5/10 to the question "What is the average pain over the last 2 days?" to be a "red flag" for CRPS.

Calcium channels have also an important role in cell working. Intracellular calcium increase contributes to depolarization processes, through kinase and determines the phosphorylation of membrane proteins that can make powerful the efficacy of the channels themselves. Following an acute injury,

AMPA receptors are stimulated which cause sharp pain. Receptors (areas in the body where biochemicals or drugs attach) are present in the spinal cord are called NMDA (N-methyl-D-aspartate) receptors and cause chronic pain.

When these NMDA receptors are stimulated, pain becomes more severe and this severe pain is maintained which implies that the pain does not decrease. The brain is responsible for the suffering associated with pain.

Pain results in bodily responses especially with respect to the cardiovascular system (heart rate increases, blood pressure increases, renal arteries constrict etc). When pain is severe, the brain can cause the body to increase both the heart rate and blood pressure.

Severe pain can also result in profuse sweating as well as nausea and vomiting. There are different types of nerve endings throughout the body. The pain nerve endings become hyper excitable when stimulated by injury, inflammation or a tumor.

Occasionally the nerve endings remain irritable even after the painful stimulus has been removed. Pain signals from areas in the body reach the brain by four processes (transduction, transmission, modulation and perception).

Axons carry pain fibers away from the neuron and direct them to the dendrites of the next neuron until they terminate in the brain or spinal cord. Remember that the axons and dendrites do not touch. They form synapses or clefts between the axon and dendrite. The synapse has chemicals in the axon nerve ending.

These chemicals allow communication between the neurons. Drugs are chemicals that can interrupt the communication between the neurons. Hypnosis and biofeedback can disrupt pain signal transmission. Injections can also inhibit transmission of pain signals from the arms or legs to the brain.

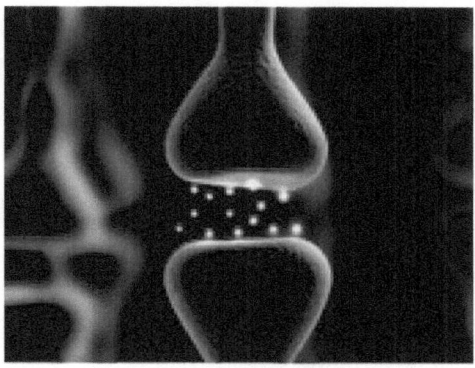

Figure 2. Chemicals are transferred between nerve endings (synapses) which cause transmission of pain signals.

A patient needs to understand that pain signals cross to the opposite side from the injury and therefore travel to the opposite side of the brain. The following illustration demonstrates by the arrows that pain signals enter the back of the spinal cord. They cross over to the other side. The pain impulses will then proceed upwards to go to the brain.

It is important to know that pain signals can be dampened by structures and chemicals that exist in the spinal cord. Pain signals as mentioned previously are transmitted from the site of injury as action potentials. Electrical and/or chemical activity between the neuron dendrites and axons propagate the axon potentials.

It is important to understand these processes in order to understand how the pain can be treated effectively. Transduction is a process where electrical signals originate in the nerve endings throughout the body. These impulses are chemically, mechanically and/or thermally mediated and transmitted to the spinal cord where they can be modulated and then sent to the brain. Tissue injury or disease (including arthritis) cause the body to release biochemicals called prostaglandins. Prostaglandins themselves do not cause pain.

Prostaglandins do however sensitize pain receptors to other chemicals in the body, which facilitate the transmission of pain impulses. Nonsteroidal drugs like ibuprofen decrease the number of prostaglandins produced in the body and may in a decrease in the pain perception. Topical creams can decrease the process of transduction at the nerve endings.

Transmission is a process where pain signals are transported to the spinal cord. Nerves in body tissues transmit impulses to the spinal cord.

Nerve blocks with anesthetics like Novicaine can interrupt the transmission of pain impulses to the spinal cord. Once pain impulses reach the spinal cord they are modulated or changed by chemicals and nerves that inhibit or lessen the number of pain impulses from going up the spinal cord to the brain.

Fibers called internuncial fibers are present within the spinal cord that can decrease pain transmission. The brain can send impulses back to these pain control fibers within the spinal cord to decrease the number of impulses that reach the pain perception center of the brain. This is the basis of hypnosis. Severe pain however, overwhelms the nerve fibers and they essentially become ineffective.

Most pain impulses cross over into the opposite side of the spinal cord from where they entered the spinal cord. The spinal cord acts like a transformer to intensify or decrease the intensity of pain impulses. Narcotics and anticonvulsants can modulate pain impulses within the spinal cord. Finally, pain impulses reach the brain where a patient perceives pain. Be aware that pain signals enter the posterior part of the spinal cord and then cross to the other side and travel upwards to the pain processing of the brain.

In CRPS I, unilateral inhibition of sympathetic vasoconstrictor neurones leads to a warmer affected limb in the acute stage. Secondary changes in neurovascular transmission may lead to vasoconstriction and cold skin in chronic CRPS I, whereas sympathetic activity is still depressed. Vascular abnormalities are dynamic.

The maximal skin temperature difference that occurs during the thermoregulatory cycle distinguishes CRPS I from other extremity pain syndromes with high sensitivity and specificity.[5]

Sympathetic neural activity might contribute to pain and sensory disturbances in CRPS by feeding into nociceptive circuits at the site of injury or elsewhere in the CRPS-affected limb, within the dorsal horn, or via thalamocortical projections.[6]

Narcotics can "numb" the brain to decrease the effects of the pain impulses on the brain by decreasing the intensity of these impulses. Higher brain centers determine how we respond to a painful stimulus. This explains why an individual can respond differently to a painful stimulus from other individuals (eg. "cry baby, whiner, vs macho man etc.). A chapter describing the anatomy and physiology of pain is not complete without an explanation of the Gate Theory of pain.

Melzak and Wall described this theory in 1965. Different types of nerve fibers (both pain and non-pain fibers) enter the spinal cord at the same time. Non-pain fibers essentially dilute out the number of pain impulses that enter the spinal cord.

An example of the Gate Control Theory is given by the following analogy. If a patient can imagine severe pain impulses represented by of multiple black balls going down a sink (analogy to spinal cord). If one adds multiple white balls (neutral non-pain transmitting entities), the number of black balls (pain impulses) is diluted. Therefore less severe impulses reach the spinal cord and the brain.

The white balls are non-pain balls and can close the gate (drain) to the number of black balls that go down the sink. To open the gate to more pain impulses, one only needs to decrease the number of white balls going to the hole in the sink. At this time, there are more black balls (pain impulses) available. The gate is now open.

Complex regional pain syndrome (CRPS) most often follows injury to peripheral nerves or their endings in soft tissue. A combination of prostanoids, kinins and cytokines cause peripheral nociceptive sensitization.7

As a patient can see, pain perception in the human body is complex. Because there are many different chemical transmitters and anatomic structures that contribute to chronic pain syndromes, each patient's treatment must be individualized. This is where the art of pain medicine is separated from pure science.

In order to understand pain transmission concepts, a patient must first become familiar with several biochemicals that are stored in the body that affect the pain signals. In order for a patient to hurt, pain-producing chemicals in the body tissue must stimulate pain fibers (Alpha-delta and C fibers). In general, the greater the tissue trauma, the more pain transmitting chemicals are produced and the worse the pain. In medical terminology, a stimulus (pin prick) produces a response (pain perception).

When a stimulus such as heat produces, tissue injury chemicals are released at the site of nerve injury, which cause pain fibers to become hyperactive. These chemicals include bradykinin, histamine, substance p, acetylcholine, serotonin and histamine. These chemicals act at the nerve endings and ultimately travel to the spinal cord and brain.

The nerves that conduct pain go to the spinal cord that allows pain signals to ultimately reach the brain. Areas of the body that have many pain receptors include the skin, the outer aspect of bone called the perios-teum, ligaments, joints, teeth and gums and the cornea of the eye.

Muscle also contains pain fibers but not as many per square meter (a measure of area) as the previously mentioned structures. Where the nerves from the body enter the spinal cord, aspartic and glutamic acid are produced. These acids increase pain impulse generation. NMDA may also be produced.

GABA (gamma-aminobutyric acid) in the spinal cord on the other hand, decreases the number of pain impulses that reach the brain. GABA inhibits pain impulse transmission. Norepinepherine and serotonin are two more chemicals in the spinal cord which attenuate the number of pain impulses which reach the brain.

The brain and spinal cord regulate pain by the production of natu-rally occurring narcotic-like substances that decrease pain transmission in specific areas of the brain. These narcotic-like drugs are called enkepha-lins, dynorphins and beta-endorphins. Some of these substances also decrease pain transmission in the spinal cord. Enkephalins are located in areas of the brain related to pain modulation.

Enkephalins inhibit pain at the spinal cord level. Enkephalins bind to narcotic receptors. When the narcotic receptors are activated, they inhibit pain signals. Dynorphins exist in both the brain and spinal cord but are more prevalent in the brain. Like enkephalins these substances bind to narcotic receptors in the brain and spinal cord.

Pain impulses that enter the spinal cord cross over to the other side and then progress upward to the brain. The natural beta-endorphins in the body exhibit morphine-like activity. They work like morphine to decrease the pain. Following injury or stress these endorphins are released into the blood stream. The effects of beta-endorphins are similar to morphine. Accumulating experimental and clinical evidence supports the hypothesis that complex regional pain syndrome type I (CRPS-I) may be a small fiber neuropathy.1

Beta-endorphins like narcotics can cause respiratory depression, constipation, euphoria, tolerance and physical dependence. The exact biochemical actions of all of the substances mentioned are complex. For a more detailed explanation of the actions of these substances one should consult a pain medicine textbook.

The purpose of this chapter is to emphasize the multiple substanc-es that can generate the transmission of pain signals. This is furthermore the reason why there are so many medications available for the management of the pain. This is also the reason why the physician may prescribe multiple medications for the management of the chronic pain.

With respect to tissue and nerve ending biochemicals, neurotransmitters and pain transduction, the physician may recommend a skin (topical) cream to decrease the transmission of pain signals to the brain. Red pepper cream decreases the pain generator called substance P. An example is Zostrix cream. Menthol containing creams (Ben Gay) also decrease pain over muscles and joints.

Non-steroidal anti-inflammatory drugs (NSAIDS) decrease the production of prostaglandin that can sensitize the body to pain mediators. Examples include Advil and Celebrex. Remember that prostaglandins sensitize pain nerve endings to pain producing tissue chemicals. Antidepressant drugs like Elavil or Prozac decrease pain by increasing norepinephrine and serotonin in the spinal cord. As previously mentioned, these two substances decrease the number of pain impulses that reach the pain perception areas of the brain.

Anticonvulsant drugs like Gabitril (tiagabine) in some instances affect GABA levels in the spinal cord and by enhancing GABA blood levels decreases the number of pain signals in the spinal cord that can go to the brain. Narcotic drugs also decrease pain impulse conduction in both the spinal cord and brain. Injections of numbing medicine (local anesthetics with steroids) can decrease pain in muscle and nerves in the arms, legs and the trunk of the body.

Epidural steroid injections can decrease pain in nerves that are buried deep within the spine. As a patient see there are multiple biochemical sources of pain and in many instances the physician may elect to prescribe multiple medications with good reason. Remember that each of these medications can have side effects that will be discussed in a later chapter.

There is an area of the brain that represents an area where a patient process pain signals. This area detects tissue injury and is a protective mechanism to alert a patient that something is wrong. A burn of the palm of the hand alerts the brain that tissue injury is occurring and initiates a reflex in the spinal cord to have a patient immediately remove the hand from the hot object. The gate control theory of pain, published in 1965, proposes that a mechanism in the dorsal horns of the spinal cord acts like a gate which inhibits or facilitates transmission from the body to the brain on the basis of the diameters of the active peripheral fibers as well as the dynamic action of brain processes.8

Without pain interpretation in the brain, a patient could sustain multiple bodily traumas and have no knowledge of its occurrence. The different dimensions of pain perception have been shown to depend on different areas of the brain. In contrast, much less is known about the neural basis of pathological chronic pain. Patients may report combinations of spontaneous pain and allodynia hyperalgesia-abnormal pain evoked by stimuli that normally induce no/little sensation of pain.

Modern neuroimaging methods (positron emission tomography (PET) and functional MRI (fMRI)) have been used to determine whether different neuropathic pain symptoms involve similar brain structures. PET studies have suggested that spontaneous neuropathic pain is associated principally with changes in thalamic activity and the medial pain system, which is preferentially involved in the emotional dimension of pain. Not only are there areas of the brain where a patient perceive pain but there are areas that are responsible for suffering as well. An area of the brain called the amygloid is associated with fear. Animals who have had their amygloid areas excised do not exhibit fear.

Fear, suffering and pain are in different areas of the brain but these areas are connected to each other. These interconnections ultimately can communicate with areas of the brain such as the midbrain that control the heart rate and respiratory rate as well. That differential activity in endogenous pain modulating systems may be not only a result of CRPS, but a potential risk factor for its development.9

If a patient has severe pain a patient may sweat profusely in addition to having increases in the heart and respiratory rates. As a patient can see, severe pain can have adverse physiologic effects on the body. RSD/CRPS may be related to an increase in the sympathetic nervous system which may cause a profound increase in the heart rate and/or the blood pressure. These bodily changes may result in anxiety with an increase in the body's sympathetic activity. These events cause a patient to be in a vicious cycle. When this occurs, consultation with a psychologist is indicated.

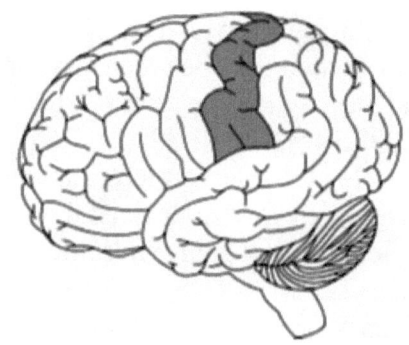

Figure 3. The brain areas (shaded) where pain signals are processed.

The transmission of pain from one part of the body to the brain is a complicated process. Remember that nerves do not touch each other. Pain signals are transmitted to the brain by chemicals that exist between the nerve endings. A patient can interrupt these pain signals by inhibiting the transfer of a chemical from one nerve to another. This can be done by medications, electrical stimulation, nerve blocks etc.

The pain of CRPS-I may depend on enhanced vasoconstrictor responsiveness, which may be relieved by blocking sympathetic efferent-dependent vasoconstriction, or by enhancing nitric oxide-dependent vasodilatation.

Glabrous and hairy skin samples from the amputated upper and lower extremity from two CRPS type I diagnosed patients were processed for double-label immunofluorescence using a battery of antibodies directed against neural-related proteins and mediators of nociceptive sensory function. In CRPS affected skin, several neuropathologic alterations were detected. The results are evidence of widespread cutaneous neuropathologic changes. Focal nerve inflammation is sufficient to cause neuronal discharge changes that are consistent with clinical findings in early CRPS.

References
1.   Baron R, Janig W. [Pain syndromes with causal participation of the sympathetic nervous system]. Anaesthesist. 1998;47(1):4-23.
2.   Bean DJ, Johnson MH, Heiss-Dunlop W, Lee AC, Kydd RR. Do psychological factors influence recovery from complex regional pain syndrome type 1? A prospective study. Pain. 2015;156(11):2310-2318.

3.   Beerthuizen A, van 't Spijker A, Huygen FJ, Klein J, de Wit R. Is there an association between psychological factors and the Complex Regional Pain Syndrome type 1 (CRPS1) in adults? A systematic review. Pain. 2009;145(1-2):52-59.

4.   Moseley GL, Herbert RD, Parsons T, Lucas S, Van Hilten JJ, Marinus J. Intense pain soon after wrist fracture strongly predicts who will develop complex regional pain syndrome: prospective cohort study. J Pain. 2014;15(1):16-23.

5.   Wasner G, Schattschneider J, Heckmann K, Maier C, Baron R. Vascular abnormalities in reflex sympathetic dystrophy (CRPS I): mechanisms and diagnostic value. Brain. 2001;124(Pt 3):587-599.

6.   Drummond PD. Sensory disturbances in complex regional pain syndrome: clinical observations, autonomic interactions, and possible mechanisms. Pain Med. 2010;11(8):1257-1266.

7.   Schwartzman RJ, Alexander GM, Grothusen J. Pathophysiology of complex regional pain syndrome. Expert Rev Neurother. 2006;6(5):669-681.

8.   Melzack R. [Acupuncture and pain mechanisms (author's transl)]. Anaesthesist. 1976;25(5):204-207.

9.   Seifert F, Kiefer G, DeCol R, Schmelz M, Maihofner C. Differential endogenous pain modulation in complex-regional pain syndrome. Brain. 2009;132(Pt 3):788-800.

14. Myofascial Pain

Complex regional pain syndrome (CRPS) remains a poorly understood chronic pain disorder. Little data has been published assessing the epidemiology of CRPS. Motor impairment is an important criterion in the Clinical Diagnostic Criteria of Complex Regional Pain Syndrome type-1 as defined by International Association for Study of Pain (IASP).[1]

An incidence rate of 5.46 per 100,000 person years at risk, and a period prevalence of 20.57 per 100,000 have been reported.[2] The female:male ratio in one study was 4:1, with a median age of 46 years at onset. The upper limb was affected twice as commonly as lower limb. All cases reported an antecedent event and fracture was the most common trigger (46%). Excellent concordance was found between symptoms and signs and vasomotor symptoms were the most commonly present.

Another study published data four years later than the above study and reported that the estimated overall incidence rate of CRPS was 26.2 per 100,000 person years (95% CI: 23.0-29.7). Females were affected at least three times more often than males (ratio: 3.4). The highest incidence occurred in females in the age category of 61-70 years. The upper extremity was affected more frequently than the lower extremity and a fracture was the most common precipitating event (44%). The observed incidence rate of CRPS is more as four times higher than the incidence rate observed in the only other population-based study, performed in Olmsted County, USA. Postmenopausal woman appeared to be at the highest risk for the development of CRPS.[3]

Three phase bone scan and autonomic testing diagnosed the condition in >80% of cases. Seventy-four percent of patients underwent resolution, often spontaneously. CRPS I is of low prevalence, more commonly affects women than men, the upper more than the lower extremity, and three out of four cases undergo resolution.

Myofascial pain syndrome is a chronic local or regional musculoskeletal pain disorder that may involve either a single muscle or a muscle group. The pain may be of a burning, stabbing, aching or nagging quality. Importantly, where the patient experiences the pain may not be where the myofascial pain generator is located. This is known as referred pain.

Following the onset of CRPS, a patient may demonstrate myofascial trigger points. A patient can develop a severe myofascial pain syndrome with reflex sympathetic dystrophy which should be addressed. The duration of CRPS symptoms and the involvement of the upper extremity was significantly associated with the presence of myofascial dysfunction.4

In another published study, fifty-one patients with a clinical diagnosis of CRPS received a bone scan, but only 53% of which were interpreted as consistent with the diagnosis of RSD/CRPS.4 Forty-seven percent had a history of physician-imposed immobilization, and 56% had a myofascial component present at evaluation.

The duration of CRPS symptoms and the involvement of the upper extremity were significantly associated with the presence of myofascial dysfunction. Thus, this study found that most CRPS patients are referred to a pain specialty clinic after several years of symptoms and many failed therapies. It is therefore recommended that a patient be referred to a pain specialist in a timely fashion.

Treatment consisting of specific myofascial trigger point (MTrP) therapy in one study was done, beginning with desensitization and gentle massage on the MTrP of the muscles noted that allodynia was remarkably reduced and further physical therapy with modalities was then administered.5 After 2 weeks of daily MTrP therapy, patients received further local steroid injection MTrP therapy 2-3 times per week. Approximately 2 months after the injections, most patients in this study were almost pain free.

If trigger points are present, treatment should consist of specific myofascial trigger point therapy, beginning with desensitization and gentle massage on the trigger points. Allodynia can be reduced and further physical therapy used to decrease the myofascial muscle pain. Trigger point injections may subsequently be effective for resolution of the extremity pain.

Almost everyone has experienced muscle pain a sometime. A patient may have had muscle pain if a patient were active playing sports or working in a a patient's garden. A myofascial pain syndrome is a soft tissue disorder of a patient's muscles that can cause a patient not only to have pain for a long time, but it can also cause a patient to on occasion, have some disability.

Myofascial dysfunction (MD) was detected in 61 % of CRPS patients in another study.6 It was more prevalent in the upper limb (70%) than in the lower limb (47%). Motor neglect was more common in those who also had MD. Patients with CRPS also may have myofascial pain syndrome as reported in a study by Rashiq and Galer who found that the myofascial pain syndrome can be treated first, and if it is treated effectively, the entire syndrome may resolve.

Myofascial pain may be treated with modalities and techniques, such as massage and myofascial release. Myofascial pathology of co-contraction appears to cause the clinical diagnostic criteria of CRPS and probable ischemic loss of myoarchitecture.1

A patient's overall activities of daily living, including work, recreation and social interaction can be significantly affected. Myofascial pain is pain related to muscle injury or overuse resulting in taut bands and palpable areas of pain that is referred to other muscular areas of a patient's body. Injury to a patient arm or leg can result in myofascial pain. CRPS is frequently caused by an injury to a patient's arm or leg. The pain can be dull, sharp or burning. A patient may suffer from sleep deprivation depression and anxiety like fibromyalgia.

Muscle strains and ligament sprains can cause pain in a patient's muscles and can contribute to the onset of a myofascial pain syndrome. The pain intensity of myofascial disorders can vary from painless decreases in range of motion about a patient's arms, legs, neck, and lower back, which are common in older individuals, to pain that is agonizing and incapacitating. This latter type of pain is seen if a patient is extremely active. Acute myofascial pain can decrease a patient's activities of daily living. If it becomes chronic, it can be a major cause of time lost at work.

Most myofascial pain can be relieved with an appropriate diagnosis and specific treatment. Pressing on the tender spots on a patient's body can identify myofascial trigger points. When a patient tender area is pressed, a patient will have pain in other areas of a patient's body that are away from the area being examined. Fibromyalgia pain does not cause referred pain when tender areas are palpated. The pains in the other areas are referred pain patterns that demonstrate trigger points. Myofascial trigger points occur when there is trauma to a patient's muscle or prolonged tension on a patient's muscle from slouching over a desk or slouching over a worktable. This slouching results in disruption of a patient's muscle cells.

When a a patient's muscle cell becomes disrupted, a patient's cells release calcium. Calcium released inside of a patient's muscle cell stimulates more contractions of a patient's muscle. A prolonged contraction will exceed the available oxygen, glucose, and other nutrients that are needed for the energy to allow a patient's muscle to continue to contract. With a sustained contraction, a patient runs out of oxygen as well as other nutrients. This allows a patient's muscle cell to build up a substance called lactic acid which stimulates muscle pain fibers.   Substances that cause a a patient's body to produce pain-causing substances are prostaglandins that sensitize pain fibers or substance P (a pain neurotransmitter) that is involved in pin transmission. Administration of Botulinism-A into the affected proximal muscles may alleviate both the myofascial pain syndrome and the distal allodynia, discoloration and, tissue swelling of the CRPS.

The pain transmitters associated with the myofascial pain syndrome stimulate nerve endings around a patient's muscle cells. These nerve endings go to other structures in a a patient's body. This is why a patient notices a referred pain pattern when a patient have a myofascial pain syndrome. A patient will notice nodular, ropelike bands under a patient's painful muscles when a patient have myofascial pain syndrome.

The lack of oxygen in a patient's muscle tissue will cause some of a a patient's muscle cells to die. This will cause scar tissue to form about a patient's muscles. This scar tissue gives a patient the nodular feeling when a patient presses over these painful areas. Not all pain in a a patient's muscles is from myofascial pain. Sometimes arthritis can cause muscle pain surrounding a a patient's joints.

Myopathy is also a disease of muscles that can occur and cause a patient to have muscle pain. If a patient has a disc herniation, a patient can have referred pain to a patient's muscles as well. Rocky Mountain spotted fever or Lyme disease can also cause a patient to have muscle pain.

A myofascial trigger point in a a patient's muscle needs to be distinguished from tender areas around a patient's ligaments as well as around a a patient's bone. The diagnosis of a patient's myofascial pain syndrome is made by a patient's health-care provider's history and physical examination and expertise. No laboratory tests are useful for the diagnosis of this syndrome.

If a patient has the myofascial pain syndrome, a patient will complain of localized muscle pain and tenderness as well as the referred pain. If a patient have myofascial trigger points around a patient's head and neck, a patient may complain of headaches as well as problems with a patient's vision. Remember that a patient can have myofascial trigger points in one muscle or many muscles.

To make a diagnosis of myofascial trigger points, a patient must have painful areas in a muscle that is noted by a patient's doctor on physical examination. These painful areas must be nodular and must be reproducible. Different amounts of pressure from a patient's examining health-care provider will give a patient referred pain. If a patient truly has myofascial pain a patient's doctor will record whether a patient have a "jump sign" noted on physical examination. This means that when a patient's doctor applies pressure on a patient's trigger point, a patient jump away from the pressure.

A patient's health-care provider will usually notice a twitch about the area that has pressure applied to it. At the time of a a patient's examination, a patient's health care provided will notice that a a patient's pain diminishes with stretching or following injection of a patient's muscle with a local anesthetic.

A patient's trigger points are classified as either active or latent. Active trigger points occur following acute muscle trauma. The latent trigger point on the other hand does not cause a patient to have pain at rest but can cause a patient to have restriction of movement about a certain part of a a patient's body. Latent trigger points are from a previous muscle injury.

A latent trigger point can persist for years after recovery from an injury. Latent trigger points can predispose a patient to have pain with overuse of a patient's previously injured muscle. Sometimes in cold weather, a patient's muscle will contract and cause a patient to have pain. Remember, only the active trigger points cause pain.

The latent trigger points cause pain when they become active. Normal muscles do not have trigger points that can be felt or have areas that can cause a patient pain when touched. A patient should feel a patient's normal muscles. Normal muscles do not have ropelike, nodular areas or tender areas to pressure and exhibit no observable twitch when a a patient's health-care provider palpates a patient's muscle. Furthermore, a patient will not have referred pain with this applied pressure.

A patient can have different degrees of severity of myofascial pain. Some trigger points are much more sensitive than others. An extremely sensitive trigger point can cause a patient to have greater referred nerve pain than a less-severe or intense trigger point. Myofascial pain is usually not symmetrical on either side of a patient's body.

However, medical conditions that cause muscle pain such as fibromyalgia are symmetrical. Trigger points are usually activated by overuse of muscles. A patient can stretch a patient's muscle beyond its normal capability, which will cause a patient's muscle to become injured.

Bleeding can occur within a patient's muscle following injury, which may cause scar formation in a patient's muscle. Active trigger points can develop in a patient's muscles following excessive, repetitive, or sustained motions. For example, if a patient work in a warehouse and load heavy boxes all day over months, a patient can begin to develop active trigger points. Common areas of trigger point pain include a patient's neck, arms, shoulders, face, back and legs.

Myofascial dysfunction is common in CRPS patients, especially in the upper limb and in those patients with motor nerve neglect.6 Emotional stress can also cause trigger points. Stress can cause a patient's muscles to stay in a contracted state.

When a patient's muscles are contracted for a length of time as previously stated, patients lose oxygen and other nutrients to a patient's muscle tissues. Heat and cold my help decrease a patient's pain.

Myofascial pain can vary in pain severity from hour by hour or from day by day. The stress required to produce pain is variable. Again, if a patient is under much stress, it does not take much additional muscle stress to produce myofascial pain. The amount of stress that is needed to make a patient's latent trigger become an active trigger point depends on a patient's degree of conditioning of a patient's muscles and a patient's exercise tolerance as well.

If a patient do not exercise and do aerobic activity and are under a lot of stress, a patient have susceptibility to develop active trigger points. If a patient's muscle is stiff, avoid placing cold packs on a muscle that may already be contracted. A patient should use heat instead of the cold. Viral illnesses can cause muscle pain.

If a patient have a virus, one should not put cold packs on a a patient's muscles. A virus will activate chemicals in a patient's body that activate pain signals. That is why a patient ache all over a a patient's body when a patient have the flu.

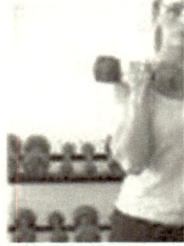

Figure 1. A muscle injury can cause myofascial pain. This pain can be superimposed with RSD/CRPS. Trigger point injections can be helpful in the injured muscle.

Myofascial pain may outlast any precipitating traumatic musculo-skeletal event. The pain duration is of myofascial pain is longer in duration than the muscle strain duration. The duration depends on a a patient's overall muscular prior to an injury. If a patient are a professional football player for example, a patient can have a muscle strain and never develop trigger points. If a patient is not physically fit, a minor muscle strain can result in myofascial pain.

A problem occurs when a patient is injured; a patient's muscles have developed a way of trying to prevent further pain. In doing so, these other muscles will cause a patient's injured muscle to be protected. Eventually a patient's active trigger points will become latent. If a patient rest a a patient's muscle and use a splint or an elastic bandage, a a patient's active trigger point may revert to become a latent trigger point.

Occasionally a patient may do an activity that will activate a a patient's latent trigger point. This not unusual and a patient should expect this occurrence on occasion. Many of a patient's muscles around a patient's active trigger point can decrease their function, causing a patient's muscles to become weak. If enough of a patient's muscles lose a significant portion of their function, a patient can develop weakness of an entire extremity.

Myofascial pain is caused by pressure over a a patient's muscles. When a patient are lying in bed, a patient may have some pressure on a a patient's body in the area of the trigger points from a patient's mattress. This pressure from a a patient's bed can cause a patient to have pain.

On the other hand, be aware that sleep disturbances can cause a patient's muscles to contract and become stiff and can worsen a patient's myofascial pain syndrome. If a patient's health-care provider does not visually notice spasms of a patient's painful muscle, this individual may snap a patient's muscle to see if a patient truly has a myofascial trigger point.

This essentially amounts to pinching and pulling a patient's muscle up. When this happens, usually a patient's muscle will demonstrate a visible muscle twitch demonstrating a myofascial trigger point. This muscle response can also be seen if a patient has latent trigger points. The highest incidence of the onset of trigger points occurs between ages thirty one and fifty.

When a patient is over 50, maximum activity could cause a patient to suffer from myofascial pain. As a patient continues to age and reduce activity as a result of pain, the patient's range of motion as a result of latent trigger points will become manifest. Many health-care providers are aware of myofascial trigger points. Muscle dysfunction is common in CRPS patients, especially in the upper limb and in those patients with muscle neglect.6

Chiropractors treat myofascial trigger points, as do physical therapists. Acupuncturists, anesthesiologists, dentists, pediatricians, rheumatologists, and specialists in physical medicine and rehabilitation all treat myofascial pain syndrome. The manner in which each of these health-care providers treats myofascial pain will vary from each of the health-care provider specialties.

If a patient's pain is not relieved with conservative measures another method that can decrease a patient's pain is a botulism toxin injection into a patient's painful muscles. This drug is a gram-negative bacterium. In small doses it can relax or even paralyze small muscle fibers. The relief from the injection of the Botox can last up to three months. Muscle dysfunction is common in CRPS patients, especially in the upper limb.

The problem with the Botox injection is that some individuals develop what appears to be fever and generalized joint pain associated with the bacteria that gets into their bloodstream. These side effects should however, subside over several days.

Prevention of myofascial trigger points should be considered. This may be accomplished by doing stretching exercises both before and immediately after engaging in strenuous exercise or after an injury to an arm or leg. This concept may also be used if a patient are not physically fit and want to work in a patient's garden for example. A patient should stretching exercises both before and after gardening. This may prevent the onset of myofascial pain.

The pathophysiology of myofascial pain remains somewhat of a mystery due to limited clinical research; however, based on case reports and medical observation, investigators think it may develop from a muscle lesion or excessive strain on a particular muscle or muscle group, ligament or tendon. It is thought that the lesion or the strain prompts the development of a "trigger point" that, in turn, causes pain.

In addition to the local or regional pain, people with myofascial pain syndrome also can suffer from depression, fatigue and behavioral disturbances, as with all chronic pain conditions. Recognition of this syndrome is difficult and requires the physician to have a precise under-standing of the body's anatomy.

Trigger points can be identified by pain produced upon digital pal-pation. In diagnosing myofascial pain syndrome, two types of trigger points can be distinguished: 1. Active trigger point; an area of exquisite tenderness that is usually located in a skeletal muscle and is associated with local or regional pain. 2. Latent trigger point; a dormant area that can potentially behave like an active trigger point.

The best treatments for myofascial pain syndrome are active and passive physical therapy methods. There is also the "stretch and spray" technique, in which the muscle with the trigger point is sprayed along its length with a coolant such as fluorimethane, and then stretched slowly.

Trigger point injection, whereby local anesthesia is injected direct-ly into the trigger point, also is used. At times, corticosteroids and botuli-num toxin can be injected. Massage therapy also can be of significant benefit in some patients. Often a combination of physical therapy, trigger point injections and massage are needed in refractory chronic cases.

The Complex Regional Pain Syndrome/Reflex sympathetic dys-trophy has sometimes been hypothesized to derive from a unique psycho-logical predisposition because of its enigmatic features, as well as the profound behavioral and emotional characteristics manifested by some patients.[7]

However, RSD and myofascial pain patients appear comparable with respect to a wide range of demographic, clinical, and psychological functioning indices. A specific psychological profile, uniquely neurotic or otherwise, has yet to be demonstrated in terms of any etiologic or mainte-nance factors in RSD patients when compared to other pain patients.

CRPS can be associated with myofascial trigger points as well. Sudden trauma to musculoskeletal tissues like muscles, ligaments, ten-dons, and bursae may cause chronic pain as well. Lack of range of motion can cause extremity myofascial pain. The fascia is a connective tissue which spreads throughout the body from a patient's head to foot.

The fascia surrounds muscles, bones, nerves, blood vessels and or-gans of the body. The fascia itself contains many pain fibers. A patient need to be aware that on occasion, trigger points can produce autonomic nervous system changes such as flushing of the skin, hypersensitivity of areas of the skin, or sweating in areas.

One study reported that hip dysfunctions may be related to tem-poromandibular dysfunction. The results of a study suggest that temporomandibular joint dysfunction plays an important role in the restriction of hip motion experienced by patients with CRPS, which indicated a connectedness between these two regions of the body.8

These symptoms are similar to those of CRPS. An active trigger point when treated will become quiet. If an injury that causes CRPS occurs, the quiet trigger points can become active. Sometimes addressing treatment of the trigger points will resolve the CRPS.

The development of a myofascial pain syndrome (MFPS) with trigger points in the proximal muscles of the patients with complex regional pain syndrome can occur and improvement of distal symptoms of CRPS can follow after successful treatment of the proximal MFPS. Furthermore, the distal allodynia, discoloration and, tissue swelling of CRPS may be eliminated as well.9

Musculoskeletal ultrasonography of muscles may be useful in the diagnosis of the CRPS. Musculoskeletal ultrasonography of muscles in CRPS in one study was characterized by a variable or/and global intramuscular structural disruption with loss of muscle bulk.

Adjacent muscles coalesced with one another to present a uniform hyper echogenic mass of tissue. Muscle edema was found in some patients. In comparison, musculoskeletal ultrasonography of muscles in muscles affected by neuropathic pain exhibited structural normalcy, but also showed considerable reduction in muscle bulk.

Another published study revealed patients who had a myofascial component present at evaluation. The duration of CRPS symptoms and the involvement of the upper extremity were significantly associated with the presence of myofascial dysfunction. Thus, this study found that most CRPS patients are referred to a pain specialty clinic after several years of symptoms and many failed therapies.

The data from this study also suggested the lack of utility of a diagnostic bone scan and highlight the prominence of myofascial dysfunction in a majority of CRPS patients.4

Musculoskeletal ultrasonography of muscles in CRPS was characterized by a variable or/and global intramuscular structural disruption with loss of muscle bulk. Adjacent muscles coalesced with one another to present a uniform hyper echogenic mass of tissue. Muscle edema was found in some patients. In comparison, musculoskeletal ultrasonography in muscles affected by neuropathic pain exhibited structural normalcy, but also showed considerable reduction in muscle bulk.1

It may be concluded that attention to myofascial trigger points with the appropriate medical treatment should be addressed in CRPS patients who have myofascial pain as well.

References

1.   Vas LC, Pai R, Pattnaik M. Musculoskeletal Ultrasonography in CRPS: Assessment of Muscles Before and After Motor Function Recovery with Dry Needling as the Sole Treatment. Pain Physician. 2016;19(1):E163-179.

2.   Sandroni P, Benrud-Larson LM, McClelland RL, Low PA. Complex regional pain syndrome type I: incidence and prevalence in Olmsted county, a population-based study. Pain. 2003;103(1-2):199-207.

3.   de Mos M, de Bruijn AG, Huygen FJ, Dieleman JP, Stricker BH, Sturkenboom MC. The incidence of complex regional pain syndrome: a population-based study. Pain. 2007;129(1-2):12-20.

4.   Allen G, Galer BS, Schwartz L. Epidemiology of complex regional pain syndrome: a retrospective chart review of 134 patients. Pain. 1999;80(3):539-544.

5.   Hong CZ. Specific sequential myofascial trigger point therapy in the treatment of a patient with myofascial pain syndrome associated with reflex sympathetic dystrophy. Australas Chiropr Osteopathy. 2000;9(1):7-11.

6.   Rashiq S, Galer BS. Proximal myofascial dysfunction in complex regional pain syndrome: a retrospective prevalence study. Clin J Pain. 1999;15(2):151-153.

7.   Nelson DV, Novy DM. Psychological characteristics of reflex sympathetic dystrophy versus myofascial pain syndromes. Reg Anesth. 1996;21(3):202-208.

8.   Fischer MJ, Riedlinger K, Gutenbrunner C, Bernateck M. Influence of the temporomandibular joint on range of motion of the hip joint in patients with complex regional pain syndrome. J Manipulative Physiol Ther. 2009;32(5):364-371.

9.   Safarpour D, Jabbari B. Botulinum toxin A (Botox) for treatment of proximal myofascial pain in complex regional pain syndrome: two cases. Pain Med. 2010;11(9):1415-1418.

15. Fibromyalgia

Fibromyalgia is a chronic pain syndrome that affects muscles, tendons, and fascia throughout the body. This disease is also referred to as fibromyositis. It affects about 5 percent of the population, 90 percent of which are women of childbearing age. Fibromyalgia causes a patient to have muscle pain throughout the body, and is associated with joint stiffness and fatigue.

CRPS is a disease that affects nerves, muscles and tendons. A patient also may experience sleep disturbances and depression if a patient have fibromyalgia. It can cause many places on a patient's body to become extremely tender.

Although fibromyalgia and complex regional pain syndrome (CRPS) have distinct clinical phenotypes, they do share many other features. Pain, allodynia and dysaesthesia occur in each condition and seem to exist on a similar spectrum. Fibromyalgia and CRPS can both be triggered by specific traumatic events, although fibromyalgia is most commonly associated with psychological trauma and CRPS is most often associated with physical trauma, which is frequently deemed routine or minor by the patient.1

Fibromyalgia and CRPS also seem to share many pathophysiological mechanisms, among which the most important are those involving central effects. Nonetheless, peripheral effects, such as neurogenic neuroinflammation, are also important contributors to the clinical features of each of these disorders.

A patient is only diagnosed with fibromyalgia after other pain-causing conditions have been eliminated as the reason for the pain. Fibromyalgia is a condition that can be painful, but it is benign and will rarely cause a patient to be totally disabled. Fibromyalgia can be quite painful but there still exists no other chronic pain syndrome that is as painful as CRPS/CRPS in its intensity.

Fibromyalgia can come and go into remission for weeks or months at a time while it is rare for that to happen for CRPS. They are still often confused in a diagnosis by some doctors as many see so little of either. The other problem that occurs is that many CRPS/CRPS patients develop fibromyalgia and end up with both to some degree.

The diagnosis of fibromyalgia includes a history of aches, pains, stiffness in eleven or more tender areas above and below the navel and to the right and left of the navel. Patients with fibromyalgia report a considerable impact on their quality of life and their perceived disability level seems influenced by their mental health condition. In comparison with patients with other pain conditions psychological distress is higher.

A patient may have a history of irritable bowel syndrome and depression as well. A patient may be depressed and suffer from sleep deprivation in addition to muscle pain. The following diagram shows common body sites where a patient might experience tender areas associated with fibromyalgia. A patient muscle will not feel contracted but will feel soft and tender to light touch.

Tender areas can also occur in patients' arms and legs. A patient should note from the diagram that these tender points occur above and below a patient's navel and occur in a plane to the right and left of a patient's navel. The main difference is how localized CRPS is. CRPS displays a kind of intense localization is not found in fibromyalgia. For instance, in CRPS the affected limb can swell up, turn colors, become stiff and develop bone loss. Swelling usually does not occur in fibromyalgia.

The common features of CRPS and fibromyalgia may suggest that a common pathway is involved, but until patients with these types of symptoms are assessed with a uniform assessment procedure, a thorough comparison cannot be made. A systematic evaluation of patients with a suspected diagnosis of CRPS or fibromyalgia, may lead to a better appreciation of the differences and similarities in these diseases and help to unravel the underlying mechanisms.[2]

The complex regional pain syndrome (CRPS) and fibromyalgia (FM) are chronic pain syndromes occurring in highly stressed individuals. Despite the known connection between the nervous system and immune cells, information on distribution of lymphocyte subsets under stress and pain conditions is limited. Future studies are warranted to answer whether such immunological changes play a pathogenetic role in CRPS and FM or merely reflect the consequences of a pain-induced neurohumoral stress response, and whether they contribute to immunosuppression in stressed chronic pain patients.[3]

Every pain syndrome has an inflammatory profile consisting of the inflammatory mediators that are present in the pain syndrome. The inflammatory profile may have variations from one person to another and may have variations in the same person at different times. The key to treatment of Pain Syndromes is an understanding of their inflammatory profile. Current evidence suggests that cytokines and especially chemokines may have a role in the pathogenesis of this syndrome.4

Cytokines are small soluble factors that work as immune system messengers. They can be classified as pro-inflammatory and anti-inflammatory cytokines. Chemokines are a special kind of pro-inflammatory cytokines that guide the movement of circulating mononuclear cells to the injured side. Some pro-inflammatory cytokine levels (i.e. IL-1RA, IL-6, and IL-8) and, recently, some chemokines' levels have been found to be increased in patients with fibromyalgia.

The unifying theory or law of pain states: the origin of all pain is inflammation and the inflammatory response. The biochemical mediators of inflammation include cytokines, neuropeptides, growth factors and neurotransmitters. 4 Irrespective of the type of pain whether it is acute or chronic pain, peripheral or central pain, nociceptive or neuropathic pain, the underlying origin is inflammation and the inflammatory response. Activation of pain receptors, transmission and modulation of pain signals, neuro plasticity and central sensitization are all one continuum of inflammation and the inflammatory response.

The pain intensity of patients with fibromyalgia has recently been reported to be correlated with the degree of small intestinal bacterial overgrowth. The small intestinal bacterial permeability in primary fibromyalgia and, unexpectedly, CRPS are increased.5 This finding should stimulate further research to determine the implication of altered IP in the disease pathophysiology of FM and CRPS.

The muscle pain that a patient experiences is probably more common in a patients neck and lower back. However, it can affect any muscle throughout a patient's body. The pain can range from sharp or cramping to a burning sensation. Pain may be worse in one specific area, even though the pain can be felt all over a patient's body. A patient also will notice that fibromyalgia pain affects tender areas on a patient body that are symmetrical, or located in the same places on the opposite side of a body.

Tenderness and swelling of a patient's hands or feet are also common. Other common areas where a patient may notice tenderness include the areas under the base of a patients skull; above the shoulder blade, elbows, the buttocks (gluteal muscle); the front of the neck midway from the chin to the collar bone; the chest; the sides of the body over the hip regions; and the inner aspects of the knees. In CRPS, the patient's pain is usually in an arm or leg. However, some CRPS patients may have generalized pain.

Patients with CRPS in one study considered their widespread pain as an important factor affecting their quality of life. For the majority of patients it was of similar severity to the original CRPS pain. Additional patients reported CRPS concomitant regional pains, most commonly headaches/migraines, lower back pain, and irritable bowel syndrome similar to fibromyalgia patients.6

It is more common for women to have an incidence of fibromyalgia and CRPS more often than men. Because of this; researchers are trying to find gender specific causes of fibromyalgia. In general the amount of pain that women can withstand is lower than the amount of pain that men can withstand. Fibromyalgia is seen mostly in women between 20 and 50 years of age. However, it can affect children and elderly people as well.

Fibromyalgia may develop after an injury, a motor vehicle accident, infection (viral or bacterial), or after an onset of rheumatoid arthritis. Stressful situations, cold weather and over exertion can worsen a patient's fibromyalgia. As a fibromyalgia sufferer, a patient may not be getting enough deep sleep. Even in normal people, not getting enough sleep can produce symptoms of fibromyalgia. It is not currently known if a lack of deep sleep is a cause of fibromyalgia. Some doctors think the loss of deep sleep can however hasten the onset of fibromyalgia.

The stress system is controlled by brain nuclei at the hypothalamus and brainstem. These nuclei interact with each other and control the HPA axis and sympathetic nervous systems, respectively. Major inputs to the stress system arise from the cerebral cortex and subcortical systems, the sensory organs and nerves, and the endocrine and immune systems.

The major peripheral effectors of the stress system are glucocorticoids and the catecholamines. Pathological hypoactivity of the stress system has been associated with atypical depression, the chronic fatigue/fibromyalgia syndromes and autoimmune inflammatory disease.

Serotonin and norepinepherine are two chemicals in a patient's central nervous system that decrease pain signals that travel to a patient's brain. Not having enough serotonin in a patient's brain and spinal cord can cause a patient lose sleep, which can cause symptoms of depression as well as fibromyalgia pain.

Fibromyalgia also affects patients' levels of norepinephrine, which is another chemical in a patient central nervous system that also modulates the number of pain signals that go to a patient's brain. Another chemical in a patient's body that causes pain is substance P. Substance P is found in all of the neurons of the central nervous system as well as nerves that go to a patient's muscles and joints. When a patients muscle tissues have been injured, substance P is released. This event can trigger burning pain sensations throughout a patient's body.

High substance P levels have been noted in the spinal fluid of patients with fibromyalgia. Endorphins, substances produced by a patient's body and deposited in the spinal cord to decrease pain transmission to a patient's brain, are known to slow down the pain-causing effects of substance P. The low levels of endorphins in a patient's brain and spinal cord when a patient has fibromyalgia may be another cause of pain associated with this condition.

It is well known that vigorous exercise can produce endorphins that are then released in a patient's body. Along with decreasing the pain signals that are sent to a patient's brain, endorphins can affect a patient's mood. It is thought that a lower than normal blood level of endorphins may be another cause of fibromyalgia.

People with and without fibromyalgia who do physical exercise have noted a decrease in their pain following aerobic exercise. Normal people usually have an increase in endorphins in their bloodstream following exercise. However, a patient may show no increase in endorphin levels after a patient exercise.

There is increased evidence that fibromyalgia can be genetically inherited. A patient may even know of a relative who has symptoms similar to a patient's. The exact gene that causes fibromyalgia has not been isolated, but several genes have been proposed as a possible explanation for the genetic inheritance of fibromyalgia and they are being studied.

Research into the causes of fibromyalgia must continue. Furthermore, CRPS can be familial and hence may have a genetic basis in some families as well.4 If a patient suffers from chronic pain, it is a good idea for a patient to keep a daily diary of his/her activities and pain levels.

It is important that a patient do exercise or some type of low-impact aerobic activity. Aerobic exercise is extremely helpful in decreasing pain and improving a patient's sleep pattern. Swimming and water aerobics are excel-lent ways for a patient to accomplish this goal. They are some of the best exercise activities for patients with fibromyalgia.

These types of nonimpact activities will help strengthen and condition patients muscles, unlike high-impact exercise that can actually do more damage to a patients muscles. Following physical exercise, almost

50 percent of people had a significant decrease in their signs and symptoms of fibromyalgia. Exercise will improve a patient's muscle range of motion. Exercise is also important in CRPS patients as well.

Most doctors agree that medications, injections, and therapy alone will not be able to eliminate a patient's pain, but rather it will help a patient to manage a patient's pain and cope with it better. Taking steroids to treat a patient's fibromyalgia will not improve patient's symptoms of pain but may decrease a patient's pain in CRPS. People with other muscle or bone conditions such as rheumatoid arthritis do respond well to steroids. However, nonsteroidal anti-inflammatory medications such as ibuprofen may relieve or at least decrease a patient's muscle pain.

The primary goal in treating a patient's fibromyalgia or CRPS is to attempt to break the pain cycle. One way of accomplishing this goal is to correct any disturbance in a patients sleep pattern. Amitriptyline (Elavil) can be an important drug in restoring a patient's sleep. Numerous studies have shown that getting enough sleep can significantly reduce a patient's pain. If a patient is allergic to amitriptyline, cyclobenzaprine (Flexeril) can be substituted.

In some people, nonsteroidal anti-inflammatory medications such as ibuprofen can be successfully used. Amantadine hydrochloride (Symmetrel) also may be used. This medication is an antiviral as well as an anti-Parkinson medication. Serotonin reuptake inhibitors (Paxil) may also have a positive effect on reducing a patient's pain. There are newer two drugs approved by the FDA for the treatment of fibromyalgia; Lyrica (an anticonvulsant) and Cymbalta (an antidepressant). Both of these medications can relieve CRPS pain.

Nerve stimulation is another method of relieving pain that a patient may find helpful. A TENS unit (Transcutaneous Electrical Nerve Stimulator) is useful in managing fibromyalgia pain in many patients. This small battery-powered instrument has two to four patches that are placed over patients painful muscle areas. Electrical impulses will stimulate the nerves around a patient's area of pain. This stimulation will cause the production of the pain-relieving chemical encephalin into a patient's spinal cord.

Enkephalin in the body will diminish the intensity of a patients pain signals that ultimately reach a patient's brain. Another useful device that is gaining in popularity is a muscle stimulator. This device has six to eight patches that are placed over a patient painful muscle area. The muscle stimulator machine will stimulate and work a patients muscle until they are fatigued and weakened. It is possible for patients' muscles that have been weakened by the fibromyalgia to be strengthened this way.

The "leaking gut" theory may be a cause of fibromyalgia. If large proteins leak into a patient's gastrointestinal circulation, a patient's immune system may become overactive. A patient can then experience an antibody response that causes a patient to have generalized body pain. Some individuals that have fibromyalgia from this cause can be treated successfully with a gluten free diet, colostrum supplements or hyper immune eggs. A psychologist can help a patient deal with the suffering aspect of a patient's pain.

A patient's psychologist also may want to teach a patient biofeed-back. This is a good way for a patient to learn relaxing techniques that can significantly reduce a patient's pain. A patient's psychologist may want a patient to listen to a CD or cassette tapes at home.

Aromatherapy also could be effective for helping a patient manage a patient's pain. This method is more effective in women because their scent perception is better than a man's. A patient may also find that hypnosis can decrease a patient's pain intensity as well. A patient may want to try self-hypnosis as another modality for the management of a patient's chronic pain.

Insomnia is common in fibromyalgia. Chronic insomnia alone impacts 10% to 15% of adults. Epidemiologic data indicate that pain, fatigue, and mood disturbance are common correlates of persistent insomnia. A patient's physician must try to correct a patient's insomnia. A good night's rest increases norepinerpherine and serotonin in a patient's central nervous system. These are two biochemicals in a patient's body that can decrease a patient's pain. Fibromyalgia is associated with insomnia.

The same is true for CRPS. Significant sleep disturbances are reported by 80% of patients with CRPS. CRPS and fibromyalgia patients have severe influences on the quality of life in these patients. Fibromyalgia is associated with significant depression. Complex regional pain syndrome like fibromyalgia is a severe disabling pain disorder that results in physical as well as emotional (depression)and financial consequences to patients.

Patients with a fibromyalgia syndrome can present with myofascial trigger points just like CRPS. Just like CRPS, fibromyalgia patients may have autonomic phenomena like skin reddening and sweating.

Fibromyalgia patients presenting with autonomic phenomena should be examined for a myofascial pain syndromes as well.

Substance P is elevated in patients suffering from fibromyalgia. A hypothesis exists that the distal tibial fracture model of a rat simulates CRPS. Leg immobilization alone can generate a syndrome resembling CRPS and substance P contributes to the vascular and pain changes observed in these models.

Substance P induced plasma protein extravasations are increased in CRPS patients on both the affected and unaffected limbs. The underlying mechanism might be impaired substance P inactivation. These findings further support the hypothesis that neurogenic inflammation plays an important role in the initiation of CRPS and possibly fibromyalgia.

Sometimes fibromyalgia can be confused with CRPS. A patient needs to be aware that CRPS can spread from the injured area to the other extremities in a patient's body. If a patients CRPS is confined to a patients arm or leg, the diagnosis of CRPS is much easier than CRPS that has spread to a patient's other three extremities. CRPS is then very difficult to distinguish from fibromyalgia.

For example, if a patient has CRPS of a hand, it can spread to the rest of the patients extremities. Therefore, it is necessary for a patient to have a basic understanding of fibromyalgia. While occasionally someone afflicted with fibromyalgia is told that he or she may have a Complex Regional Pain Syndrome (CRPS), it is not uncommon for someone with CRPS to be told he/she has Fibromyalgia. Unfortunately, this only adds confusion to those with either of these disorders.

The hallmark of CRPS is cold sensitivity in the presence of blood vessel and sweat changes in addition to an abnormal skin color. Symptoms usually begin after an identifiable, causative event. It has been shown that barometric changes can sensitize pain fibers. As a result of this increased sensation, a patient's pain can significantly increase.

In patients with CRPS, the weather-sensitive component may manifest itself as pain that increases with barometric changes. This is a noticeable worsening and a major feature in those with CRPS. In contrast, Fibromyalgia patients may also have weather sensitivity; however, this problem is not a hallmark feature of the disorder. Fibromyalgia patients tend to have more generalized pain, earlier complaints of fatigue, and a history of immune system over-activity or persistent infection when compared to the CRPS patient.

Fibromyalgia patients are less likely to have an inciting event that they can relate their symptoms to. Despite these variations, there may be considerable overlap between the two diagnostic groups. For example, a CRPS patient whose symptoms seem to have spread may look very much as if they have Fibromyalgia. This is because the new areas of pain may have no obvious inciting event, are less likely to be associated with contracture or bone loss, and are often associated with increasing fatigue.

While it is important to evaluate new symptoms to determine if there has been a progression of CRPS, spread can usually be proven in only a minority of cases. New symptoms may: represent an unrelated problem, provide evidence that the disease has developed into Chronic Regional Pain Syndrome (CRPS) that is independent of sympathetic pain or be a clue that there is an infection or immunologic compromise.

If the previously mentioned hallmark changes for CRPS occur, or if thermographic or bone scan findings suggest objective findings then a true spread of CRPS can be diagnosed. Likewise it should be recognized that a Fibromyalgia patient's symptoms might progressively worsen to the point that the sympathetic component becomes dominant and CRPS features develop.

While this is not common, if it does happen, treatment should be aggressive. Although there can be considerable overlap between patients with sympathetic pain who do not develop full blown CRPS and fibromyalgia patients who are weather-sensitive, a skilled clinician should be able to differentiate between the two conditions in the majority of cases.

The complex regional pain syndrome (CRPS) and fibromyalgia (FM) are chronic pain syndromes occurring in highly stressed individuals. Future studies are warranted to answer whether such immunological changes play a pathogenetic role in CRPS and FM or merely reflect the consequences of a pain-induced neurohumoral stress response, and whether they contribute to immunosuppression in stressed chronic pain patients.

Neurogenic neuroinflammation might contribute to the multifactorial pathogenesis of both fibromyalgia and CRPS, and suggests that this mechanism is an important link between the two disorders.

Seemingly inexplicit adverse reactions have been described after the injection of the newer vaccines vs. human papillomavirus (HPV). Different isolated cases and small series have described the development of complex regional pain syndrome (CRPS), postural orthostatic tachycardia syndrome (POTS), and fibromyalgia after HPV vaccination. Neuroin-flammation in fibromyalgia and CRPS is multifactorial.

What is helpful is that the treatments for both entities are similar other than spinal cord stimulators or sympathetic injections are not indicated for the treatment of fibromyalgia. In CRPS patients, muscle cramps (spasms and dystonia) can be treated with clonazepam and baclofen. Muscles stiffness may be treated with muscle relaxants such as Tizanidine (Zanaflex), Baclofen or Clonazepam (Klonopin).

Sometimes fibromyalgia can be confused with CRPS. A patient needs to be aware that CRPS can spread from the injured area to the other extremities in a patient's body. For example, if a patient has CRPS of a patient's hand, it can spread to the rest of a patient's extremities. Therefore, it is necessary for a patient to have a basic understanding of fibromyalgia. While occasionally someone afflicted with fibromyalgia is told that he or she may have Reflex Sympathetic Dystrophy (CRPS), it is not uncommon for someone with CRPS to be told he has Fibromyalgia. Unfortunately, this only adds confusion to those with either of these disorders.

The hallmark of CRPS is cold sensitivity in the presence of blood vessel and sweat changes in addition to an abnormal skin color. Symptoms usually begin after an identifiable, causative event. It has been shown that barometric changes can sensitize pain fibers. As a result of this increased sensation, a patient's pain can significantly increase. In patients with CRPS, the weather-sensitive component may manifest itself as pain that increases with barometric changes. This is a noticeable worsening and a major feature in those with CRPS.

In contrast, Fibromyalgia patients may also have weather sensitivity; however, this problem is not a hallmark feature of the disorder. Fibromyalgia patients tend to have more generalized pain, earlier complaints of fatigue, and a history of immune system over-activity or persistent infection when compared to the CRPS patient. Fibromyalgia patients are less likely to have an inciting event that they can relate their symptoms to.

Previous published findings suggest that the longer the patients have CRPS the more likely they are to report symptoms suggestive of centralized pain. These data may explain why some patients with a longer duration of CRPS as well as fibromyalgia do not respond to peripherally directed therapies.7

Despite these differences, there may well be considerable overlie between the two diagnostic groups. For example, a CRPS patient whose symptoms seem to have spread may appear as if he/she has fibromyalgia. This is because the new areas of pain may have no apparent provocative occurrence, are less likely to be linked with muscle contractures or bone loss, and can be associated with chronic fatigue.

While it is important to evaluate new symptoms to determine if there has been a succession of CRPS, spread of CRPS can usually be verified in only a minority of cases. New symptoms in a CRPS patient may represent an unrelated problem, provide evidence that the disease has developed into chronic CRPS that is independent of sympathetic pain, or be a suspicion that there is unknown infection or immunologic compromise.

The pain intensity of patients with FM has recently been reported to be correlated with the degree of small intestinal bacterial overgrowth (SIBO). SIBO is often associated with an increased intestinal permeability. The pain intensities in primary FM and, unexpectedly, CRPS are increased. This should stimulate further research to determine the implication of altered intestinal permeability in the disease pathophysiology of FM and CRPS.8

A study published in 2014 is itself a major update of previous reviews published in 2005 and 2000, investigating the effects of gabapentin in chronic neuropathic pain.9 It investigated the effects of gabapentin in chronic neuropathic pain. This is important data because many insurance carriers prefer gabapentin over pregabilin for pain management. Antiepileptic drugs are used to manage chronic neuropathic pain. CRPS and fibromyalgia.

The outcome of at least 50% pain intensity reduction in this study is regarded as a useful outcome of treatment by patients, and the achievement of this degree of pain relief is associated with important beneficial effects on sleep interference, fatigue, and depression, as well as quality of life, function, and work. About 35% achieved this degree of pain relief with gabapentin, compared with 21% for placebo. Over half of those treated with gabapentin will not have worthwhile pain relief. Results might vary between different neuropathic pain conditions, and the amount of evidence for gabapentin in neuropathic pain conditions except postherpetic neuralgia and painful diabetic neuropathy, and in fibromyalgia, is very limited.9

If the hallmark changes for CRPS occur, or if thermographic or bone scan findings confirm objective findings, then true spread of CRPS can be diagnosed. Similarly it should be accepted that a fibromyalgia patient's symptoms might progressively worsen to the point that the sympathetic element becomes dominant and CRPS features develop.

Although there can be considerable overlap between patients with sympathetic pain who do not develop CRPS, and fibromyalgia patients who are weather responsive, a capable physician should be able to differentiate between the two diseases.

Fibromyalgia can be quite painful there still exists no other chronic pain syndrome that touches RSD/CRPS in its intensity; Fibromyalgia can come and go into remission for weeks or months at a time while it is much rarer for that to happen for RSD/CRPS. The other problem that occurs is that many RSD/CRPS patients develop Fibromyalgia and end up with both to some degree.

The common features of CRPS and FM may suggest that a common pathway is involved, but until patients with these types of symptoms are assessed with a uniform assessment procedure, a thorough comparison cannot be made. Neuroinflammation in fibromyalgia and CRPS is multifactorial.10,11

Apart from some obvious differences between CRPS and fibromyalgia, the similarities are conspicuous. The common features of CRPS and fibromyalgia may suggest that a common pathway is involved, but until patients with these types of symptoms are assessed with a uniform assessment procedure, a thorough comparison cannot be made.2

References
1.   Littlejohn G. Neurogenic neuroinflammation in fibromyalgia and complex regional pain syndrome. Nat Rev Rheumatol. 2015;11(11):639-648.

2.   Marinus J, Van Hilten JJ. Clinical expression profiles of complex regional pain syndrome, fibromyalgia and a-specific repetitive strain injury: more common denominators than pain? Disabil Rehabil. 2006;28(6):351-362.

3.   Kaufmann I, Eisner C, Richter P, et al. Lymphocyte subsets and the role of TH1/TH2 balance in stressed chronic pain patients. Neuroimmunomodulation. 2007;14(5):272-280.

4.   Omoigui S. The biochemical origin of pain: the origin of all pain is inflammation and the inflammatory response. Part 2 of 3 - inflammatory profile of pain syndromes. Med Hypotheses. 2007;69(6):1169-1178.

5.   Goebel A, Buhner S, Schedel R, Lochs H, Sprotte G. Altered intestinal permeability in patients with primary fibromyalgia and in patients with complex regional pain syndrome. Rheumatology (Oxford). 2008;47(8):1223-1227.

6.   Tajerian M, Sahbaie P, Sun Y, et al. Sex differences in a Murine Model of Complex Regional Pain Syndrome. Neurobiol Learn Mem. 2015;123:100-109.

7.   Golmirzaie G, Holland LS, Moser SE, Rastogi M, Hassett AL, Brummett CM. Time Since Inciting Event Is Associated With Higher Centralized Pain Symptoms in Patients Diagnosed With Complex Regional Pain Syndrome. Reg Anesth Pain Med. 2016;41(6):731-736.

8.   Goebel A. Immunoglobulin responsive chronic pain. J Clin Immunol. 2010;30 Suppl 1:S103-108.

9.   Moore RA, Wiffen PJ, Derry S, Toelle T, Rice AS. Gabapentin for chronic neuropathic pain and fibromyalgia in adults. Cochrane Database Syst Rev. 2014(4):CD007938.

10.   Littlejohn G. Neuroinflammation in fibromyalgia and CRPS: top-down or bottomup? Nat Rev Rheumatol. 2016;12(4):242.

11.   Vasquez A. Neuroinflammation in fibromyalgia and CRPS is multifactorial. Nat Rev Rheumatol. 2016;12(4):242.

16. Anticonvulsant Medication

The Complex Regional Pain Syndrome (CRPS) poses a dilemma for many clinicians due to its unknown etiology and largely unsuccessful treatment modalities.1 The Complex regional pain syndrome (CRPS) represents a state of constant and often disabling pain, affecting one region (usually hand) and often occurs after a trauma whose severity does not correlate with the level of pain.

Chronic pain, whether arising from viscera, bone, or any other tissue or structure, is, more often than commonly thought, the result of a mixture of pain mechanisms, and therefore there is no simple formula available to manage chronic complex pain states.

Aversion to addiction and diversion remains a potent force that shapes prescribing profiles. Patients often convey that different medications will impart distinct analgesic benefits.

Antidepressants, antiepileptic drugs and opioids are the most important drug classes for alleviating neuropathic pain whereas acute nociceptive pain may be positively influenced by non-steroidal anti-inflammatory drugs and steroids.2

CRPS is a chronic neuropathic pain syndrome. It causes nerve pain. The pharmacological approach to its management is mainly symptomatic, including analgesics, glucocorticoids, baclofen, bisphosphonates and prophylactic administration of vitamin C.3

The relative benefit of oral medications compared with the widely used treatments of intensive physical therapy, nerve blocks, sympathectomy, intraspinally administered drugs, and neuromodulatory therapies (eg, spinal cord stimulation) remains however uncertain.

Another pharmacologic treatment of CRPS pain is utilization of an anticonvulsant medication. Anticonvulsant drugs have been used for the management of neuropathic (damaged nerve) pain since the 1960s. These drugs interfere with the total number of pain signals that travel to patient's brain. This type of drug seems to be especially effective for managing sharp, shooting and lancinating pain.

It is possible that anticonvulsants stabilize excitable nerve membranes, limit neuronal hyper excitability, and inhibit trans synaptic neuronal impulses in the CNS. Gabapentin (Neurontin), a GABA-mimetic, seems currently (since 1994) to be the anticonvulsant used most widely in

North America in the treatment of RSD. Gabapentin might be considered in the treatment and prevention of CRPS I.4

An 84-year-old woman was treated because of aches and pain in her left hand and foot. Three months before her symptoms occurred, a pacemaker had been implanted for the treatment of a 2:1 atrioventricular block with bradycardia.

In an X-ray examination, prominently decreased bone density was noted in her left fingers and toes. She was diagnosed to have CRPS-I, which was considered to have been induced by the pacemaker implantation. After treatment with methylprednisolone and Neurotropin, her symptoms dramatically improved.5

The outcome of at least 50% pain intensity reduction is regarded as a useful outcome of treatment by patients, and the achievement of this degree of pain relief is associated with important beneficial effects on sleep interference, fatigue, and depression, as well as quality of life, function, and work.

In one study, about 35% of patients with neuropathic pain achieved this degree of pain relief with gabapentin, compared with 21% for placebo. Over half of those treated with gabapentin will not have worthwhile pain relief.

Results might vary between different neuropathic pain conditions, and the amount of evidence for gabapentin in neuropathic pain conditions except postherpetic neuralgia and painful diabetic neuropathy, and in fibromyalgia, is very limited.6

Lyrica (pregabilin is however becoming very popular). Detailed psychological and psychiatric evaluation is however, recommended in individuals with CRPS because psychiatric support and improvement of associated psychosocial concerns in addition to pregabalin seems to facilitate treatments in some patients.7

Gabapentin binds in the outer layer of the neocortex (outer layer of patientr brain) of patientr brain and the hippocampus. At one time it was thought that gabapentin's anticonvulsant effects may be mediated by increasing the promoted release of GABA.

When GABA is released within a patient's spinal cord, pain signals going toward patient's brain are decreased. It has both analgesic and antianxiety effects. In the formalin test with mice, gabapentin selectively blocks nociception associated with inflammation, suggesting a central site of action, perhaps by blocking the sensitization of dorsal horn neurons that occurs during inflammation.

Neuropathic pain is a prominent feature of CRPS I, and is often refractory to treatment. Since gabapentin is an anticonvulsant with a proven analgesic effect in various neuropathic pain syndromes, we sought to study the efficacy of the anticonvulsant gabapentin as treatment for pain in patients with CRPS I.8

It is now known that gabapentin and pregabilin act on voltage sensitive alpha 2 delta receptors to decrease pain. Gabapentin appears to differ from the other anticonvulsants in its mechanism of action. Gabapentin is not metabolized by the liver and can therefore safely be given with other anticonvulsants.

It is well tolerated and has few adverse effects (mostly drowsiness, fatigue and dizziness). These side effects these tend to decrease with continued usage. Other anticonvulsants used for RSD are phenytoin (Dilantin), carbamezapine (Tegretol) and valproic acid (Depakot).

The clinical impression of these drugs is that they are useful for chronic neuropathic (nerve damage) pain, especially when the pain is lancinating or burning. Remember that RSD pain is burning.

Pain is usually the natural consequence of tissue injury resulting in approximately forty million medical appointments per year. In general, following most injuries, as the healing process commences, the pain and tenderness associated with the patient's injury will resolve.

Unfortunately, some individuals experience pain without an obvious injury or suffer pain that persists for months or years after their initial injury. This pain condition is neuropathic in nature and accounts for a large number of patients presenting to pain clinics with chronic pain.

Following any tissue injury (nerve, muscle, bone, etc.) a patient's nervous system sounds an alarm to a patient's brain to make patient aware that patient have been injured. Rather than a patient's nervous system functioning properly to sound an alarm regarding tissue injury, in neuropathic pain, the peripheral or central nervous systems are malfunctioning and become the cause of the pain.

In other words, after a nerve has healed it may still transmit pain signals. An example is a car alarm. The alarm will sound if patient's vehicle is being tampered with. This is normal. Now imagine that patient's alarm sounds when no one is near patient's car. Somehow there is a short circuit. The same occurs within a patient's nervous system.

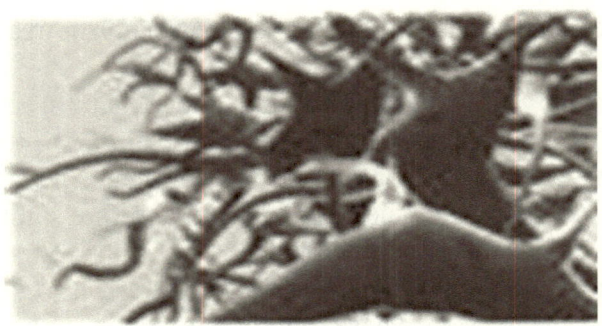

Figure 1. Neurons are intertwined in patients' nervous systems.

Pain signals are transmitted between gaps between patients' axons and dendrites. Anticonvulsant medications can interrupt pain signals by blocking transmission of these pain signals.

Neuropathic pain is a complex, pain state that usually is accompanied by nerve injury. With neuropathic pain the nerve fibers themselves may be damaged, dysfunctional or injured. These damaged nerve fibers send incorrect signals to other pain centers.

The impact of nerve injury includes a change in nerve function both at the site of injury and areas around the injury. Symptoms may include: shooting and burning pain and tingling and numbness. In order to understand the effects of anti-seizure drugs, patient need to be aware that these drugs can block the ion (calcium and sodium) channels that are present throughout patient's nervous system.

Ion channels are pore-forming proteins that help to establish and control a small electrical gradient between the inside and outside of nerve cells. When ions flow in and out of a neuron, this electrical gradient ceases and pain signals subsequently cease to be transmitted to a patient's brain. Calcium and sodium channel anticonvulsant drugs block the pores or channels. When these drugs drop off of these channels, patient will experience pain again.

Antiseizure drugs are frequently used in pain management. It is not known exactly how anticonvulsants work to reduce pain. They may block the flow of pain signals from patient's brain and spinal cord. Some anticonvulsant drugs may work better than others for certain conditions.

Neuropathic pain is a form of chronic pain caused by an injury to or a disease of patient's peripheral or central nervous system. It does not respond well to traditional pain therapies like opioids or nonsteroidal anti-inflammatory drugs.

In neuropathic pain, it has shown that a number of pathophysiological and biochemical changes take place in patientr nervous system as a result of an insult to a nerve. This property of the nervous system to adapt to external stimuli plays a crucial role in the onset and maintenance of pain symptoms.

Carbamazepine (Tegretol), the first anticonvulsant studied in clinical trials, probably alleviates pain by decreasing conductance in sodium channels and inhibits ectopic nerve discharges. Results from clinical trials have been positive in the treatment of trigeminal neuralgia, painful diabetic neuropathy and post herpetic neuralgia with this medication.

Gabapentin (Neurontin) and pregabilin (Lyrica) have the most clearly demonstrated analgesic effects for the treatment of neuropathic pain, specifically for the treatment of painful diabetic neuropathy and postherpetic neuralgia. Based on the positive results of these studies and its favorable adverse effect profile, gabapentin or pregabilin should be considered the first choice of therapy for neuropathic pain.

Evidence for the efficacy of phenytoin as an antinociceptive agent is, at best, weak to modest. Lamotrigine on the other hand has good potential to modulate and control neuropathic pain.

Detailed psycological and psychiatric evaluation is recommended in individuals with CRPS because psychiatric support and improvement of associated psychosocial concerns in addition to pregabalin seems to facilitate treatments in some patients.

There is a potential for phenobarbital, clonazepam, valproic acid, topiramate, pregabalin and tiagabine to have antihyperalgesic and antinociceptive activities based on result in animal models of neuropathic pain, but the efficacy of these drugs in the treatment of human neuropathic pain has not yet been fully determined in clinical trials.

The role of anticonvulsant drugs in the treatment of neuropathic pain is evolving and has been clearly demonstrated with gabapentin and carbamazepine. Further advances in our understanding of the mechanisms underlying neuropathic pain syndromes and well-designed clinical trials should further the opportunities to establish the role of anticonvulsants in the treatment of neuropathic pain.

If patient have had a direct injury to one of patientr nerves, patient may benefit from an anticonvulsant drug. The clinical impression is that these drugs are useful for the treatment of chronic neuropathic pain, especially when the pain is lancinating or burning.

There are seven drugs that are useful in neuropathic (nerve injury) pain; pregabilin (Lyrica),gabapentin (Neurontin), carbamazipine (Tegretol (valproic acid (Depakote), clonazepam (Klonopin), phenytoin (Dilantin) ,zonisamide (Zonegran)) and lamotrigine (Lamictal).

Neurontin is an effective drug for the treatment of neuropathic pain but Lyrica is becoming widely used as previously mentioned in the management of many pain syndromes. It has fewer side effects than other anticonvulsant drugs. These drugs can be useful for the treatment of shingles, diabetic neuropathy and fibromyalgia.

Reflex Sympathetic Dystrophy, diabetic neuropathy migraine headaches, sciatica, radiculitis, and pain associated with multiple sclerosis may respond to either of these drugs.

If patient experience sharp shooting pain, these drugs may be helpful in decreasing the pain. If a patient experiences side effects from either drug, other anticonvulsant medications are available. Oxcarbazepine (Trileptal), lamotrigine (Lamictal), topiramate (Topamax), and zonisamide (Zonegran) may also be effective in reducing pain caused by diabetic neuropathy and postherpetic neuralgia.

Lyrica is FDA approved for the treatment of fibromyalgia. Anticonvulsant drugs are effective in the treatment of chronic neuropathic pain but were not initially thought to be useful in the management of postoperative pain. However, similar to any nerve injury, surgical tissue injury is known to produce neuroplastic changes leading to spinal sensitization and the expression of nerve induced pain.

The pharmacological effects of anticonvulsant drugs, which may be important in the modulation of these postoperative neural changes, include suppression of sodium channel, calcium channel and glutamate receptor activity at peripheral, spinal and supraspinal sites.

Gabapentin and pregabalin reduce pain and opioid consumption after surgery.9Gabapentin and pregabalin are anticonvulsant agents that may decrease perioperative central sensitization and early post-surgical neuropathic pain. Gabapentin and pregabalin effectively relieved neuropathic pain and prevented the conversion of acute pain to chronic pain in one study.10

A doctor may obtain a complete blood count and liver tests before prescribing some of these anticonvulsant drugs (e.g. Tegretol). A patient's doctor will give patient a 4 to 6 week trial of the drug. It may take the medication this length of time to exert its effects. Therefore, if patient have no pain relief after several days patient should not stop the drug that was prescribed to patient.

Because it takes patient's body time to adjust to one of these medications, patientr doctor must adhere to the phrase "begin low and proceed slow" which means that patient should be prescribed a low dose and this dose may be increased gradually over days to weeks.

Anticonvulsant drugs are effective in the treatment of chronic pain but may also be useful for pain management following surgery. Be aware that CRPS complicating antiepileptic drug (AED) therapy is not well acknowledged in the neurologic literature.

CRPS may occur while taking antiepileptic drug therapy.11 The mechanisms for this observation are not known. Similar to any nerve injury, surgical tissue injury is known to produce tissue changes leading to spinal cord sensitization which can cause patient to have pain after surgery. Gabapentin and pregabilin have been shown to decrease post-surgery pain.12

Pregabilin is effective for the treatment of diabetic neuropathy and shingles. Pregabilin binds to calcium channels of nerves, which results in a reduction of patientr pain.

Some health insurance plans do not pay for Lyrica because it is relatively expensive. However, it has been shown to be more cost effective than gabapentin. In other words, it is more effective than gabapentin for RSD pain control. However, this drug can cause dizziness, blurred vision, drowsiness, weight gain and swelling of the patient's legs. This medication may decrease the platelet count as well.

Some anticonvulsant medicines can cause a decrease in platelets which can interfere with a patient's ability to form a blood clot. If the platelets are too low, a patient will bruise easily. Gabapentin is effective for the management of oral phantom pain following a tooth extraction. Gabapentin binds to nerve calcium channels. Gabapentin has a mild effect on pain in CRPS. It can significantly reduce a sensory deficit in the affected limb.

A subpopulation of CRPS patients may therefore, benefit from gabapentin. Gabapentin is useful for the management of CRPS pain as well as facial RSD. The drug is useful in most nerve injury pain disorders.

An average dose is 300 mg taken three times a day. Gabapentin produced dose-related inhibition of mechanical hyperalgesia over a 3-week period, but this effect was blocked by concomitant caffeine.13

Gabapentin might be considered in the treatment and prevention of CRPS I. In an animal study, gabapentin produced dose-related inhibition of mechanical hyperalgesia over a 3-week period, and this effect was blocked by concomitant caffeine.13

A rare side effect has however, also been reported with gabapentin use. A 35-year-old woman suffered a traumatic injury to her right sciatic nerve. She developed a complex regional pain syndrome and was treated with gabapentin for pain control.

Three months after the initiation of gabapentin therapy (1800 mg/day), the patient reported complete cessation of her menses. The patient was weaned off the gabapentin over 6 days with return of her menses 2 weeks later. It was conclude that gabapentin has the potential to cause amenorrhea with return of menses occurring after discontinuation of the drug.14

Tegretol is a drug that is chemically related to amitriptyline. It prevents repetitive discharges of patient's nerves. This medication works on sodium channels in patient's painful nerves. Inhibition of these sodium channels can decrease patient's pain sensations. An average dose is 200 mg every day. Side effects include dizziness, drowsiness, blurred vision and nausea. This medication can cause various forms of anemia and liver damage. As a result, patient's doctor will obtain a blood count and liver tests.

Tegretol is rarely used today for RSD pain because of the side effects associated with this drug. Tegretol has been shown to be effective for the treatment of trigeminal neuralgia (facial pain). Some physicians use this drug for RSD pain.

Depakote is given in a dose of 250 mg twice a day. This medication can cause patient to have liver failure. A patient's doctor will monitor patient's liver function closely. This medicine is used when the other anti convulsant medications have been tried but failed to provide pain relief. Side effects of this drug include nausea, vomiting loss of appetite and diarrhea. Tremors and sedation may also be associated with this medication.

Klonipin is useful also for the treatment of lancinating pain associated with the phantom limb syndrome. The drug may also be useful for migraine headache prophylaxis and for the treatment of trigeminal neural-gia (facial pain) as well as RSD.

The usual dose is 1 mg per day. Side effects include mood dis-turbances and delirium. Lethargy and sedation may also be seen. This drug has a significant sedative effect. It should be initially only taken at bedtime. It is prescribed by some neurologists for RSD pain.

Dilantin alters sodium, calcium and potassium channels in patientr nerves. An average dose is 300 mg three times a day. The number of side effects associated with this drug is significant. Liver damage can occur and the drug can decrease a patient's folic acid level in the bloodstream. A decrease in the folic acid blood level may actually cause nerves in the arms and legs to have burning sensations.

Zonegran 's mechanisms of action suggest that it could be effective in controlling neuropathic pain symptoms. It can be effective in the management of CRPS pain. It also decreases sodium channel activity on the sodium channels of some nerves.

Side effects can include a decrease in blood sodium levels, kidney stones, visual difficulties and secondary angle-closure glaucoma. A typical dose of this medication is 300 mg per day. Side effects related to this drug include agitation, anxiety, ataxia, confusion, depression, difficul-ty concentrating, headache, difficulty sleeping, memory problems, stom-ach pain as well as liver pathology. This medication may also cause weight loss. A dry mouth and flu like syndrome may also be associated with this drug.

Lamictal also exerts its effects on sodium channels. This drug de-creases the release of some pain-causing chemical from the ends of patientr nerves. The reason why patient develop chronic pain after having acute nerve injury pain remains unclear. However, it is believed that Lamictal in addition to some of the other drugs mentioned may prevent this transformation.

A typical dose will be 200 mg twice a day after starting at a low dose and going to 200 mg slowly. Adverse effects related to this drug include headaches, dizziness, blurred vision and nausea and vomiting. This medication may be of benefit for the treatment of pain associated with Reflex Sympathetic Dystrophy.

Lamictal also can be effective for many kinds of neuropathic pain including that which comes from CRPS, AIDS and central brain pain as a result of a stroke. Lamictal is a seizure medicine that acts as a sodium channel blocker as previously mentioned but may exhibit some calcium channel blockade as well.

In one study with patients who had severe refractory neuropathic pain who had failed at least two other treatments, there was an average 70% decrease in pain in 14 of 21 patients. This medication is not commonly prescribed for the treatment of CRPS because there other drugs that have fewer side effects like gabapentin which are effective for CRPS pain management.

Reflex sympathetic dystrophy (RSD) complicating barbiturates therapy is not well acknowledged in the neurologic literature in spite of the fact that barbiturates are present in 17% of the cases of RSD.15 The association of RSD and barbiturates affects predominantly upper limbs and is often accompanied by other fibrosing musculoskeletal disorders.

Treatment recommendations based on the literature findings were formulated and formally approved by all Dutch professional associations involved in CRPS-I treatment. For pain treatment, the WHO analgesic ladder is advised with the exception of strong opioids. For neuropathic pain, anticonvulsants and tricyclic antidepressants may be considered. For inflammatory symptoms, free-radical scavengers (dimethylsulphoxide or acetylcysteine) are advised.

To promote peripheral blood flow, vasodilatory medication may be considered. Percutaneous sympathetic blockades may be used to increase blood flow in case vasodilatory medication has insufficient effect. To decrease functional limitations, standardized physiotherapy and occupational therapy are advised.

To prevent the occurrence of CRPS-I after wrist fractures, vitamin C is recommended. Adequate perioperative analgesia, limitation of operating time, limited use of tourniquet, and use of regional anesthetic techniques are recommended for secondary prevention of CRPS-I.16

Bisphosphonates appear to be the treatment of choice in early stages of CRPS 1.17 The effects of calcitonin surpass that of bisphosphonates and other substances as a short-term medication in more chronic stages of the illness. While most medications showed some efficacy on short-term follow-up, only bisphosphonates, NMDA analogs, and vasodilators showed better long-term pain reduction than placebo.

For pain treatment, the WHO analgesic ladder is advised with the exception of strong opioids. For neuropathic pain, anticonvulsants and tricyclic antidepressants may be considered. For inflammatory symptoms, free-radical scavengers (dimethylsulphoxide or acetylcysteine) are advised.

Ketamine hydrochloride, an agent used for general anesthesia, has local anesthetic effects and N-methyl-D-aspartate receptor antagonist action.18 Palmitoylethanolamide and topical ketamine could be a combination therapy option for treating CRPS patients.19

A sub-anesthetic low-dose ketamine has shown promise in advanced CRPS. The efficacy of ketamine in anesthetic was studied dosage in chronic, refractory CRPS patients that had failed available standard therapies. The patients received 1-5 ketamine courses for 10 days.

The effect of gradual pain reduction was observed beginning on the 4th-5th day of treatment, associated with a decrease in the intensity of the allodynia. No improvement in function of the affected hands was noted in any patient. This beneficial analgesic effect was confined to 1.5-2.5 months after treatment and then pain relapsed to the baseline level.20 The results of this study show a short-term analgesic effect for this therapy.

Another study showed promise for the use of topical ketamine as opposed to parenteral and oral forms which often result in undesirable side effects.21 Systemic effects of the ketamine are unlikely to account for this as the plasma levels were below detectable limits. Patients in the palliative care and hospice setting, especially the one at the end of their lives, may benefit from oral ketamine even if an intravenous trial is not feasible.22

Ketamine is efficacious in the chronic, but not acute, stage of CRPS, suggesting that the centrally acting drug is relatively ineffective in early CRPS when peripheral mechanisms are more critical for supporting nociceptive sensitization.23

In summary, chronic pain, whether arising from nerve or any other tissue or structure, is, more often than commonly thought, the result of a mixture of pain mechanisms, and therefore there is no simple formula available to manage chronic complex pain states. Patients often convey that different medications will impart distinct analgesic benefits.

The presence of disabling non-painful complaints and the need to manage symptoms such as insomnia, depression, anxiety, and fatigue that all cause worsening of the patient's quality of life and function need to be addressed by physicians as well. The major rationale for introducing anti convulsion adjuvants and other medications is to better balance the efficacy and adverse effects of single drugs.

References

1.   Lee SK, Yang DS, Lee JW, Choy WS. Four treatment strategies for complex regional pain syndrome type 1. Orthopedics. 2012;35(6):e834-842.

2.   Ruegg S. [Drug treatment of CRPS]. Handchir Mikrochir Plast Chir. 2010;42(1):19-29.

3.   Blazekovic I, Bilic E, Zagar M, Anic B. [Complex Regional Pain Syndrome]. Lijec Vjesn. 2015;137(9-10):297-306.

4.   Akkus S, Yorgancigil H, Yener M. A case of recurrent and migratory complex regional pain syndrome type I: Prevention by gabapentin. Rheumatol Int. 2006;26(9):852-854.

5.   Okada M, Suzuki K, Hidaka T, et al. Complex regional pain syndrome type I induced by pacemaker implantation, with a good response to steroids and neurotropin. Intern Med. 2002;41(6):498-501.

6.   Moore RA, Wiffen PJ, Derry S, Toelle T, Rice AS. Gabapentin for chronic neuropathic pain and fibromyalgia in adults. Cochrane Database Syst Rev. 2014(4):CD007938.

7.   Saltik S, Sozen HG, Basgul S, Karatoprak EY, Icagasioglu A. Pregabalin Treatment of a Patient With Complex Regional Pain Syndrome. Pediatr Neurol. 2016;54:88-90.

8.   van de Vusse AC, Stomp-van den Berg SG, Kessels AH, Weber WE. Randomised controlled trial of gabapentin in Complex Regional Pain Syndrome type 1 [ISRCTN84121379]. BMC Neurol. 2004;4:13.

9.   Dauri M, Faria S, Gatti A, Celidonio L, Carpenedo R, Sabato AF. Gabapentin and pregabalin for the acute post-operative pain management. A systematic-narrative review of the recent clinical evidences. Curr Drug Targets. 2009;10(8):716-733.

10.   Dolgun H, Turkoglu E, Kertmen H, et al. Gabapentin versus pregabalin in relieving early post-surgical neuropathic pain in patients after lumbar disc herniation surgery: a prospective clinical trial. Neurol Res. 2014;36(12):1080-1085.

11.   Falasca GF, Toly TM, Reginato AJ, Schraeder PL, O'Connor CR. Reflex sympathetic dystrophy associated with antiepileptic drugs. Epilepsia. 1994;35(2):394-399.

12.   Dahl JB, Nielsen RV, Wetterslev J, et al. Post-operative analgesic effects of paracetamol, NSAIDs, glucocorticoids, gabapen-

tinoids and their combinations: a topical review. Acta Anaesthesiol Scand. 2014;58(10):1165-1181.

13.   Martins DF, Prado MR, Daruge-Neto E, et al. Caffeine prevents antihyperalgesic effect of gabapentin in an animal model of CRPS-I: evidence for the involvement of spinal adenosine A1 receptor. J Peripher Nerv Syst. 2015;20(4):403-409.

14.   Berger JJ. Amenorrhea in a patient after treatment with gabapentin for complex regional pain syndrome type II. Clin J Pain. 2004;20(3):192-194.

15.   Olazaran J, Farcha I. [Reflex sympathetic dystrophy due to phenobarbital: a frequent and treatable condition]. Neurologia. 1997;12(8):365-367.

16.   Perez RS, Zollinger PE, Dijkstra PU, et al. Evidence based guidelines for complex regional pain syndrome type 1. BMC Neurol. 2010;10:20.

17.   Wertli MM, Kessels AG, Perez RS, Bachmann LM, Brunner F. Rational pain management in complex regional pain syndrome 1 (CRPS 1)--a network meta-analysis. Pain Med. 2014;15(9):1575-1589.

18.   Ushida T, Tani T, Kanbara T, Zinchuk VS, Kawasaki M, Yamamoto H. Analgesic effects of ketamine ointment in patients with complex regional pain syndrome type 1. Reg Anesth Pain Med. 2002;27(5):524-528.

19.   Keppel Hesselink JM, Kopsky DJ. Treatment of chronic regional pain syndrome type 1 with palmitoylethanolamide and topical ketamine cream: modulation of nonneuronal cells. J Pain Res. 2013;6:239-245.

20.   Puchalski P, Zyluk A. Results of the Treatment of Chronic, Refractory CRPS with Ketamine Infusions: a Preliminary Report. Handchir Mikrochir Plast Chir. 2016;48(3):143-147.

21.   Finch PM, Knudsen L, Drummond PD. Reduction of allodynia in patients with complex regional pain syndrome: A double-blind placebo-controlled trial of topical ketamine. Pain. 2009;146(1-2):18-25.

22.   Soto E, Stewart DR, Mannes AJ, et al. Oral ketamine in the palliative care setting: a review of the literature and case report of a patient with neurofibromatosis type 1 and glomus tumor-associated complex regional pain syndrome. Am J Hosp Palliat Care. 2012;29(4):308-317.

23.   Tajerian M, Leu D, Yang P, Huang TT, Kingery WS, Clark JD. Differential Efficacy of Ketamine in the Acute versus Chronic Stages

of Complex Regional Pain Syndrome in Mice. Anesthesiology. 2015;123(6):1435-1447.

17. Muscle Relaxants

Complex Regional Pain Syndrome (CRPS) is a multifactorial and disabling disorder with complex etiology and pathogenesis. Goals of therapy in CRPS should be pain relief, functional restoration, and psychological stabilization, but early interventions are needed in order to achieve these objectives.

Several drugs have been used to reduce pain and to improve functional status in CRPS, despite the lack of scientific evidence supporting their use in this scenario. They include anti-inflammatory drugs, analgesics, anesthetics, anticonvulsants, antidepressants, oral muscle relaxants, corticosteroids, calcitonin, bisphosphonates, calcium channel blockers and topical agents.[1]

Numerous oral drugs, including muscle relaxants, benzodiazepines, antidepressants, anticonvulsants, and opioids, have been reported on anecdotally. NSAIDs showed no value in treating CRPS. Glucocorticoids are the only anti-inflammatory drugs for which there is direct clinical trial evidence in early stage of CRPS.

Opioids are a reasonable second or third-line treatment option, but tolerance and long term toxicity are unresolved issues. The use of anticonvulsants and tricyclic antidepressants has not been well investigated for pain management in CRPS.[2]

Muscle cramps (spasms and dystonia) associated with CRPS can be treated with clonazepam and baclofen as well as with other muscle relaxants. Antispasmodics, also called muscle relaxants, are helpful in treating the symptoms of CRPS.

Many patients with CRPS experience muscle spasms which aggravate the pain. Medications such as benzodiazepine, clonazepam and tizanidine are prescribed to alleviate these spasms and aid in pain control.

Muscle relaxants are effective for short-term symptomatic relief in patients with acute and chronic low back pain as well as those patients suffering from CRPS. Remember, that myofascial pain is not uncommon. Baclofen a muscle relaxant may help with muscle spasms associated with CRPS in some cases.

However, the incidence of drowsiness, dizziness and other side effects is high. Muscle relaxants must be used with caution. Muscle relaxants are a useful adjunct in the treatment of patients with chronic and persistent pain. There are a number of categories in muscle relaxants, but one may broadly divide them into centrally acting muscle relaxants and peripherally acting muscle relaxants.

Muscle relaxants are effective for short-term symptomatic relief in patients with acute and chronic low back pain as well as with some CRPS pain. However, the incidence of drowsiness, dizziness and other side effects is high. Muscle relaxants must be used with caution.

Muscle relaxants are a useful adjunct in the treatment of patients with chronic and persistent pain. There are a number of categories in muscle relaxants, but one may broadly divide them into (1) centrally acting muscle relaxants and (2) peripherally acting muscle relaxants.

If a patient's muscles are tense, a patient can have decreased oxygen in a patient's muscle tissue that can cause a patient to experience pain. Muscle relaxants are drugs that decrease tension in a patient r muscles. These drugs can be useful in pain management.

Muscle relaxants are not really a single class of drugs, but are a group of different drugs and each of these drugs can have an overall sedative effect on a patient's body. These drugs other than dantrolene do not act directly on a patient's muscles, but they act in a patient's brain and are more of a total body relaxant.

Skeletal muscle relaxants are drugs that relax striated muscles (those that control a patient's skeleton). Skeletal muscle relaxants may be used for relief of spasticity in neuromuscular diseases, such as multiple sclerosis, as well as for spinal cord injury and stroke. They may also be used for pain relief in minor strain injuries and control of the muscle symptoms of tetanus.

The muscle relaxants may be divided into only two groups, centrally acting and peripherally acting. The centrally acting group, which appears to act on the central nervous system, while only dantrolene has a direct action at the level of the nerve-muscle connection.

Strains, sprains, and other muscle and joint injuries that may occur in CRPS patients can result in pain, stiffness, and muscle spasms. Muscle relaxants do not heal the injuries, but they do relax muscles and help ease discomfort. Muscle relaxants exert their effects by acting on the central nervous system. In the United States, they are available only with a physician's prescription. Several examples include; carisoprodol (Soma), cyclobenzaprine (Flexeril), and methocarbamol (Robaxin).

Most drugs come only in pill form. However, methocarbamol (Robaxin) is available in both tablet and injectable forms. Muscle relaxants are usually prescribed along with rest, exercise, physical therapy, or other treatments.

One muscle relaxant, Zanaflex (tizanidine) does provide pain relief by decreasing Substance P which is one of the body's pain signal transmitters. Substance P has been implicated in CRPS pain. This medication is also helpful in decreasing pain associated with fibromyalgia.

Although the muscle relaxant drugs may provide a patient with pain relief, they should never be considered a substitute for other forms of treatment like physical therapy. Because muscle relaxants exert their effects on a patient's central nervous system, they may potentate the effects of alcohol and other drugs.

They may also add to the effects of anesthetics, including those used for dental procedures. For this reason, anyone taking these medications should not drive; operate machinery, or any activity that might be dangerous.

People with certain medical conditions or who are taking certain other medicines can have problems if they take muscle relaxants. Diabetics should be aware that metaxalone (Skelaxin) may cause false test results on one type of test that detects sugar in a patient's urine. Patients with epilepsy should be cautioned that taking the muscle relaxant methocarbamol might increase the likelihood of seizures.

Common side effects of muscle relaxants are visual changes, such as double vision or blurred vision; dizziness; lightheadedness; drowsiness; and dry mouth. These problems usually go away as a patient r body adjusts to the drug and do not require medical treatment.

Other side effects are stomach cramps, nausea and vomiting, constipation, diarrhea, hiccups, clumsiness or unsteadiness, confusion, nervousness, restlessness, irritability, flushed or red face, headache, heartburn, weakness, trembling, and sleep problems.

More serious side effects are not common, but may occur. Anyone who experiences breathing problems, facial swelling, fainting, unusually fast or unusually slow heartbeat, fever, tightness in the chest, rash, itching, hives, burning, stinging, red, or bloodshot eyes, or unusual thoughts or dreams after taking muscle relaxants should seek medical help promptly.

Parafon Forte can cause liver pathology (injury) in some individuals. The reaction is rare, but a patient can develop the following symptoms: fever, rash, loss of appetite, nausea, vomiting, fatigue, pain in the upper right part of the abdomen, dark urine, or yellow skin or eyes.

Muscle relaxants may interact with some other medicines. The effects of a drug may either be lessened or potentiated.

When this occurs, the effects of one or both of the drugs may change or the risk of side effects may be greater with either drug. Anyone taking muscle relaxants should let their physician know all other medicines, including over-the-counter or nonprescription medicines that he or she is taking.

Some of the muscle relaxant drugs are antispasticity medications used to treat muscle spasms and are usually associated with disorders of a patient r nervous system. A muscle spasm is an involuntary increase in a patient's muscle tone that that occurs when a patient stretch a patient's muscle. The cause of the spasm is not known but may be related to a decrease in a patient's body's nervous system's ability to be able to control muscle contractions.

Drugs that decrease spasms are called antispasmodic drugs and include drugs like Valium (benzodiazepine), baclofen (Lioresal), Zanaflex (tizanidine) or dantrolene. Each of these drugs can exert their effects for a long time. Shorter acting medications will be described below.

Botulism toxin administered into a patient r muscle can decrease pain from muscle spasms or muscle dysfunction. These toxins (7 total A-G) prevent release of a chemical called acetylcholine from the nerve ending that goes to a patient r muscle. This action can stop muscle spasms.

Botulism toxins A and B are commonly used in a medical practice. These toxins can be used to manage pain associated with whiplash disorders, some headaches, torticollis and low back pain.

Botulism toxin can relieve a patient's pain for 3 months. It can take two weeks for the toxin to exert its effects. Botulism toxin injections can cause a patient to experience mild side effects. These effects may be a fever or mild joint pain.

Benzodiazepines are used for anxiety and seizure treatment, but Valium and Klonopin can both be used for muscle relaxation. Klonopin is used for the treatment of CRPS. These drugs exert their effects by acting in a patient's spinal cord. These drugs are useful if a patient has a history of a spinal cord injury.

These drugs can last for a long time once they have been introduced into a patient's body. Valium should not be used long term. A patient should know Valium is a depressant and can worsen depression associated with chronic pain.

Carisoprodol (Soma) has sedative properties as well as muscle relaxant properties. This drug should be used for muscle pain. It will not however, relieve muscle spasms. This drug furthermore, may decrease a patient's ability to fall asleep. Methocarbamol (Robaxin) is a sedative and decreases muscle pain by its sedative action. It has no muscle relaxant effects.

Dantrolene has a possibility to cause liver damage. The incidence of hepatitis is related to the amount of drug that a patient has taken, but may occur even with a short period of small doses.

Hepatitis has been most frequently observed between the third and twelfth months of therapy. The risk of liver injury appears to be greater in women, in patients over 35 years of age and in patients taking other medications in addition to dantrolene.

Drugs that inhibit the metabolism of Valium in a patient's liver may increase the activity of the diazepam (Valium). These drugs include: cimetidine, oral contraceptives, disulfiram, fluoxetine, isoniazid, ketoconazole, metoprolol, propoxyphene, propranolol, and valproic acid.

In females dantrolene may have an interaction with estrogens. The rate of liver damage in women over the age of 35 who were taking estrogens is higher than in other groups.

Antispasmodics, also called muscle relaxants, are helpful in treating the symptoms of CRPS. Many patients with CRPS experience muscle spasms which aggravate the pain.

Medications such as benzodiazepine, clonazepam and Zanaflex are prescribed to alleviate these spasms and aid in pain control. Muscle relaxants are effective for short-term symptomatic relief in patients with acute and chronic low back pain as well as those patients suffering from CRPS.

Skeletal muscle relaxants are drugs that relax striated muscles (those that control a patient's skeleton). Skeletal muscle relaxants may be used for relief of spasticity in neuromuscular diseases, such as multiple sclerosis, as well as for spinal cord injury and stroke. They may also be used for pain relief in minor strain injuries and control of the muscle symptoms of tetanus.

The muscle relaxants may be divided into only two groups, centrally acting and peripherally acting. The centrally acting group, which appears to act on the central nervous system, while only dantrolene has a direct action at the level of the nerve-muscle connection.

Strains, sprains, and other muscle and joint injuries that may occur in CRPS patients can result in pain, stiffness, and muscle spasms. Muscle relaxants do not heal the injuries, but they do relax muscles and help ease discomfort.

Muscle relaxants exert their effects by acting on the central nervous system. In the United States, they are available only with a physician's prescription. Several examples include; carisoprodol (Soma), cyclobenzaprine (Flexeril), and methocarbamol (Robaxin).

One muscle relaxant, Zanaflex (tizanidine) does provide pain relief by decreasing Substance P which is one of a patient r body's pain signal transmitters. Substance P has been implicated in CRPS pain. This medication is also helpful in decreasing pain associated with fibromyalgia.

Although the muscle relaxant drugs may provide a patient with pain relief, they should never be considered a substitute for other forms of treatment like physical therapy.

Because muscle relaxants exert their effects on a patient's central nervous system, they may potentate the effects of alcohol and other drugs. They may also add to the effects of anesthetics, including those used for dental procedures. For this reason, anyone who takes these drugs should not drive; operate machinery, or any activity that might be dangerous.

People with certain medical conditions or who are taking certain other medicines can have problems if they take muscle relaxants. Diabetics should be aware that metaxalone (Skelaxin) may cause false test results on one type of test that detects sugar in a patient's urine. Patients with epilepsy should be cautioned that taking the muscle relaxant methocarbamol might increase the likelihood of seizures.

Anyone who experiences breathing problems, facial swelling, fainting, unusually fast or unusually slow heartbeat, fever, tightness in the chest, rash, itching, hives, burning, stinging, red, or bloodshot eyes, or unusual thoughts or dreams after taking muscle relaxants should seek medical help promptly.

Parafon Forte can cause liver pathology (injury) in some individuals. The reaction is rare, but a patient can develop the following symptoms: fever, rash, loss of appetite, nausea, vomiting, fatigue, pain in the upper right part of the abdomen, dark urine, or yellow skin or eyes.

Muscle relaxants may interact with some other medicines. The effects of a drug may either be lessened or potentiated. When this occurs, the effects of one or both of the drugs may change or the risk of side effects may be greater with either drug.

Anyone taking muscle relaxants should let their physician know all other medicines, including over-the-counter or nonprescription medicines that he or she is taking. Some patients for example, receive muscle relaxants from an emergency department. They may not tell their treating physician.

A muscle spasm is an involuntary increase in a patient's muscle tone that that occurs when a patient stretches a muscle. The cause of the spasm is not known but may be related to a decrease in a patient's body's nervous system's ability to be able to control muscle contractions.

Drugs that decrease spasms are called antispasmodic drugs and include drugs like Valium (benzodiazepine), baclofen (Lioresal), Zanaflex (tizanidine) or dantrolene. Each of these drugs can exert their effects for a long time. Shorter acting medications will be described below.

Drugs that inhibit the metabolism of Valium in a patient's liver may increase the activity of the diazepam (Valium). These drugs include: cimetidine, oral contraceptives, disulfiram, fluoxetine, isoniazid, ketoconazole, metoprolol, propoxyphene, propranolol, and valproic acid.

In females dantrolene may have an interaction with estrogens. The rate of liver damage in women over the age of 35 who were taking estrogens is higher than in other groups.

Focal dystonia, often affecting part of a limb, is a manifestation of the complex regional pain syndrome. This can be difficult to diagnose and treat. Furthermore, there may be significant latency between the onset of dystonia after the diagnosis of CRPS. Intrathecal baclofen therapy can be effective in the management of focal dystonia after rigorous preoperative testing and counseling of adolescents with CRPS.3

Given its therapeutic utility in the control of neuromuscular transmission, Botulism toxin has been utilized to treat diseases related to muscular hyperactivity, such as dystonia and spasticity.4

Furthermore, it has been recognized that Botulism toxin is also useful in controlling the neurotransmitter release of sensory and autonomic nerve terminals as well.5   Muscle relaxants, benzodiazepines, antidepressants, anticonvulsants, and opioids, have been reported anecdotally for CRPS treatment.

Numerous oral drugs, including muscle relaxants, benzodiaze-pines, antidepressants, anticonvulsants, and opioids, have been reported on anecdotally. Gabapentin, tricyclic antidepressants, and opioids have been proven effective for chronic pain in disorders other than CRPS. Each has shown a broad enough spectrum of analgesic activity to be cautiously recommended for treatment of CRPS until adequate randomized con-trolled trials settle the issue.

The relative benefit of oral medications compared with the widely used treatments of intensive physical therapy, nerve blocks, sympathec-tomy, intraspinally administered drugs, and neuromodulatory therapies (eg, spinal cord stimulation) remains uncertain. In summary, treatment of CRPS has received insufficient study and remains largely empirical.

Permanent delivery of baclofen by implantation of an intrathecal drug delivery pump has been reported however, to result in resolution of the dystonia associated with CRPS.

With this drug delivery system a patient is was able to receive bo-lus doses of intrathecal baclofen.3

In another study, investigators evaluated the differential effects of central gamma-aminobutyric acid receptor stimulation on the different pain qualities in CRPS patients with dystonia.6 Intrathecal baclofen has been shown to exert differential antinociceptive effects on specific pain qualities in CRPS patients with dystonia.

References
1.   Rowbotham MC. Pharmacologic management of complex regional pain syndrome. Clin J Pain. 2006;22(5):425-429.
2.   Resmini G, Ratti C, Canton G, Murena L, Moretti A, Io-lascon G. Treatment of complex regional pain syndrome. Clin Cases Miner Bone Metab. 2015;12(Suppl 1):26-30.
3.   Bahl A, Tripathi C, McMullan J, Goddard J. Novel use of intrathecal baclofen drug delivery system for periodic focal dystonia in a teenager. Neuromodulation. 2013;16(3):273-275.
4.   Wertli MM, Kessels AG, Perez RS, Bachmann LM, Brun-ner F. Rational pain management in complex regional pain syndrome 1 (CRPS 1)--a network meta-analysis. Pain Med. 2014;15(9):1575-1589.
5.   Nodera H. [Use of botulinum toxin for pain therapy]. Brain Nerve. 2008;60(5):503-508.

6.   van der Plas AA, van Rijn MA, Marinus J, Putter H, van Hilten JJ. Efficacy of intrathecal baclofen on different pain qualities in complex regional pain syndrome. Anesth Analg. 2013;116(1):211-215.

18. Anti-inflammatory Medication

The Complex regional pain syndrome (CRPS) is characterized by signs and symptoms of peripheral inflammation, which leads to peripheral neural sensitization associated most frequently (in about 70%) with blunt pressure hyperalgesia.1 When there is an injury, inflammatory substances such as bradykynins and prostaglandin are released in the area of the injury.

Aversion to addiction and diversion remains a potent force that shapes medication prescribing profiles. Chronic pain, whether arising from viscera, bone, or any other tissue or structure, is, more often than commonly thought, the result of a mixture of pain mechanisms, and therefore there is no simple formula available to manage chronic complex pain states.

The main symptoms of excruciating pain, trophic and inflammatory changes, as well as functional impairment of limbs are the hallmark of the complex regional pain syndrome (CRPS).

While functional impairments have to be treated by physical and occupational therapy, the former three symptoms are amendable to drug treatment: antidepressants, antiepileptic drugs and opioids are the most important drug classes for alleviating neuropathic pain whereas acute nociceptive pain may be positively influenced by non-steroidal anti-inflammatory drugs and steroids.2

The efficacy of oral corticosteroids is reported to be limited in treating CRPS of more than 3 months duration who did not respond to previous non-steroid treatment.3 Published randomized controlled trials can only provide limited evidence to formulate recommendations for treatment of CRPS I.4

These chemicals are synthesized by activity between the tissues and white blood cells that come to heal the injury. There are large lists of chemicals, (serotonin, hydrogen ions, potassium) which are released in the area of an injury. Sensitizations of C nociceptor nerve fibers cause the threshold to be lowered. The lowered threshold make these nerve fibers fire more frequently causing more intense pain.

The biochemical mediators of inflammation include cytokines, neuropeptides, growth factors and neurotransmitters. Irrespective of the type of pain whether it is acute or chronic pain, peripheral or central pain, nociceptive or neuropathic pain, the underlying origin is inflammation and the inflammatory response. Cytokines and oxygen free radicals have been implicated in the potential pathogenic development of complex regional pain syndrome.5

Early in the course of the disease patients demonstrate prominent inflammatory signs and symptoms that include neurogenic edema, erythema and an increased temperature of the affected extremity while long standing patients suffer pain spread and an apparent centralization of the process with concomitant severe generalized autonomic motor and trophic changes of skin, nails, bone and muscle.

CRPS is therefore believed to be an inflammatory disease. As a result many patients are prescribed nonsteroidal anti-inflammatory drugs. Cyclooxygenase, an enzyme involved in inflammation can be inhibited by anti-inflammatory drugs like ibuprofen. Cyclooxygenase-2 has been implicated in the development of CRPS and may be inhibited by celecoxib.

In CRPS, the hyperactive sympathetic response is provoked by an exaggerated inflammatory response. A soft tissue injury causes local inflammation and excitation of sensory nerve fibers. In the spinal cord, the sensory nerve fibers release inflammatory neuropeptides which increase the rate of firing of the sympathetic nerves to the injured extremity.

Increased sympathetic firing to the extremity is associated with excessive sweating, temperature instability, and vasoconstriction, which causes additional sensitization of pain receptors, causing allodynia.

The main symptoms of excruciating pain, trophic and inflammatory changes, as well as functional impairment of limbs are the hallmark of the complex regional pain syndrome (CRPS).2 Antidepressants, antiepileptic drugs and opioids are the most important drug classes for alleviating neuropathic pain whereas acute nociceptive pain may be positively influenced by non-steroidal anti-inflammatory drugs and steroids.

One of the medications effectively used to stop RSD during the very early stages are steroids. They reduce the inflammation and take away the inflammatory chemicals that begin the whole process of RSD.2 Acute nociceptive pain may be positively influenced by non-steroidal anti-inflammatory drugs and steroids.

A short-term oral prednisolone therapy significantly reduced the symptoms and signs of CRPS, and improved the functional abilities and quality of life.6 Prednisolone in another study resulted in significant improvement in the symptoms and signs of CRPSI following stroke, compared to piroxicam.7

Steroids are drugs used to reduce inflammatory pain such as arthritic joint pain. However, steroids may have significant side effects associated with their use. For example, steroids can cause weight gain, osteoporosis, avascular necrosis of your hips etc. Nonsteroidal anti-inflammatory drugs are commonly used to treat painful conditions.

These may include a sprain strain injury, a headache, a toothache etc. Many individuals believe that these drugs are safe because many of them are sold over the counter. However, these drugs may have serious side effects in some individuals.

The first types of painkillers that are often used to treat the pain of CRPS are nonsteroidal anti-inflammatory drugs (NSAIDs such as ibuprofen. People are often surprised that their use is recommended to treat severe pain, but they have proved to be very effective in relieving the symptoms of CRPS in many people. They can also help to reduce any associated swelling and may help relieve pain and redness.

Nonsteroidal anti-inflammatory drugs inhibit prostaglandins. Prostaglandins are a related family of chemicals that are produced by the cells of your body and have several important functions. They promote inflammation, pain, and cause fevers.

They are involved with the function of platelets that are necessary for the clotting of your blood, and protect the lining of your stomach from the damaging effects of acid. Prostaglandins are produced within your body's cells by the enzyme cyclooxygenase (COX).

There are two of these enzymes, Cox 1 and Cox 2. However, only Cox-1 produces prostaglandins that support platelets and protect the stomach. Nonsteroidal anti-inflammatory drugs (NSAIDs) block the Cox enzymes and reduce prostaglandins throughout your body. As a consequence, ongoing inflammation, pain, and fever are reduced.

Since the prostaglandins that protect the stomach and support the platelets and blood clotting also are reduced, NSAIDs can cause ulcers in the stomach and cause bleeding. NSAIDs differ in how strongly they inhibit Cox-1 and, therefore, in their tendency to cause ulcers and promote bleeding.

Another important difference between the two enzymes is their ability to cause ulcers and bleeding. The more an NSAID blocks Cox-1, the greater is its tendency to cause ulcers and bleeding. One NSAID called Celebrex, blocks Cox-2, but has little effect on Cox-1. This drug is referred to as one of the selective Cox-2 inhibitors and therefore causes less bleeding and fewer ulcers than other NSAIDs.

Aspirin is the only NSAID that is able to inhibit the clotting of blood for a prolonged period (4 to 7 days). This prolonged effect of aspirin makes it an ideal drug for preventing the blood clots that cause heart attacks and strokes. COX-2 inhibitors do not cause your blood to not clot. This is one reason why COX-2 inhibitors are implicated in heart attacks. You should be aware that the FDA issued a public health advisory concerning use of non-steroidal anti-inflammatory drug products including those known as COX-2 selective agents.

The COX-2 selective agents like Celebrex may be associated with an increased risk of serious cardiovascular events especially when they are used for long periods of time or in very high-risk settings. Preliminary results from a long-term clinical trial suggest that long-term use of a non-selective NSAID; naproxen may be associated with an increased cardiovascular risk compared to placebo.

Non-steroidal anti-inflammatory drugs (NSAIDs) have shown to be effective in treating both the pain and inflammation of CRPS. Commonly prescribed NSAIDs include Celebrex and Feldine. It is important to understand that NSAIDs have not been consistently effective for treating neuropathic pain during CRPS studies.

Celebrex and other anti-inflammatory coxib medications may counter the positive effects of aspirin in preventing blood clots. Physical therapies remain the lynchpin of management of CRPS but the roles of anti-inflammatory medication, sympathectomies and a team approach are emphasized.8

The research, published in the Proceedings of the National Academy of Sciences (PNAS), indicates that people who are taking aspirin and coxibs together are in fact inhibiting the aspirin's effectiveness in preventing heart attacks and strokes. It is suggested that patients who are consuming coxibs and a low dose of aspirin simultaneously are exposed to a greater risk of cardiovascular events.

In the past decade, a new group of anti-inflammatory drugs, coxibs, which include Celebrex was developed to treat arthritis pain as well as other pain such as CRPS. Arthritis patients who take Celebrex are instructed to take low-dose aspirin to counteract Celebrex's own potential clot-promoting effect.

Aspirin is the oldest and one of the most effective non-steroidal anti-inflammatory drugs. It is also well known for its ability to prevent the blood clots that can potentially lead to heart attack and stroke. Therefore, doctors often advise patients who are more prone to heart-related illnesses to take a daily tablet of low dose aspirin (81 mg). Approximately, 50 million Americans take aspirin every day to reduce their risk of cardiovascular diseases.

The FDA (Federal Drug Administration) stated that patients who are at a high risk of gastrointestinal bleeding, have a history of intolerance to non-selective NSAIDs, or are not doing well on non-selective NSAIDs may be appropriate candidates for COX-2 selective agents. Non-selective NSAIDs are widely used in both over-the-counter and prescription settings.

As prescription drugs, many are approved for short-term use in the treatment of pain and menstrual discomfort, and for longer-term use to treat the signs and symptoms of osteoarthritis and rheumatoid arthritis. NSAIDS are classified as non-opioid analgesic drugs and are aspirin like drugs.

Although the pharmacologic and toxicological properties of these compounds are similar and all possess analgesic activity, only certain drugs are indicated specifically for the relief of pain (eg. Feldene, Voltaren, Advil, Naprosyn, Celebrex etc,).

NSAIDS stop the production of prostaglandin production. Since prostaglandins are formed and released in response to cell membrane injury, these substances have become associated with pain reactions that accompany tissue injury and inflammation. Prostaglandins sensitize pain receptors (mostly C fibers) by lowering the threshold to thermal, mechanical and chemical stimuli.

Thus, the increased pain sensations induced by prostaglandins is a localized event that allows the mediators of pain such as bradykinin, histamine and substance p, to exert a greater effect on pain receptors. The receptors are stimulated to a greater extent causing more pain. All of the

NSAIDS analgesics prevent the biosynthesis and release of prostaglandins by inhibition of prostaglandin cyclooxygenase, a cell membrane enzyme that is present in almost all cells. Therefore, the NSAIDS reduce the formation of prostaglandins and decrease the pain sensitivity caused by these substances. NSAIDS have analgesic, fever reducing, and anti-inflammatory effects.

Not all of the drugs are equally active, nor are all clinically useful, with respect to these effects. Dolobid (diflunisal) for example, is used exclusively as an analgesic but does not decrease a fever. With the exception of acetaminophen, aspirin, and ibuprofen, none of the other compounds are used to reduce fever.

NSAIDS are used in the treatment of various arthritic conditions such as rheumatoid arthritis, ankylosing spondylitis, osteoarthritis and acute gouty arthritis. As the particular inflammatory condition being treated is alleviated, the pain associated with the disease is also decreased. Pain associated with inflammatory diseases is effectively reduced by all of these NSAID drugs. Aspirin is the oldest NSAID.

Toradol (ketolorac) has minimal antiinflammatory effects but has significant pain relieving effects. This observation suggests that anti-inflammatory effects are not related to pain relieving effects. NSAIDS have a ceiling affect. This means that when you take a certain dose of an NSAID, more of the NSAID will not give you more pain relief. This affect is opposite to that of opioid analgesics. They have no ceiling effects. This means that more of an opioid will increase your pain relief.

Research studies have concluded that IV parecoxib is an effective anti-inflammatory drug combined with clonidine/lidocaine loco-regional block in CRPS type 1. However, the FDA will not permit this drug to be marketed. In some cases of RSD anti-inflammatory agents have no effects on CRPS pain. These results indicate a non-inflammatory pathogenesis in CRPS presumably central in origin.

The Bayer Company in Germany discovered aspirin in the late 1800's. Aspirin is the prototype to which other NSAIDS are compared. The side effects of the NSAIDS should be briefly discussed. Serious side effects are rare. The liver and kidneys can be affected by high doses of NSAIDS prescribed over a long duration. Patients with forms of arthritis will require NSAIDS long term for the anti-inflammatory properties of the NSAIDS.

Gastrointestinal toxicity can occur with all NSAIDS that can lead to bleeding from the stomach and may lead to hospitalization and surgery as well as blood transfusions. Localized irritation of the stomach lining constitutes the most common adverse reaction associated NSAIDS.

Although epigastric distress is common at the lower doses, gastric and/or intestinal ulceration and bleeding will occur in only a small percentage of patients. At higher doses of aspirin, erosive gastritis and gastrointestinal hemorrhage is observed more often. These effects are the result of the inhibition of cyclo-oxygenase 1 (COX-1).

You need cyclo oxygenase 1 to form protective prostaglandins that reduce acid secretion by your stomach and promote the secretion of protective intestinal mucus. Aspirin and other compounds with high anti-inflammatory activity, such as indomethacin, tend to elicit the highest incidence of gastrointestinal reactions. Other NSAIDS like naproxen are considered to produce fewer and less intense gastrointestinal reactions than aspirin.

Acetaminophen is essentially devoid of these effects. Acetaminophen has some anti-inflammatory affects.   Newer NSAIDS that are specific for cyclo oxygenase 2 enzymes are safer than the rest of the NSAIDS that inhibit both cyclooxygenase 1 and 2. Celebrex is safer on your stomach. With respect to the heart and lungs all of the NSAIDS can cause swelling in your extremities as well as increase your blood pressure.

It should be noted that all NSAIDS including ibuprofen and naproxen could be linked to an increased risk of a heart attack. Because of this research, it is advisable to use the lowest effective dose of NSAID for the shortest time necessary, NSAIDS can cause clotting problems and make you prone to bleeding or bruising. This is due to the inhibition of thromboxane A, formation in thrombocytes (cells in the bloodstream associated with clotting). However, Celebrex does not cause this problem. In other words, Celebrex is the only NSAID that does not adversely affect the blood thinning effects of aspirin.

With respect to your kidneys, sodium and water retention with extremity swelling are seen with NSAID use. The higher the dose, the more prone you are for these side effects. Ask your doctor about the lowest effective dose that can be prescribed for you. If you are over sixty years of age you should be prescribed lower doses, as you may be more sensitive to NSAIDS than younger patients.

NSAIDS are excellent analgesic medications for pain in extremities, as well as for dental pain and headaches. They are furthermore, non-addicting. NSAIDS should be used with caution in elderly patients.   If you are significantly sick (such as an intensive care patient, an NSAID can adversely affect your kidneys. In some instances NSAIDS can cause kidney failure.

Nonsteroidal anti-inflammatory drugs (NSAIDs are commonly used in the elderly for the treatment of fever, pain, pain associated with inflammation in rheumatoid arthritis and osteoarthritis, neuromuscular disorders, headache, and musculoskeletal conditions. In another study however, anti-inflammatory agents had no effect on CRPS pain. These results indicate a non-inflammatory pathogenesis in CRPS presumably central in origin.9

Inflammation may be reduced with the use of a steroid drug. Prednisone is the most commonly prescribed corticosteroid to treat CRPS, and may also help improve limb mobility and function. Since prednisone does not offer pain relief, this is usually prescribed in addition to other medications. Prednisolone a steroid, was compared to piroxicam, an anti-inflammatory medication for the treatment of CRPS pain.[7] Prednisolone resulted in a significant improvement in the symptoms and signs of CRPS I, compared to piroxicam.

Each year in the United States, people spend 5 to 10 billion dollars to purchase prescription and over-the-counter NSAIDs. Gastrointestinal side effects such as ulcers and bleeding are the most prevalent and life-threatening problems associated with NSAIDs in elderly individuals. Specifically in the elderly, NSAIDs have become a leading cause of hospitalization in this age group and may increase the risk of death from ulceration more than four fold.

NSAIDs and the new class of cyclooxygenase-2 selective NSAIDs continue as drugs of choice for analgesia and anti-inflammatory effects in patients with CRPS. Physiological changes of aging worsen the side-effect profile of NSAIDs in the elderly. These side effects, when added to the increased potential for drug interactions, lead to a much greater risk for adverse outcomes when NSAIDs are used in the elderly patient.

NSAIDS should be used with caution in pregnant patients as well. These drugs are not recommended during pregnancy, especially in the third trimester. NSAIDs as a class are not direct congenital malformation drugs. They may however, cause premature closure of the fetal ductus arteriosus and also cause a reduction in maternal amniotic fluid. As a result, pregnant patients taking NSAIDS may require ultrasound monitoring by the treating obstetrician. In addition NSAIDS may cause premature birth.

Aspirin should not be used during pregnancy. Fetal bleeding could occur as a result of the inhibitory effects on the fetal platelets. Acetaminophen which does have slight anti-inflammatory properties is safe and well-tolerated during pregnancy.

References
1.   Breuer AJ, Mainka T, Hansel N, Maier C, Krumova EK. Short-term treatment with parecoxib for complex regional pain syndrome: a randomized, placebo-controlled double-blind trial. Pain Physician. 2014;17(2):127-137.

2.   Ruegg S. [Drug treatment of CRPS]. Handchir Mikrochir Plast Chir. 2010;42(1):19-29.

3.   Barbalinardo S, Loer SA, Goebel A, Perez RS. The Treatment of Longstanding Complex Regional Pain Syndrome with Oral Steroids. Pain Med. 2016;17(2):337-343.

4.   Tran DQ, Duong S, Bertini P, Finlayson RJ. Treatment of complex regional pain syndrome: a review of the evidence. Can J Anaesth. 2010;57(2):149-166.

5.   Miclescu AA, Nordquist L, Hysing EB, et al. Targeting oxidative injury and cytokines' activity in the treatment with anti-tumor necrosis factor-alpha antibody for complex regional pain syndrome 1. Pain Pract. 2013;13(8):641-648.

6.   Atalay NS, Ercidogan O, Akkaya N, Sahin F. Prednisolone in complex regional pain syndrome. Pain Physician. 2014;17(2):179-185.

7.   Kalita J, Vajpayee A, Misra UK. Comparison of prednisolone with piroxicam in complex regional pain syndrome following stroke: a randomized controlled trial. QJM. 2006;99(2):89-95.

8.   Bushnell TG, Cobo-Castro T. Complex regional pain syndrome: becoming more or less complex? Man Ther. 1999;4(4):221-228.

9.   Sieweke N, Birklein F, Riedl B, Neundorfer B, Handwerker HO. Patterns of hyperalgesia in complex regional pain syndrome. Pain. 1999;80(1-2):171-177.

19. Opioids

Despite being a recognized clinical entity for over 140 years, the complex regional pain syndrome (CRPS) remains a difficult-to-treat condition. The complex regional pain syndrome remains a challenging condition to diagnose and treat for many physicians. There are few large-scale, randomized trials of pharmacologic agents.1 Pain medications drugs may on occasion be ineffective for the management of RSD/CRPS pain. The therapeutic approach often calls for a combination of treatments. Medications such as antiepileptics, opioids, antidepressants, and topical agents along with a rehabilitation medicine program can help a major portion of patients suffering from these disorders.2

RSD pain is called neuropathic pain meaning nerve fiber pain. Narcotic drugs on the other hand, are prescribed for postoperative pain, cancer pain and for some chronic pain syndromes which is called nociceptive pain. Narcotic drugs can relieve moderate to severe pain.

While narcotic pain medications and opiate medications can help some patients, for others, they don't make a dent on the degree of pain they are experiencing. The medications in this class are most effective when used with other medications.

The term narcotic refers to agents that benumb or deaden nerves, causing loss of feeling or paralysis. Psychodelic drugs like LSD, contrary to popular belief are not narcotics. Many law enforcement officials in the United States inaccurately use the word "narcotic" to refer to any illegal drug or any unlawfully possessed drug.

Some physicians prescribe narcotics for CRPS pain. It has been stated that neuropathic pain is less sensitive to opioids, meaning higher doses are required compared to known non-neuropathic pain. Thus, observation that higher doses of opioids are needed in neuropathic pain to provide pain relief has been confirmed by many studies. It has been established that higher doses of narcotics produce a better effect on pain relief in neuropathic pain.

Most medical professionals prefer the term opioid which refers to natural, semi-synthetic and synthetic substances that behave pharmacologically like morphine. The Opioids are a class of controlled pain-management drugs that contain natural or synthetic chemicals based on morphine, the active component of opium. These narcotics effectively mimic the pain-relieving chemicals that the body produces naturally. Opioids are the most often prescribed pain-relievers because they are so effective. Morphine is the standard to which other opioid drugs are compared. Morphine is frequently prescribed to alleviate severe pain after surgery.

Codeine can be helpful in soothing somewhat milder pain, as are oxycodone (OxyContin, an oral, controlled-release form of the drug), propoxyphene (Darvon), hydrocodone (Norco), hydromorphone (Dilaudid and meperidine (Demerol), which is used less often because of its side effects. Diphenoxylate or Lomotil can also relieve severe diarrhea, and codeine can ease severe coughs.

The primary medical use of opioids is to relieve pain. Other medical uses include control of coughs and diarrhea, and the treatment of addiction to other opioids. Opioids can produce euphoria, making them prone to abuse. Opioids should only be used for moderate to severe pain that has not responded to non-narcotic drugs like aspirin or ibuprofen.

Several synthetic opioids function additionally as NMDA-antagonists, such methadone and tramadol. The combination of morphine with an NMDA-receptor antagonist significantly affects the cerebral processing of nociceptive information in CRPS.3 The correlation of pain relief and decrease in cortical activity in cS1 and cS2 is in accordance with the expected impact of the NMDA-receptor antagonist on cerebral pain processing with emphasis on sensory-discriminative aspects of pain.

There has been an analgesic algorithm published for difficult-to-treat pain syndromes. Pharmacological Iiterventions for moderate to severe pain/functional impairment; pain with a score of > 4 on the brief pain inventory. 1.Gabapentinoid (gabapentin, pregabalin)+/-Opioid/opioid rotation or 2. Antidepressant (TCA, duloxetine, venlafaxine venlafaxine)+/-Opioid/opioid rotation or 3. Gabapentinoid+antidepressant + Opioid/opioid rotation.3

Mild to moderate cases may require adjuvant analgesics, such as anticonvulsants and/or antidepressants. An opioid should be added to the treatment regimen if these medications do not provide sufficient analgesia to allow the patient to participate in physical therapy.4

Narcotics can be used alone like oxycodone or used in combination with aspirin, ibuprofen or acetaminophen (Tylenol). Some narcotics like oxycodone or morphine are available as an extended release tablet that must be swallowed whole. Valid and high quality evidence to treat

RSD / CRPS with narcotics is still missing. Butorphanol may be helpful for the control of CRPS pain as well.

When used appropriately, opioids may be very effective in controlling certain types of chronic pain. They tend to be less effective or require higher doses in nerve type pain. For pain is present all day and night, a long acting opioid is usually recommended. One of the most frequent side effects is constipation.

Even without solid scientific support, though, most experts believe that opioids should be given as part of a comprehensive pain treatment program for CRPS. Opioids should be prescribed immediately if other medications do not provide sufficient analgesia if a patient has severe pain. .

Tablets, which are not extended release, may be split. In 1914, the Federal Government passed a law that prohibited prescribing opioid drugs for recreational use.   The Federal Controlled Substances Act of 1970 formulated schedules for drugs.

Patients need to be aware of three of five schedules; I; has no current accepted medical use like heroin or marijuana II; high abuse and dependence potential like morphine, codeine or oxycodone, and III; includes drugs with a lesser dependence and abuse liability. Hydrocodone (Norco) is a schedule III drug. Valium, a relaxant is a schedule IV drug and some cough medicines are schedule V drugs. Oxycodone (Oxycotin) is a schedule II drug which means that it is potentially more habit forming than higher schedule drugs.

There is a difference between the descriptions of narcotic drugs and opioids. Opioids are drugs like morphine, hydrocodone etc. Narcotics are extremely addictive drugs and include heroin and other drugs that can cause significant sedation.

These drugs act by attaching to a group of proteins called opioid receptors found in the brain, spinal cord and gastrointestinal tract. When these drugs link to certain opioid receptors in the brain and spinal cord they can block the transmission of pain messages to the brain. Furthermore, they can cause constipation my affecting mu receptors in the gastrointestinal tract.

For the purposes of discussion in outlining the pharmacologic activity of these compounds, the opioids will be classified as (1) agonists, (2) antagonists, and (3) mixed agonist-antagonists. All drugs bind to receptors that exist on the outer membrane of the cells. Narcotics bind to narcotic receptors on cells in the brain and spinal cord.

Opioid receptors may also be recruited on tissue cells outside of the central nervous system such as the knee following an injury. An injection of morphine into the knee may alleviate the pain. When opioids turn on a receptor, that receptor decreases pain signals usually in the spinal cord that prevents pain signals from going to the brain.

As a result, a patient's pain perception is decreased. Experimental studies involving binding of opioids to specific receptors in the brain and spinal cord have substantiated the hypothesis that these receptors exist which mediates the actions of the opioid drugs to stop pain signals to the brain.

There are two basic classes of opioid receptors called mu and kappa receptors. Other classes exist (e.g. delta) but are not important for the discussion of patient's pain in this chapter.

These receptors also appear to be the site of action of the endogenous (pain drugs produced by the patient's body) opioid-like substances and have been divided into three major categories, designated mu, delta and kappa. It has also been proposed that at least two subtypes of each category of opioid receptors exist.

Experimental evidence suggests that activation of mu receptors (found principally at sites in the brain) is associated with analgesia, respiratory depression, euphoria, and physical dependence. The kappa receptors (located within the spinal cord) are believed to mediate spinal analgesia, constriction of the pupil size and sedation.

The other receptors may influence affective behavior, and although some physicians believe that activation of these receptors do play a role in opioid-induced analgesia. Since a number of different compounds, (e.g., certain antihistamines, some steroids, and anti-psychotics have phencyclidine) none of which are opioid in structure but can affect binding affinity for these sites.

Agonistic (stimulating) opioids act as analgesics by binding to and activating both mu and kappa receptors in the brain and spinal cord. The opioid antagonists bind to all categories of opioid receptor sites throughout the body, but fail to activate them. These compounds are not used for pain control; rather, the utility of these drugs lies in their ability to reverse an overdose of opioids including narcotics.

The compounds that comprise the mixed agonist-antagonist group are more recent additions to the clinically important opioids. These drugs are semi-synthetic derivatives of morphine, the chemical structures of which have agonistic activity at some kappa receptors but antagonistic activity at mu receptors, e.g., butorphanol, or partial agonistic activity at mu receptors and antagonistic activity at kappa receptors, eg. buprenorphine.

All are effective analgesics since they stimulate either mu or kappa receptors. The use of pain medication in long term pain narcotic patients should be limited to the non-addicting type of pain medications (such as Stadol or Ultram). N-methyl-D-aspartate antagonists have recently gained in popularity as well for CRPS patients.1

Chemically, the opioid agonists include a number of classes of drugs, all of which have pharmacologic effects similar to those of morphine. Morphine is the oldest known drug of this class. It remains as the prototype for the opioid group and is the standard to which all other opioid analgesic drugs are compared.

Opioid drugs decrease pain but also affect all organ systems. The pituitary gland in patient's brain can be adversely affected by chronic narcotic use. For example in males opioids can decrease testosterone that can cause depression and erectile dysfunction. Drowsiness and blurred vision can occur. Changes in mood can occur. An inability to concentrate can occur as well.

Euphoria can be experienced in 20% of individuals taking opioid drugs. Euphoria can be the cause of addiction. Opioids can stop patient's respiratory drive that can cause patients to stop breathing. Narcotics affect patient's stomach by slowing down the passage of food in combination with patient's brain to cause nausea and vomiting. Opioids can cause a significant decrease in patient's blood pressure that may cause patients to fall.

Opioids decrease movement of the bowel resulting in constipation. Morphine can make gall bladder disease worse by contracting a valve where the gall bladder meets the intestine called the sphincter of Oddi. Opioid drugs can result in a release of histamine from certain cell in the body that can cause itching and a rash.

Tolerance, addiction and physical dependence can occur with opioid drugs. Tolerance occurs when it takes more drugs to cause the same decrease in patientsr pain. This is not addiction.

Patients may find that they develop tolerance to opioid pain medications and may need to have their doses increased in order to be effective. Tolerance has not been shown to lead to drug addiction.

Physical dependence is a condition that occurs when continued use of the drug is needed to prevent a withdrawal reaction. Steady use of opioids can result in tolerance to the drugs so that higher doses must be taken to achieve the same effects. Long-term use also can lead to physical dependence which means that the body adapts to the presence of the drug and withdrawal symptoms occur if use is reduced abruptly.

Treatment with intravenous ketamine appears to be effective in completely resolving intractable pain caused by severe refractory CRPS I in some patients.5 Ketamine initiates a cascade of events, including desensitization of excitatory receptor systems in the central nervous system, which persisted but slowly abated when ketamine molecules were no longer present.6

A four-hour ketamine infusion escalated from 40-80 mg over a 10-day period can result in a significant reduction of pain with increased mobility and a tendency to decreased autonomic dysregulation.7

Ketamine may be administered topically.8 Ketamine 10%, pentox-ifylline 6%, clonidine 0.2%, and dimethyl sulfoxide 6% to 10% combined in a cream is reported to be effective. Another report also described a compound analgesic cream consisting of ketamine 10%, pentoxifylline 6%, clonidine 0.2%, and dimethyl sulfoxide 6% to 10% has been reported to decrease CRPS pain as well.9

Sub anesthetic inpatient infusions of ketamine may offer a promising therapeutic option in the treatment of appropriately selected patients with intractable CRPS. The data available reveal ketamine as a promising treatment for CRPS. The optimum dose, route and timing of administration remain to be determined.

Addiction is an intense craving for an opioid and is often associated with recreational use. Signs and symptoms of addiction include yawning, sweating, restlessness, irritability, anxiety, nasal discharge, tearing, dilated pupils, gooseflesh, tremors, loss of appetite, body aches, nausea and vomiting, fever and chills and an increase in heart rate and blood pressure. These symptoms last for 7-10 days.

Minor symptoms can begin in 8-12 hours after the last dose of the opioid. The more severe symptoms like nausea and vomiting begin 48-72 hours after the last dose of the drug.

With respect to agonist drugs, morphine is the prototype. It can be administered by mouth, rectum or by injection into muscle or vein. It is prepared in a capsule, tablet or a liquid. It is available by a rectal suppository as well. This route of administration is used for those patients who cannot swallow or are having severe vomiting. Hydromorphone and oxymorphone also come in the form of rectal suppositories.

The duration of action of opioids varies from drug to drug. Sustained release morphine and oxycodone give a longer duration of action. Immediate release drugs (eg. OXIR) give a faster onset but have a shorter duration of action.

Fentanyl, which is 75 times more potent than morphine is available in a patch and sucker, forms. The fentanyl patch is used for severe constant pain. The pain relief is continuous. The sucker, which only comes in a raspberry flavor, is used for severe cancer pain in instances where the severe pain fluctuates. Fentora is another oral form of fentanyl.

With respect to the fentanyl pain patch, the amount of drug released is controlled by small holes in a membrane in the patch. A larger hole permits the release of fentanyl into patient's body. The patches are available in different doses.

The fentanyl is released from the patch for 48-72 hours. Patients with a fever can be at a risk for an overdose as the amount of fentanyl administered to patient's body can increase by 25% for every 30 C increase in body temperature. The advantage of the patch is that patients do not have to take frequent pills during the night. The patch should be applied to a hairless surface.

The Food & Drug Administration granted marketing approval to oxymorphone immediate-release and oxymorphone extended-release tablets (Opana/Opana ER, Endo Pharmaceuticals). Opana is approved for relief of moderate to severe acute pain where the use of an opioid is appropriate.

Opana ER is approved for relief of moderate to severe pain in patients requiring round-the-clock opioid treatment for an extended period. This approval marks the first time oxymorphone will be available in an oral and extended-release formulation. Opana ER is now available in most retail pharmacies.

The adverse-effect profiles of Opana and Opana ER are comparable to those of other opioids. Darvon (propoxyphene) and codeine are weaker opioids that are used to treat mild pain. They may be combined with acetaminophen to make each more potent. Patients need to be aware that smoking tobacco can decrease the potency of Darvon and hydrocodone.

Tramadol (Ultram) is an interesting drug and may be used for moderate to moderately severe pain. It has a low abuse potential. It is not a scheduled drug. It activates mu and kappa receptors. The side effects are minimal when compared to opioid drugs.

Tramadol does not produce withdrawal symptoms like opioids. The advantage of tramadol over other drugs is that tramadol inhibits noreoinepherine and serotonin release from patientsr brain and spinal cord. The two substances in the brain and spinal cord also decrease pain.

The opioid drugs do not have this effect. Tramadol can cause nausea dizziness and headaches. Tramadol does not lower the heart rate or blood pressure.

Tramadol provides pain relief similar to codeine and propoxyphene. Ryzolt (tramadol hydrochloride extended-release tablets) is a centrally acting analgesic composed of a dual-matrix delivery system with both immediate-release and extended-release characteristics.

Naloxone and naltrexone are drugs that reverse the respiratory effects of opioids. Naltrexone can be given orally. The only time that these drugs are given is to treat opioid intoxication.

Butorphanol (Stadol) and pentazocine (Talwin) are called mixed agonist-antagonists drugs. These drugs show receptor selectivity and these two drugs stimulate kappa receptors.

These drugs have less opioid abuse tendencies than the agonist drugs. Opioids on the other hand work on both mu and kappa receptors. Strong opioids exist which are usually reserved for cancer patients or other patients with severe pain.

Hydromorphone (Dilaudid and levorphanol (Levo-Dromanare eight and five times more potent than morphine. Meperidine (Demerol is an opioid that is weaker than morphine. It is used infrequently in pain management as it can cause tremors or seizures if used on a chronic basis. Methadone is a synthetic drug similar to morphine.

The advantage of methadone for patient's pain management is that it does not cause euphoria. Methadone however, can cause a conduction problem in patient's heart. Consequently, patients have died from heart problems after being prescribed methadone.

Hydrocodone and oxycodone are two opioids used for moderate to moderately severe pain. These drugs are usually combined with aspirin and acetaminophen which can potentiate the analgesic efficacy of these drugs.

In some individuals some narcotic drugs do not provide pain relief. This happens in 20-30% of patients. This is because some narcotics like hydrocodone, codeine, oxycodone and tramadol need to be converted by an enzyme in patient's body called CYP 34A.

The drugs themselves only decrease pain after each is converted to another chemical in a patient's body. The drug that patients are prescribed is converted to a pain relieving drug in patient's body. For example, hydrocodone is converted to morphine. The morphine provides patients pain relief not the hydrocodone itself.

If a patient has a genetic abnormality, the CYP 450 enzyme does not convert hydrocodone to morphine. Therefore, a patient feels no pain relief. Antidepressant drugs, benzodiazepine drugs like Valium can inhibit the cytochrome p 450 enzyme which in turn inhibits the CYP 34A enzyme.

Drugs like fentanyl, morphine, dilaudid and oxymorphone do not need this enzyme activity to provide pain relief. Many patients are terminated from pain practices because their narcotics like hydrocodone provide no pain relief. Some doctors unfortunately believe that the patients are drug seeking and the doctors terminate patients from their practice.

Another fact to know is that opioid drugs can actually cause increased pain in some instances. This observation is called opioid induced pain. Many physicians are unaware of this fact. In this situation, a reduction in the dose of a patient's medicine or stopping it can actually decrease pain. This phenomenon can also be seen in patents that have spinal morphine drug delivery systems.

Another fact that patients need to be aware of is that smoking cigarettes can affect the absorption of some narcotics from the stomach to the blood stream. Drugs have to get to the brain to become effective for pain relief.

As one can see, there are many opioids that can be used for the management of acute and chronic pain. The proper choice of a medication is dependent upon the magnitude of the pathology, the side effects of the drug prescribed, the effectiveness of the drug and the overall health.

In general, opioids are not always useful for the management of RSD pain because RSD is primarily nerve pain. However, when bone, muscles and ligaments are involved in an injury, narcotic drugs may be indicated.

Few randomized controlled trials of oral pharmacotherapy have been performed in patients with complex regional pain syndrome (CRPS). The relative benefit of oral medications compared with the widely used treatments of intensive physical therapy, nerve blocks, sympathectomy, intraspinally administered drugs, and neuromodulatory therapies (eg, spinal cord stimulation) remains uncertain.

In summary, treatment of CRPS has received insufficient study and remains largely empirical.10 In general, the evidence level for treatment strategies specifically for the complex regional pain syndrome is very poor; most recommendations and algorithms rely on results derived from studies testing drugs against other conditions where chronic (neuropathic) pain is prevalent, like diabetic polyneuropathy or postherpetic neuralgia, or medications are used on the basis of pathomechanistic considerations.11

Aversion to addiction and diversion remains a potent force that shapes prescribing profiles.

References
1. Mackey S, Feinberg S. Pharmacologic therapies for complex regional pain syndrome. Curr Pain Headache Rep. 2007;11(1):38-43.
2. Pappagallo M, Rosenberg AD. Epidemiology, pathophysiology, and management of complex regional pain syndrome. Pain Pract. 2001;1(1):11-20.
3. Gustin SM, Schwarz A, Birbaumer N, et al. NMDA-receptor antagonist and morphine decrease CRPS-pain and cerebral pain representation. Pain. 2010;151(1):69-76.
4. Rho RH, Brewer RP, Lamer TJ, Wilson PR. Complex regional pain syndrome. Mayo Clin Proc. 2002;77(2):174-180.
5. Shirani P, Salamone AR, Schulz PE, Edmondson EA. Ketamine treatment for intractable pain in a patient with severe refractory complex regional pain syndrome: a case report. Pain Physician. 2008;11(3):339-342.
6. Dahan A, Olofsen E, Sigtermans M, et al. Population pharmacokinetic-pharmacodynamic modeling of ketamine-induced pain relief of chronic pain. Eur J Pain. 2011;15(3):258-267.
7. Goldberg ME, Domsky R, Scaringe D, et al. Multi-day low dose ketamine infusion for the treatment of complex regional pain syndrome. Pain Physician. 2005;8(2):175-179.
8. Keppel Hesselink JM, Kopsky DJ. Treatment of chronic regional pain syndrome type 1 with palmitoylethanolamide and topical ketamine cream: modulation of nonneuronal cells. J Pain Res. 2013;6:239-245.

9.   Russo MA, Santarelli DM. A Novel Compound Analgesic Cream (Ketamine, Pentoxifylline, Clonidine, DMSO) for Complex Regional Pain Syndrome Patients. Pain Pract. 2016;16(1):E14-20.

10.   Rowbotham MC. Pharmacologic management of complex regional pain syndrome. Clin J Pain. 2006;22(5):425-429.

11.   Ruegg S. [Drug treatment of CRPS]. Handchir Mikrochir Plast Chir. 2010;42(1):19-29.

Chronic opioid therapy (defined as greater than 3 months on opioids) is a common practice for those with non-cancer pain, cancer survivors with treatment-related pain, and individuals with cancer undergoing disease-modifying therapy with a survival that can be for a year or more. Drugs are chemicals that have a profound impact on the neurochemical balance in the brain.1

The risk of addiction, depression, central hypogonadism, sleep-disordered breathing, impaired wound healing, infections, cognitive impairment, falls, non-vertebral fractures, and mortality are increased in populations on long-term opioids.

Chronic pain, whether arising from bone, or any other tissue or structure, is, more often than commonly thought, the result of a mixture of pain mechanisms, and therefore there is no simple formula available to manage chronic complex pain states. One possible explanation for the severe pain described in some patients is opioid induced hyperalgesia induced by high doses of opioids.

Patients receiving chronic opioid treatment who develop paradoxical pain sensations, as well as worsening existing pain, can be diagnosed as suffering from opioid-induced hyperalgesia.2 As the worldwide population expands so too does the proportion of patients who experience pain that requires a strong opioid.

Opioid-induced hyperalgesia is a phenomenon associated with the long term use of opioids such as morphine, hydrocodone, oxycodone, and methadone. This entity may mimic addiction.

Identifying the development of hyperalgesia is of great clinical importance since patients receiving opioids to relieve pain may paradoxically experience more pain as a result of treatment.

As a result he/she takes more pain medication and subsequently appears to be addicted. Ketamine has been shown to be significantly beneficial in patients who require large amounts of opioid medications or exhibit some degree of opioid tolerance. Methadone is also effective in reducing high-dose opioid OIH.

The clinical use of opioids is further complicated by an increasingly deleterious profile of side effects beyond addiction, including tolerance and opioid-induced hyperalgesia (OIH), where OIH is defined as an increased sensitivity to already painful stimuli.

This paradoxical state of increased nociception results from acute and long-term exposure to opioids, and appears to develop in a substantial subset of patients using opioids.3 As more opioids are prescribed, especially to treat chronic nonmalignant pain, OIH becomes more of a relevant and significant issue.4

In the last decade, a significant number of preclinical studies have investigated the factors that modulate OIH development as well as the cellular and molecular mechanisms underlying OIH. Several factors have been shown to influence OIH including the genetic background and sex differences of experimental animals as well as the opioid regimen.

Mu opioid receptor variants and interactions with different proteins were shown to be important.5 Furthermore, at the cellular level, both neurons and glia play a major role in OIH development.

People who are suffering emotionally use drugs to escape from their problems and this can lead to drug abuse and addiction. While progress is being made in treating patients with CRPS, it is important to remember that the goals of care are always to: 1) perform a comprehensive diagnostic evaluation, 2) be prompt and aggressive in treatment interventions, 3) assess and reassess the patient's clinical and psychological status, 4) be consistently supportive, and 5) strive for the maximal amount of pain relief and functional improvement.6

The annual number of US deaths from prescription-opioid overdose quadrupled between 1999 and 2010 and in 2010 alone reached 16,651. Deaths from opioid overdose have now surpassed the historic death toll from another drug-related epidemic - anesthesia mortality.7

Repeated, or chronic, use of opioids induces adaptive or allostatic changes that modify neuronal circuitry and create an altered normality.8 Patients receiving long-term opioid therapy often transitioned to chronic use after starting opioids.9

Ongoing opioid analgesic use in patients suffering from chronic non-malignant pain (CNMP) has been associated with the development of opioid misuse, abuse, addiction, and overdose.10 Some physicians are afraid to prescribe scheduled drugs because of the possibility of causing addiction.

Chronic pain, whether arising from viscera, bone, or any other tissue or structure, is, more often than commonly thought, the result of a mixture of pain mechanisms, and therefore there is no simple formula available to manage chronic complex pain states.

It has been shown previously that the risk of true addiction in chronic pain patients was approximately 0.3%. Accurate anatomical diagnosis can be provided in only 15% of the patients utilizing traditional medical technology. The question of, "Why not relief?" should be raised in our society on a daily basis.

It is imperative to understand the true nature of pain by separating the myth of psychological pain from the reality of organic pain and manage it appropriately utilizing all available means, not only narcotics and interventional technology, but also behavioral therapy.11

Prescription monitoring programs and using urine toxicology to monitor opioid use may decrease opioid abuse. CRPS patients may request opioids to control the severe pain.

Addiction is a chronic relapsing brain disease. Brain imaging shows that addiction severely alters the brain's areas critical to decision-making, learning and memory, and behavior control, which may help to explain the compulsive and destructive behaviors of addiction.

An addiction is a recurring problem by an individual to engage in some specific activity, despite harmful consequences to the individual's health, mental state or social life. An addiction can occur with drugs, gambling, overeating etc. Drugs can make one euphoric. As a result, one may request more and more drugs to maintain this euphoria.

Moreover, aversion to addiction and diversion remains a potent force that shapes prescribing profiles.1 Addiction is a hindrance in the long term treatment of complex regional pain syndrome (CRPS) because addiction in itself aggravates CRPS, causes stress in the sympathetic nervous system resulting in more severe sympathetic dysfunction.

Drug abuse or substance abuse, involves the repeated and excessive use of prescription or street drugs. In one way or another, almost all drugs over stimulate the pleasure center of the brain, flooding it with the neuro-transmitter dopamine which produces euphoria. That heightened sense of pleasure can be so compelling that the brain wants that feeling back, again and again.

Addiction is frequently found in people with a wide variety of mental illnesses, including anxiety disorders, unipolar and bipolar depression, schizophrenia, and borderline and other personality disorders.

Long term pain narcotic patients should be limited to the nonaddicting pain medications (such as Stadol or Ultram) or at least to the less addicting pain medications such as Stadol or Buprenorphine (Buprenex). Methadone may be considered in severe pain that is refractive to these drugs.

Methadone can be used for the treatment of pain in addicted patients. Methadone is also an opiate that prevents users from getting high on heroin by competing with the much more potent opiates for the body's opiate receptors. Buprenophrine is another drug that is effective for the treatment of addiction and is also an analgesic.

Addiction and drug dependence occur when drugs become so important that a patient is willing to sacrifice his/her work, home and even the family. Once a patient's brain and body get used to the substances a patient is taking, a patient begins to require increasingly larger and more frequent doses, in order to achieve the same effect.

Narcotics such as Heroin may over-stimulate the pleasure centers of the brain producing euphoric effects that cause compulsive drug-seeking behaviors. The severities of withdrawal symptoms associated with narcotics include chills, shakes, muscle pain, nausea, vomiting, and headaches and cravings.

A clinician must be able to distinguish between legitimate patients with chronic pain and individuals engaged in non-therapeutic drug seeking behavior. Physicians have for years recognized the value of opioid analgesics in relieving chronic pain.

Unfortunately, drug seekers may also request opioid analgesics. They do this by feigning illnesses, and seek controlled substances from multiple doctors and by forge prescriptions. Drug seekers may be difficult to distinguish from true chronic pain sufferers.

In general, drug seekers prefer illicit drugs such as heroin and cocaine to prescription drugs. Prescription drugs however, have advantages over illicit drugs. Third-party insurers or welfare-entitlement programs may pay for prescribed drugs. Prescription pharmaceuticals are obtained in the safety of the physician's office.

Drug abuse and addiction have a devastating impact on society. Her-oin use alone is responsible for the epidemic number of new cases of HIV/AIDS and hepatitis. Drug abuse is responsible for decreased job productivity and attendance, increased healthcare costs, and an escalation of domestic violence and violent crimes.

An estimated 20 percent of people in the United States have used prescription drugs for nonmedical reasons. Central nervous stimulants, depressants and opioids are prescription drugs that are frequently abused.

Central nervous system depressants are used to treat anxiety, panic attacks, and sleep disorders.

Examples are Nembutal (pentobarbital sodium), Valium (diazepam), and Xanax (alprazolam). Long-term use can lead to physical dependence and addiction.

Central nervous system stimulants are used to treat narcolepsy and the attention-deficit/hyperactivity disorder. Examples include Ritalin (methylphenidate) and Dexedrine (dextroamphetamine). Opioids, also known as narcotic analgesics are used to treat pain. Opioids are the most commonly abused prescription drugs. Examples include morphine, codeine, OxyContin (oxycodone), Vicodin (hydrocodone) and Demerol (meperidine).

One may obtain drugs by the following means: prescription forgery, by telephone (faking to be a physician's office), multiple doctors, and indiscriminate prescribing by physicians. Pain clinicians who prescribe chronic opioids are aware that there is an illicit market for opioid analgesics. For example OxyContin can be sold for $1.00 per milligram.

One 80 mg pill can be sold on the street for $80.00. Telephone scams occur when the drug seeker claims to be a patient of one of the other physicians in the on-call group, and asks for a prescription for an analgesic to last until they can see their regular physician.

Sometimes, the drug seeker uses a telephone to impersonate a practicing physician. Prescription forgery is a common activity among drug seekers.

Drug seekers can modify a legitimate prescription to increase the dosage or quantity of an opioid. The easiest method is to increase the number of tablets on the prescription.

Multiple episodes of noncompliance raise an alert of drug seeking behavior as well as multiple episodes of prescription loss. The patient with chemical dependency loses control over drug taking. The patient cannot take medications as prescribed. The patient repeatedly reports lost or stolen medications.

The physician will notice that the drug seeker frequently requests early renewals of prescriptions. A pain physician must however, be aware that aggressive complaining about the need for more drugs may indicate inadequate pain management as opposed to drug seeking behavior.

A patient should not be allowed to suffer. It should be understood that substance abusers can suffer from chronic pain which should be treated in a humane manner. Unapproved use of opioids to treat another symptom such as sleep deprivation should not be tolerated.

However, the pain management physician must objectively identify a patient's pain complaint with the appropriate medical test before prescribing an opioid. Opioid analgesics are powerful tools in the armamentarium of the pain clinician. Criminal and chemically dependent drug seekers may attempt to obtain such drugs from the physician. A pain medicine physician must therefore, use safe prescribing strategies.

A physician has no legal obligation to prescribe opioid analgesics on demand. A reasonable precaution to be taken by the pain medicine physician with an unfamiliar patient is to establish a policy of not prescribing opioid analgesics pending a complete assessment including corroboration of the patient's history.

Some patients or patient families are afraid of addiction. However, a significant number of individuals do not understand the difference between addiction and tolerance.

The American Academy of Pain Medicine, the American Pain Society, and the American Society of Addiction Medicine recognize the following definitions and recommend their use.

I. Addiction

Addiction is a primary, chronic, neurobiologic disease, with genetic, psychosocial, and environmental factors influencing its development and manifestations. It is characterized by behaviors that include one or more of the following: impaired control over drug use, compulsive use, continued use despite harm, and craving.

An entity termed pseudo-addiction exists which is not true addiction. Pseudo-addiction occurs when pain is under treated. Pseudoaddiction resolves when the pain resolves. Addictive behavior on the other hand, persists in spite of increasing the patient's pain medication.

II. Physical Dependence

Physical dependence is a state of adaptation that is manifested by a drug class specific withdrawal syndrome that can be produced by abrupt cessation, rapid dose reduction, decreasing blood level of the drug, and/or administration of an antagonist.

III. Tolerance

Tolerance is a state of adaptation in which exposure to a drug induces changes that result in a diminution of one or more of the drug's effects over time. Most specialists in pain medicine and addiction medicine agree that patients treated with prolonged opioid therapy usually do develop physical dependence and sometimes develop tolerance, but do not usually develop addictive disorders.

Addiction is a primary chronic disease and exposure to opioid medications is only one of the etiologic factors in its development. Therefore, good clinical judgment must be used in determining whether the pattern of behaviors signals the presence of addiction or reflects a different issue.

Drug overdose has become the leading cause of injury death in the United States. More than half of those deaths involve prescription drugs, specifically opioids. A key component of addressing this national epidemic is improving prescriber practices.12

References
1.   Davis MP, Mehta Z. Opioids and Chronic Pain: Where Is the Balance? Curr Oncol Rep. 2016;18(12):71.
2.   Bannister K. Opioid-induced hyperalgesia: where are we now? Curr Opin Support Palliat Care. 2015;9(2):116-121.
3.   Arout CA, Edens E, Petrakis IL, Sofuoglu M. Targeting Opioid-Induced Hyperalgesia in Clinical Treatment: Neurobiological Considerations. CNS Drugs. 2015;29(6):465-486.
4.   Yi P, Pryzbylkowski P. Opioid Induced Hyperalgesia. Pain Med. 2015;16 Suppl 1:S32-36.
5.   Roeckel LA, Le Coz GM, Gaveriaux-Ruff C, Simonin F. Opioid-induced hyperalgesia: Cellular and molecular mechanisms. Neuroscience. 2016;338:160-182.
6.   Pappagallo M, Rosenberg AD. Epidemiology, pathophysiology, and management of complex regional pain syndrome. Pain Pract. 2001;1(1):11-20.
7.   Kissin I. Opioid prescriptions for pain and epidemic of overdose death: can the dramatic reduction in anesthesia mortality serve as an example? J Pain Res. 2016;9:453-456.
8.   Evans CJ, Cahill CM. Neurobiology of opioid dependence in creating addiction vulnerability. F1000Res. 2016;5.
9.   Callinan CE, Neuman MD, Lacy KE, Gabison C, Ashburn MA. The initiation of chronic opioids: a survey of chronic pain patients Characterizing Chronic Opioid Use. J Pain. 2016.
10.   Chaudhary S, Compton P. Use of Risk Mitigation Practices by Family Nurse Practitioners Prescribing Opioids for the Management of Chronic Non-Malignant Pain. Subst Abus. 2016:0.

11.   Dotson DA. Why not relief? Pain Physician. 2000;3(1):65-68.

12.   Antman KH, Berman HA, Flotte TR, Flier J, Dimitri DM, Bharel M. Developing Core Competencies for the Prevention and Management of Prescription Drug Misuse: A Medical Education Collaboration in Massachusetts. Acad Med. 2016;91(10):1348-1351.

21. Topical Medications

While progress is being made in treating patients with CRPS, it is important to remember that the goals of care are always to: 1) perform a comprehensive diagnostic evaluation, 2) be prompt and aggressive in treatment interventions, 3) assess and reassess the patient's clinical and psychological status, 4) be consistently supportive, and 5) strive for the maximal amount of pain relief and functional improvement.1

Pain relievers that can be applied directly to a patient's skin are available for the control of a variety of a patient's pain syndromes. These topical pain relievers are a noninvasive and convenient method for delivering pain-relieving medication to a patient.

This is especially important and beneficial if a patient is not able to take medications by mouth. Topical pain relievers include complementary and alternative medications as well as conventional medications. Topical forms of analgesics, or pain relievers, have been used throughout human history.

The use of ointments for medicinal purposes is mentioned in the Bible on many occasions. The purpose of a topical analgesic is to transmit a medication through a patient's skin for the effect of pain relief.

The amount of drug that actually gets through a patient's skin is determined by the amount of pressure applied as a patient rub it over a patient's skin, the area of a patient's skin covered by the drug, the way in which the drug is dissolved, and the use of dressings over a patient's skin. Analgesics are available in ointments, creams, and gels. They also may be placed in patches that may be applied to a patient's skin.

Ointments are semisolid preparations that melt at body temperature and spread easily. Ointments are not routinely used in the practice of pain medicine unless the ointment is specially compounded by a pharmacy. Ointments are defined in three categories based on a patient's skin penetration.

One type of ointment does not penetrate beyond the external layer of a patient's skin called the epidermis. Ointments of this class can be used for the treatment of sunburn. A second type of ointment penetrates to the internal layer of a patient's skin called the dermis. The third type of ointment actually goes through a patient's skin to the nerves and ligaments and in some instances into a patient's bloodstream.

Substances applied on a patient's skin can evaporate. A patient does not want a patient's analgesic drug evaporating from a patient's skin. A patient's pharmacist will add substances such as glycerin to the ointment to keep this evaporation from happening.

Ointments can be prepared by a patient's pharmacist or purchased over the counter or by prescription. Some ointment preparations will contain absorption enhancers. Absorption enhancers make it easier for the drug to be absorbed through a patient's skin. Azone and DMSO can both enhance the absorption of ointments through a patient's skin. Ointments should be packaged in tubes.

Neuropathic pain is often resistant to opioids, so other medication classes, such as tricyclic antidepressants, anticonvulsants, and local anesthetics, are often used. Central sensitization, or pain 'wind-up', may perpetuate chronic neuropathic pain even when ongoing peripheral sensory input is absent. Wind-up is thought to cause allodynia, hyperalgesia, and hyperpathia.[2]

Receptors such as NMDA, AMPA, and M-glu have recently been identified for their role in central sensitization or pain 'wind-up'. Ketamine has been proposed for neuropathic pain secondary to its NMDA receptor activity. The current application as a topical gel stems from the theory that ketamine has peripheral action at opioid and Na+-K+ channels. Ketamine Gel may provide clinicians with a new option in the battle against chronic neuropathic pain.

Creams are opaque, thick, liquid substances that consist of medications dissolved in a cream base that usually vanishes through the skin. They are less of a liquid consistency than ointments. The term cream is used to describe a soft type of preparation that is less affected by a patient's body temperature than ointments. Gels are a delivery system that usually contain penetration enhancers and are usually used for administering anti-inflammatory medications.

The anti-inflammatory medication must be absorbed through a patient's skin to provide a patient with pain relief. Gels are useful treatment methods if a patient have arthritic and/or muscle pain. There is a certain activity of DMSO 50% cream in patients suffering from RSD. [3]

Gels usually are thicker than creams or ointments and are usually clear, unlike creams and ointments. The concentration of medication in gels is usually no greater than 2 percent. For example, lidocaine, which is a numbing medicine for the control of pain, is dispensed as a 2 percent gel. However, the cream is available in a 5 percent concentration.

This is because medications are usually absorbed through the skin better if used in gel form. Gels usually have clarity and sparkle. They maintain their thickness even with an elevated body temperature. Some gels have been developed to be given nasally. Some drugs are absorbed better through the nose than through the skin. Gels are usually dispensed in tubes or squeeze bottles.

Growing evidence indicates that patients with complex regional pain syndrome (CRPS) exhibit tissue abnormalities caused by microvascular dysfunction in the blood vessels of skin, muscle, and nerve. Allodynia in an animal model of CRPS has been shown to be effectively relieved by topical combinations of alpha2A receptor agonists or nitric oxide.[4]

This suggests that topical treatments aimed at improving microvascular function by increasing both arterial and capillary blood flow produce effective analgesia for CRPS.

Another delivery system for analgesics is a transdermal patch, which contains medication that is transmitted directly through a patient's skin. A patch containing a medication is placed on a patient's skin and remains there for a specified time so that the drug within the patch can be delivered through a patient's skin to a patient's bloodstream.

Local anesthetics such as lidocaine, capsaicin cream, and fentanyl (discussed in the narcotic drugs chapter), a potent opioid medication, are some of the medicines that can be delivered through a patient's skin using a transdermal drug delivery system.

These patches should be applied only to areas on a patient's skin that have no blisters or open areas such as a cut. The patches are made of adhesive materials. A patient should not use the patch if a patient is allergic to some adhesives.

With respect to the patches, the amount of drug that is absorbed from the patch is directly related to the length of the application of the patch, as well as the area of a patient's skin to which it is applied.

The advantage of the patch is that it gives a patient a continuous flow of analgesic medications. When a patient takes a pill, after it leaves a patient's stomach or intestine and enters into a patient's bloodstream, a patient receives a high concentration of the drug initially. As the drug is distributed to other tissues in a patient's body, a patient's blood level concentration of the drug decreases.

Once a patient's body breaks down the drug, a patient will no longer have an analgesic effect of that particular drug. However, when using a patch, a patient will have a continuous release of the drug from the patch into a patient's bloodstream. A patient will have constant pain relief without the peaks and valleys of the drug concentration in a patient's bloodstream associated with oral medications.

Natural compounds such as herbs or leaves and roots also can be used to treat a patient's pain topically. Aloe Vera can be used to decrease a patient's pain if a patient has sunburn. Use of this natural topical product for the treatment of various medical conditions was discovered in 1935. This drug is effective for the treatment of skin inflammation as well as minor burns. There are no side effects nor are there are any known drug interactions. Some patients use it for RSD/CRPS pain.

Capsaicin is a drug that has been extensively studied in both the clinical and laboratory settings. Capsaicin is the active component of chili or red peppers. Capsaicin can be put on a patient's skin over a patient's joints if a patient has joint pain. The capsaicin first stimulates the small pain-transmitting fibers by depleting them of the neurotransmitter substance P.

After the substance P has been depleted, a patient will have a block of the pain fibers that cause burning pain sensations. Observations in Hispanic individuals demonstrated that they did not have mouth or stomach pain after ingesting red peppers. The reason is the depletion of the substance P in the nerve endings in these areas following continual exposure to red peppers.

Substance P also is present in a patient's joints throughout a patient's body. For this reason, capsaicin can be an effective pain reliever for the treatment of pain associated with osteoarthritis and rheumatoid arthritis. It may take a week for a patient to feel the pain-relieving effects of capsaicin.

As substance P is being depleted from a patient's nerve endings, a patient nerve endings still manufacture substance P. As a result, it will take several days to deplete enough of the substance P to provide a patient with pain relief. Once a patient discontinues use of this cream, a patient's nerves will replenish substance P and a patient's pain may return.

Some studies have shown that if a patient has a neuropathy related to a patient's diabetes a patient could have significant pain relief with topical capsaicin. Some pain-medicine physicians have used topical capsaicin to relieve the pain associated with shingles. A patient may have a brief burning sensation following the use of capsaicin.

A patient should be warned to avoid contact with the eyes and genital areas. It is recommended that a patient use rubber gloves when applying the capsaicin cream. A patient should use the capsaicin cream no more than three times a day. Various concentrations of capsaicin exist. Begin with a small concentration that contains 0.025 percent capsaicin. A patient may eventually increase a patient's capsaicin dose to 0.075 percent capsaicin.

Menthol is oil that is one component of peppermint oil. This oil in a cream base can significantly decrease a patient's pain. When a patient places a menthol preparation on a patient's skin, the menthol will feel cold to a patient's nerve endings. While a patient feel the cold, a patient's pain-stimulating nerves will be depressed. Following the initial cool sensation, a patient will feel a period of warmth.

Menthol products can be used for the treatment of pain associated with arthritis, muscle pain, and tendonitis. Application of a menthol-containing cream may be of benefit to a patient if a patient suffers from tension headaches. It can be rubbed around the neck muscles just below the skull. It can be an extremely effective method for the treatment of a patient's headaches.

Allergic reactions with menthol have been reported. It is recommended that a patient test a small amount of menthol on a patient's skin before applying it extensively to assure a patient's self that a patient are not allergic it.

A patient should not use the menthol preparation more than three times a day. Do not use a heating pad or a cold pack over the area of a patient's skin where the menthol substance was placed.

Some natural herbs and vegetables can be used as a topical analgesic. One example is an onion. It is reported by some doctors that spreading the juice of a sliced onion over one of a patient's painful areas could reduce a patient's pain.

A tincture can be made by putting 100 grams of minced onions in 30 grams of ethanol for a 70 percent solution. There are no hazards or side effects associated with the topical administration of an onion. However, frequent contact with the onion over time could possibly lead to an allergic reaction.

The bark of a poplar tree also can be used for relieving a patient's pain. The bark can be used for control of a patient's pain over a patient's joints or nerves or if a patient has rheumatoid arthritis. A patient should not use the bark if a patient is allergic to aspirin. When externally applied using the poplar bark and leaves, a patient should use no more than five grams of the drug per day.

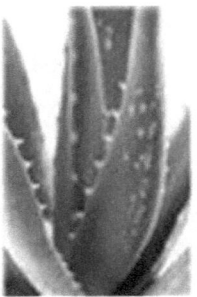

Figure 1. Some plant extracts may be helpful in controlling RSD/CRPS pain.

Another topical medication used to prevent pain is EMLA cream. It is used as a numbing agent more than it is used for reducing pain. This is a cream consisting of lidocaine and prilocaine, which are both numbing agents. This local anesthetic combination is packaged in tubes.

There also is an EMLA cellulose disc that can be applied over a patient's painful area. The purpose of this medication is to provide pain relief over the area of the skin. It is used in children to reduce the pain of starting intravenous lines.

Some pain-management doctors advocate its use to decrease the pain associated with reflex sympathetic dystrophy or the pain associated with shingles. This cream should be placed on an intact skin area. The EMLA should be applied under a bandage for at least 60 minutes to provide relief over the painful area of a patient's skin.

This cream is not recommended if a patient have an allergy to lidocaine or prilocaine. If a patient has the blood disorder methemoglobinemia, a patient should not use this cream. A patient should not exceed the recommended dose prescribed by a patient's physician.

The problem with this cream as opposed to the Lidoderm patches is that it does provide pain relief for a patient's skin. This means that a patient have a block of all sensation in the skin treated with this cream.

A patient should avoid causing any trauma to the area, including scratching a patient's skin or rubbing or exposing a patient's skin to extreme hot or cold temperatures until a patient have complete return of sensation to a patient's skin.

It is recommended that a patient not use this medication if a patient are taking heart medication. The local anesthetics in this cream can interact with some heart medicines.

Another analgesic cream that is available is a combination of methyl salicylate and menthol. This is a cream that is effective for the temporary relief of arthritis and pain in a patient's muscles. A patient should not use this medicine if a patient's skin is sensitive to the oil of wintergreen.

A patient should apply this cream around the sore areas on a patient's body. A patient should not apply this cream more than three times a day. Do not place this cream over areas of the skin that are broken

Steroid creams are sometimes used for the treatment of joint pain. Topical steroids are anti-inflammatory agents. Pramoxine hydrochloride is a topical anesthetic agent that sometimes is combined with steroids to attempt to manage pain. This cream provides a temporary relief from pain.

A patient should not use this cream if a patient is allergic to any of the substances in the cream such as the steroid or the pramoxineIf a patient develop a rash or blistering, a patient must stop using the cream. A patient should not use this cream more than three times a day.

Furthermore, do not use this steroid preparation for more than five days. Do not reuse this cream until a patient has discussed the situation with the patient's doctor.

Nonsteroidal anti-inflammatory agents (NSAIDS) that are commonly taken by mouth for the treatment of bone, joint, and muscle pain may be placed into a cream by a patient's pharmacist. For these drugs to give a patient pain relief, they must penetrate a patient's skin and enter a patient's bloodstream.

These creams should not be used more than three times a day. Side effects with the nonsteroidal anti-inflammatory creams are the same as with the NSAIDs taken by mouth.

However, the side effects of the topical NSAIDS are less than the oral NSAIDS. The side effects of any NSAID can include stomach upset and allergic reactions. If the dose is high enough, it could affect a patient's liver and kidneys. The Voltaren gel and the Flector patch are two examples of topical NSAIDs.

These NSAIDs can be very effective for the management of a patient's pain when applied over a patient's skin. The use of a ketoprofen gel and a diclofenac gel, both NSAIDs, were compared at painful sites in a four-week study.

The ketoprofen gel gave positive results for the treatment of knee pain and was shown to be better at relieving pain than the diclofenac gel. If a patient has joint pain, a patient may want to discuss these facts with a patient's pain-medicine doctor or orthopedic doctor. Aspirin creams also may provide a patient with some pain relief when applied over a patient's painful joints or muscles.

New research is being done into the topical administration of amitriptyline and ketamine. Ketamine is a potent analgesic that can cause a patient to hallucinate if the dose is too high. A study in animals has used both of these agents together to treat pain in the laboratory setting.

Currently available therapies are limited. However, the intermittent application of large-dose topical capsaicin may provide significant pain relief, decrease chronic analgesic dependence, and decrease aggregate health care expenditures.5

Amitriptyline, which is an antidepressant, has recently been shown to have pain-relieving properties when applied topically. Amitriptyline cream may be advantageous if a patient do not want to take amitriptyline pills by mouth.

The amitriptyline cream will not help a patient if a patient are suffering from significant depression, but can be helpful in decreasing a patient's pain. Some people complain of being tired while taking amitriptyline.

However, amitriptyline can contribute to pain relief in fibromyalgia and the topical application may be a way of avoiding significant side effects that can be associated with oral use. There is ongoing research in this area. A patient may want to keep informed of the research on both of these drugs through the National Library of Medicine website at www.nlm.nih.gov.

Another popular patch that is readily available by prescription from a patient's pain-management doctor is the lidocaine-containing patch called Lidoderm. The Lidoderm transdermal drug-delivery system exerts a significant amount of its pain-relieving effects by releasing a small amount of lidocaine into a patient's bloodstream.

There also is an effect on the nerves under a patient's skin that are transmitting pain. The Lidoderm patch contains 5 percent lidocaine. The lidocaine essentially does not reach a patient's bloodstream like fentanyl does in the fentanyl transdermal patch delivery system.

The lidocaine penetrates a patient's skin just enough to reach the nerve endings that are transmitting a patient's pain. As a result, there are minimal side effects from the use of this patch other than from the adhesive layer of the patch.

The amount of the lidocaine that is absorbed from the Lidoderm is related to the length of application over a patient's skin.

The patch should be used for 12 hours over a patient's painful area and then removed for 12 hours. If an irritation or a burning sensation occurs around the adhesive aspect of the patch, a patient should discontinue use of the patch. None of the patches mentioned in this chapter should ever be reused.

The Lidoderm patch has a polyester felt backing covered with a polyethylene film release liner. Prior to applying the patch on a patient's skin, the release liner must be removed. Be aware that the patch does contain methylparaben, which is found in many suntan lotions and can cause an allergic reaction.

Do not use the Lidoderm patch if a patient has allergies to any suntan lotions that contain this chemical. Support for improved pain and functional outcome with early adjunct treatment of CRPS with topical lidocaine ointment.6

Clonidine is another transdermal medication. This patch is applied weekly to an area of a patient's skin. The clonidine patch inhibits the release of norepinephrine, which is a RSD/CRPS pain transmitter. The clonidine patch also is used for the treatment of hypertension.

If a patient have neuropathic (nerve injury) pain or reflex sympathetic dystrophy, the clonidine patch may provide a patient with significant pain relief. It can significantly decrease the burning component of a patient's pain.

Topical treatments aimed at improving microvascular function by increasing both arterial and capillary blood flow produce effective analgesia for CRPS.4 The use of topical ketamine as opposed to parenteral and oral forms which often result in undesirable side effects.7

Topical application of ketamine appears to be beneficial for the patients with acute early dystrophic stage of CRPS I because of either its local anesthetic effect or NMDA receptor antagonist action. Patients with chronic atrophic stage of CRPS I and CRPS II patients do not appear to respond to this treatment.8

Chronic pain, whether arising from viscera, bone, or any other tissue or structure, is, more often than commonly thought, the result of a mixture of pain mechanisms, and therefore there is no simple formula available to manage chronic complex pain states.9

A multimodal stepped care approach has been successfully applied to a patient with complex regional pain syndrome type 1 and severe intractable pain, not responding to regular neuropathic pain medications.

The choice to administer drugs in creams was made because of the intolerable adverse effects to oral medication. With this method, peak-dose adverse effects did not occur. The multimodal stepped care approach resulted in considerable and clinically relevant decrease in pain after every step, using topical amitriptyline, ketamine, and dimethylsulphoxide.10

Physicians have been drawn to the adjuvant treatments secondary to new realities of clinical practice. Moreover, aversion to addiction and diversion remains a potent force that shapes prescribing profiles.9

The relative benefit of oral medications compared with the widely used treatments of intensive physical therapy, nerve blocks, sympathectomy, intraspinally administered drugs, and neuromodulatory therapies (eg, spinal cord stimulation) remains uncertain.

In summary, treatment of CRPS has received insufficient study and remains largely empirical.11 A patient can conclude however that some topical drugs may be effective for control of his/her RSD/CRPS pain. In summary, treatment of CRPS has received insufficient study and remains largely empirical.11

There are however, no good studies to date which indicate complete resolution of CRPS however with the use of topical analgesic agents.

Studies do however; demonstrate promise for topical medicine combinations as a useful treatment in multimodal therapy for patients with CRPS, with the potential to resolve pain/symptoms in early CRPS patients.

Growing evidence indicates that patients with complex regional pain syndrome exhibit tissue abnormalities caused by microvascular dysfunction in the blood vessels of skin, muscle, and nerve.

Animal studies suggests that topical treatments aimed at improving microvascular function by increasing both arterial and capillary blood flow produce effective analgesia for CRPS.4

Driven by these findings, researchers assessed the outcomes of CRPS patients treated with a compound analgesic cream (CAC) consisting of ketamine 10%, pentoxifylline 6%, clonidine 0.2%, and dimethyl sulfoxide 6% to 10%.

Results of this study demonstrated promise for this topical combination as a useful treatment in multimodal therapy for patients with CRPS, with the potential to resolve pain/symptoms in early CRPS patients.12

References
1.   Pappagallo M, Rosenberg AD. Epidemiology, pathophysi-ology, and management of complex regional pain syndrome. Pain Pract. 2001;1(1):11-20.
2.   Gammaitoni A, Gallagher RM, Welz-Bosna M. Topical ketamine gel: possible role in treating neuropathic pain. Pain Med. 2000;1(1):97-100.
3.   Zuurmond WW, Langendijk PN, Bezemer PD, Brink HE, de Lange JJ, van loenen AC. Treatment of acute reflex sympathetic dystrophy with DMSO 50% in a fatty cream. Acta Anaesthesiol Scand. 1996;40(3):364-367.
4.   Laferriere A, Abaji R, Tsai CY, Ragavendran JV, Coderre TJ. Topical combinations to treat microvascular dysfunction of chronic postischemia pain. Anesth Analg. 2014;118(4):830-840.
5.   Robbins WR, Staats PS, Levine J, et al. Treatment of in-tractable pain with topical large-dose capsaicin: preliminary report. Anesth Analg. 1998;86(3):579-583.
6.   Hanlan AK, Mah-Jones D, Mills PB. Early adjunct treat-ment with topical lidocaine results in improved pain and function in a patient with complex regional pain syndrome. Pain Physician. 2014;17(5):E629-635.
7.   Finch PM, Knudsen L, Drummond PD. Reduction of allo-dynia in patients with complex regional pain syndrome: A double-blind placebo-controlled trial of topical ketamine. Pain. 2009;146(1-2):18-25.
8.   Ushida T, Tani T, Kanbara T, Zinchuk VS, Kawasaki M, Yamamoto H. Analgesic effects of ketamine ointment in patients with complex regional pain syndrome type 1. Reg Anesth Pain Med. 2002;27(5):524-528.
9.   Knotkova H, Pappagallo M. Adjuvant analgesics. Med Clin North Am. 2007;91(1):113-124.
10.   Kopsky DJ, Keppel Hesselink JM. Multimodal Stepped Care Approach Involving Topical Analgesics for Severe Intractable Neuropathic Pain in CRPS Type 1: A Case Report. Case Rep Med. 2011;2011:319750.
11.   Rowbotham MC. Pharmacologic management of complex regional pain syndrome. Clin J Pain. 2006;22(5):425-429.

12.   Russo MA, Santarelli DM. A Novel Compound Analgesic Cream (Ketamine, Pentoxifylline, Clonidine, DMSO) for Complex Regional Pain Syndrome Patients. Pain Pract. 2016;16(1):E14-20.

22. Other Medications

Chronic pain, whether arising from viscera, bone, or any other tissue or structure, is, more often than commonly thought, the result of a mixture of pain mechanisms, and therefore there is no simple formula available to manage chronic complex pain states.

Few randomized controlled trials of oral pharmacotherapy have been performed in patients with complex regional pain syndrome (CRPS). The prevalence of CRPS is uncertain. Severe and advanced cases of CRPS are easily recognized but difficult to treat and constitute a minority compared with those who meet minimum criteria for the diagnosis.1

Various drug strategies in the treatment of the complex regional pain syndrome (CRPS) type I, i.e. NSAIDs, corticosteroids, free radical scavengers, antidepressants, anticonvulsants, local anesthetics, opioid analgesics, clonidine, capsaicin, NMDA receptor antagonists, calcitonin, bisphosphonates, GABA(B)-agonists, alpha-blockers, IV (bretylium/ketanserin), IV (clonidine), IVSB, local anesthetics sympathetic blockade, and iloprost have all been reported .2 However no consistent efficacy has been reported with these therapies.

Fibromyalgia syndrome (FMS) a central nervous system entity is currently perceived by rheumatologists and pain physicians alike as representing the classic condition of central sensitization. This term has come to denote a condition in which chronic, widespread pain is attributed mainly to an increase in the processing and handling of pain by the central nervous system.3 CRPS (complex regional pain syndrome) is also a condition of the central nervous system. Some medication (pregabilin) is helpful in reducing pain in both entities.

Both the dorsal root ganglia and the spinal cord are important sites contributing to CB(2) receptor-mediated analgesia and that the changes in CB(2) receptor expression play a crucial role for the sites of action in regulating pain perception. Cannabinoid CB(2) receptor activation by selective agonists has been shown to produce analgesic effects in preclinical models of inflammatory and neuropathic pain.4

The experience of chronic pain is one of the commonest reasons individuals seek medical attention, making the management of chronic pain a major issue in clinical practice. Drug metabolism and responses are affected by many factors, with genetic variations offering only a partial explanation of an individual's response. There is a paucity of evidence for the benefits of pharmacogenetic testing in the context of pain management.5

Over the past five years, there has been a considerable increase in clinical research on cannabinoid use for a range of pain syndromes. Cannabinoid products are becoming available for research and clinical use. Clinical trial data in the field of pain management and suggests that the potential for cannabinoid therapy for chronic pain states is encouraging.6

Medical marijuana has been approved for use in 23 states, and the law in Illinois allows patients with one of 40 specified medical conditions, including complex regional pain syndrome/reflex sympathetic dystrophy (CRPS/RSD), to get a doctor's recommendation to buy marijuana from one of the state's approved dispensaries. Physicians involved in the treatment of CRPS patients are required to keep up-to-date on these promising avenues of progress and to be ready to incorporate them into clinical use.

Despite the benefits, medical marijuana still faces a great deal of opposition. It remains illegal under federal law and is classified, along with heroin and LSD, as Level I, the most dangerous level of drug. The American Psychiatric Association (APA) has stated that there is no scientific evidence that marijuana use benefits a psychiatric disorder, and the American Medical Association (AMA) does not advocate the use of marijuana as medicine.

The U.S. Food and Drug Administration (FDA) is currently reviewing all of the medical literature pertaining to the medicinal use of marijuana, and could recommend the rescheduling or descheduling of marijuana, opening the door for research and better access.

Mammalian tissues contain at least two types of cannabinoid receptor, CB(1), found mainly on neurones and CB(2), found mainly in immune cells. Endogenous ligands for these receptors have also been identified. These endocannabinoids and their receptors constitute the endogenous cannabinoid system.

The contribution of CB1-type receptors expressed on the peripheral terminals of nociceptors to cannabinoid-induced analgesia is paramount, which should enable the development of peripherally acting CB1 analgesic agonists without any central side effects.7

Future research is likely to be directed at characterizing the endogenous cannabinoid system more completely, at obtaining more conclusive clinical data about cannabinoids with regard to both beneficial and adverse effects, at developing improved cannabinoid formulations and modes of administration for use in the clinic and at devising clinical strategies for separating out the sought-after effects of CB(1) receptor agonists from their psychotropic and other unwanted effects.8

There are at least two types of cannabinoid receptors, CB(1) and CB(2), both coupled to G proteins. CB(1) receptors exist primarily on central and peripheral neurons, one of their functions being to modulate neurotransmitter release. CB(2) receptors are present mainly on immune cells.9

Strong laboratory evidence now underwrites anecdotal claims of cannabinoid analgesia in inflammatory and neuropathic pain. Sites of analgesic action have been identified in brain, spinal cord and the periphery, with the latter two presenting attractive targets for divorcing the analgesic and psychotrophic effects of cannabinoids.10 Such inhibitors have therapeutic potential as animal data suggest that released endocannabinoids mediate reductions both in inflammatory pain and in the spasticity and tremor of multiple sclerosis.

A study evaluated the safety of cannabis use by patients with chronic pain over 1 year. The study found that there was a higher rate of adverse events among cannabis users compared with controls but not for serious adverse events at an average dose of 2.5 g herbal cannabis per day.11 Preliminary studies suggest that the synthetic cannabinoid nabilone might be an effective therapy in patients with neuropathic pain.12

Although there is still a need for randomized controlled trials, preliminary studies have suggested that medical marijuana and related cannabinoids may be beneficial in treating people with chronic pain, inflammation, spasticity, and other conditions seen commonly in physical therapist practice. Clinicians however, should be aware that marijuana can produce untoward effects on cognition, coordination, balance, and cardiovascular and pulmonary function and should be vigilant for any problems that may arise if patients are using cannabinoids during physical rehabilitation.13

Cannabinoids appear to be safe in low and medium doses. Methodological limitations of the trials limited the ability to make sound conclusions. Further research is warranted before efficacy, safety, and utility of cannabinoids for chronic pain can be determined.

Ketamine hydrochloride (KET), an agent used for general anesthesia, has local anesthetic effects and N-methyl-D-aspartate (NMDA) receptor antagonist action. Because recent studies emphasized the role of peripherally distributed NMDA receptors in processing the nociceptive information, a study investigated whether peripheral application of the ointment containing KET is able to attenuate the symptoms of local neuropathic pain.14

Findings suggest in another study that at a 6-week follow up: (1) deep ketamine therapy is effective for relief of pain CRPS I and (2) there were no adverse cognitive effects of extended treatment with deep ketamine infusion. No definitive conclusions could be drawn about the relationship between mood and personality factors and the presence of CRPS I.15

Patients with chronic atrophic stage of CRPS I and CRPS II patients did not appear to respond to this treatment. Chronic, refractory complex regional pain syndrome remains very difficult to treat. However, a sub-anesthetic low-dose ketamine has shown promise in advanced CRPS.16 Furthermore, treatment with intravenous ketamine appeared to be effective in completely resolving intractable pain caused by severe refractory CRPS I.17

The synergistic effect of the ketamine and dexmedetomidine together is shown to provide excellent symptom relief while decreasing the total ketamine administered. The combination minimized unwanted side effects and eliminated the need for intensive care unit admission secondary to anesthetic doses of ketamine.18

Patients with CRPS receiving long-term frequent ketamine treatment showed impairment in cognitive function (specifically executive function) compared with those who do not. These findings may have implications for clinical assessment and rehabilitation of cognitive function in CRPS patients.19

Sympathetic ganglion block (SGB) or intravenous regional block (IVRB) has been recommended for pain management in patients with complex regional pain syndrome type I (CRPS-I). Drowsiness, the most frequent side effect, and dry mouth occurred only in patients submitted to SGB with lidocaine combined with clonidine. However, IVRB seems to be preferable to SGB due to its easier execution and lower risk of undesirable effects.20

In a population of mostly chronic CRPS-1 patients with severe pain at baseline, a multiple day ketamine infusion resulted in significant pain relief without functional improvement. Treatment with ketamine was safe with psychomimetic side effects that were acceptable to most patients.21

Data indicated that while ketamine's effect on acute experimental pain is driven by pharmacokinetics, its effect on CRPS pain persisted beyond the infusion period when drug concentrations were below the analgesia threshold for acute pain. This indicates a disease modulatory role for ketamine in CRPS-1 pain, possibly via desensitization of NMDAR in the spinal cord or restoration of inhibitory sensory control in the brain.22

Long-term ketamine treatment is effective in causing pain relief in CRPS-1 patients with analgesia outlasting the treatment period by 50 days. These data suggest that ketamine initiated a cascade of events, including desensitization of excitatory receptor systems in the central nervous system, which persisted but slowly abated when ketamine molecules were no longer present.23

There is an increased risk for development of ketamine-induced liver injury when the infusion is prolonged and/or repeated within a short time frame. Regular measurements of liver function are therefore required during such treatments.24 Some patients are resistant to multiple therapies but responsive to oral ketamine. With respect to oral ketamine, this drug should be administered after an intravenous trial to monitor response and side effects in patients with an adequate functional status. 25

Intra thecal baclofen appears to be an option for patients with intractable CRPS who have failed other modalities, including IT morphine.26 There is evidence to support the use of IV bisphosphonates, immunoglobulin, ketamine, or lidocaine as valuable interventions in selected patients with CRPS. However, high-quality studies are required to further evaluate the safety, efficacy, and cost-effectiveness of IV therapies for CRPS.27

A previous suggests however, that limited subanesthetic inpatient infusions of ketamine may offer a promising therapeutic option in the treatment of appropriately selected patients with intractable CRPS.28 Current literature on the other hand supports the effectiveness of ketamine in blocking central sensitization through its effects on the NMDA receptor. Mre study is needed to further establish the safety and efficacy of this novel approach.

Intravenous infusions of certain pharmacologic agents have been known to provide substantial pain relief in patients with various chronic painful conditions. Some of these infusions are better, and although not necessarily the first therapeutic choice, have been widely used and extensively studied.

Non-opiate intravenous infusions that have been utilized for chronic painful disorders such as fibromyalgia, neuropathic pain, phantom limb pain, post-herpetic neuralgia, complex regional pain syndromes (CRPS), diabetic neuropathy, and central pain related to stroke or spinal cord injuries.

The management of patients with chronic pain conditions is challenging and continues to evolve as new treatment modalities are explored and tested. The following intravenous infusions used to treat chronic pain conditions include lidocaine, ketamine, phentolamine, dexmedetomidine, and bisphosphonates.29

References

1. Rowbotham MC. Pharmacologic management of complex regional pain syndrome. Clin J Pain. 2006;22(5):425-429.

2. Von Eisenhart-Rothe R, Rittmeister M. [Drug therapy in complex regional pain syndrome type I]. Orthopade. 2004;33(7):796-803.

3. Ablin JN, Buskila D. Emerging therapies for fibromyalgia: an update. Expert Opin Emerg Drugs. 2010;15(3):521-533.

4. Hsieh GC, Pai M, Chandran P, et al. Central and peripheral sites of action for CB(2) receptor mediated analgesic activity in chronic inflammatory and neuropathic pain models in rats. Br J Pharmacol. 2011;162(2):428-440.

5. Kapur BM, Lala PK, Shaw JL. Pharmacogenetics of chronic pain management. Clin Biochem. 2014;47(13-14):1169-1187.

6. Ware M, Beaulieu P. Cannabinoids for the treatment of pain: an update on recent clinical trials. Pain Res Manag. 2005;10 Suppl A:27A-30A.

7. Agarwal N, Pacher P, Tegeder I, et al. Cannabinoids mediate analgesia largely via peripheral type 1 cannabinoid receptors in nociceptors. Nat Neurosci. 2007;10(7):870-879.

8. Pertwee RG. Neuropharmacology and therapeutic potential of cannabinoids. Addict Biol. 2000;5(1):37-46.

9. Pertwee RG, Ross RA. Cannabinoid receptors and their ligands. Prostaglandins Leukot Essent Fatty Acids. 2002;66(2-3):101-121.

10. Beaulieu P, Rice AS. [The pharmacology of cannabinoid derivatives: are there applications to treatment of pain?]. Ann Fr Anesth Reanim. 2002;21(6):493-508.

11.   Ware MA, Wang T, Shapiro S, Collet JP, team Cs. Cannabis for the Management of Pain: Assessment of Safety Study (COMPASS). J Pain. 2015;16(12):1233-1242.

12.   Staud R, Koo EB. Are cannabinoids a new treatment option for pain in patients with fibromyalgia? Nat Clin Pract Rheumatol. 2008;4(7):348-349.

13.   Ciccone CD. Medical Marijuana: Just the Beginning of a Long, Strange Trip? Phys Ther. 2016.

14.   Ushida T, Tani T, Kanbara T, Zinchuk VS, Kawasaki M, Yamamoto H. Analgesic effects of ketamine ointment in patients with complex regional pain syndrome type 1. Reg Anesth Pain Med. 2002;27(5):524-528.

15.   Koffler SP, Hampstead BM, Irani F, et al. The neurocognitive effects of 5 day anesthetic ketamine for the treatment of refractory complex regional pain syndrome. Arch Clin Neuropsychol. 2007;22(6):719-729.

16.   Puchalski P, Zyluk A. Results of the Treatment of Chronic, Refractory CRPS with Ketamine Infusions: a Preliminary Report. Handchir Mikrochir Plast Chir. 2016;48(3):143-147.

17.   Shirani P, Salamone AR, Schulz PE, Edmondson EA. Ketamine treatment for intractable pain in a patient with severe refractory complex regional pain syndrome: a case report. Pain Physician. 2008;11(3):339-342.

18.   Nama S, Meenan DR, Fritz WT. The use of sub-anesthetic intravenous ketamine and adjuvant dexmedetomidine when treating acute pain from CRPS. Pain Physician. 2010;13(4):365-368.

19.   Kim M, Cho S, Lee JH. The Effects of Long-Term Ketamine Treatment on Cognitive Function in Complex Regional Pain Syndrome: A Preliminary Study. Pain Med. 2016;17(8):1447-1451.

20.   Nascimento MS, Klamt JG, Prado WA. Intravenous regional block is similar to sympathetic ganglion block for pain management in patients with complex regional pain syndrome type I. Braz J Med Biol Res. 2010;43(12):1239-1244.

21.   Sigtermans MJ, van Hilten JJ, Bauer MC, et al. Ketamine produces effective and long-term pain relief in patients with Complex Regional Pain Syndrome Type 1. Pain. 2009;145(3):304-311.

22.   Sigtermans M, Noppers I, Sarton E, et al. An observational study on the effect of S+-ketamine on chronic pain versus experimental

acute pain in Complex Regional Pain Syndrome type 1 patients. Eur J Pain. 2010;14(3):302-307.

23.   Dahan A, Olofsen E, Sigtermans M, et al. Population pharmacokinetic-pharmacodynamic modeling of ketamine-induced pain relief of chronic pain. Eur J Pain. 2011;15(3):258-267.

24.   Noppers IM, Niesters M, Aarts LP, et al. Drug-induced liver injury following a repeated course of ketamine treatment for chronic pain in CRPS type 1 patients: a report of 3 cases. Pain. 2011;152(9):2173-2178.

25.   Soto E, Stewart DR, Mannes AJ, et al. Oral ketamine in the palliative care setting: a review of the literature and case report of a patient with neurofibromatosis type 1 and glomus tumor-associated complex regional pain syndrome. Am J Hosp Palliat Care. 2012;29(4):308-317.

26.   Zuniga RE, Perera S, Abram SE. Intrathecal baclofen: a useful agent in the treatment of well-established complex regional pain syndrome. Reg Anesth Pain Med. 2002;27(1):90-93.

27.   Xu J, Yang J, Lin P, Rosenquist E, Cheng J. Intravenous Therapies for Complex Regional Pain Syndrome: A Systematic Review. Anesth Analg. 2016;122(3):843-856.

28.   Correll GE, Maleki J, Gracely EJ, Muir JJ, Harbut RE. Subanesthetic ketamine infusion therapy: a retrospective analysis of a novel therapeutic approach to complex regional pain syndrome. Pain Med. 2004;5(3):263-275.

29.   Kosharskyy B, Almonte W, Shaparin N, Pappagallo M, Smith H. Intravenous infusions in chronic pain management. Pain Physician. 2013;16(3):231-249.

23. Sympathetically Maintained Pain

Complex regional pain syndrome (CRPS) is clinically characterized by pain, abnormal regulation of blood flow and sweating, edema of skin and subcutaneous tissues, trophic changes of skin, appendages of skin and subcutaneous tissues, and active and passive movement disorders. The changes suggest that the CNS representations of the systems have been altered.

Acute Complex Regional Pain Syndrome (CRPS) is associated with signs of inflammation such as increased skin temperature, edema, skin color changes and pain. Patients with CRPS also have peripheral changes (eg, edema, signs of inflammation, sympathetic-afferent coupling (the basis for sympathetically maintained pain), and trophic changes) that cannot be explained by central changes.[1]

Two types of CRPS have been recognized: type I, corresponds to RSD and occurs without a definable nerve lesion, and type II, formerly called causalgia refers to cases where a definable nerve lesion is present.

The term sympathetically maintained pain (SMP) was also evaluated and considered to be a variable phenomenon associated with a variety of disorders, including CRPS types I and II. These revised categories have been included in the 2nd edition of the IASP Classification of Chronic Pain Syndromes.[2]

The "sympathetically maintained pain" (SMP) is a symptom (and not a clinical entity) that can principally also be present in other pain syndromes.[3] Recent experimental investigations on rats show that the sympathetic nervous system is possibly also causally involved in the generation of inflammation and inflammatory pain.

The mechanisms by which this occurs are different from those operating in SMP during CRPS.

Pro-inflammatory cytokines (tumor necrosis factor-alpha (TNF-alpha), interleukin-2 (IL-2), IL-1beta, IL-6) are up-regulated, whereas anti-inflammatory cytokines (IL-4, IL-10) are diminished.

CRPS is accompanied by increased neurogenic inflammation which depends mainly on neuropeptides such as CGRP and Substance P. Besides inflammatory signs, sympathetic nervous system involvement in CRPS results in cool skin, increased sweating and sympathetically-maintained pain.[4]

The term "sympathetically maintained pain" (SMP) describes a symptom that might accompany a variety of diseases (CRPS, (post-) herpetic and post-injury neuralgia), which might transform into sympathetically independent pain (SIP) after some time. Patients with SMP present a bunch of disorders of the autonomic and sensory system, but the only reliable way to diagnose a pain as SMP is a positive response to an intervention at the sympathetic nervous system.

The sympathetic nervous system makes an unknown contribution to CRPS/RSD, but it is not known whether this is a cause or an effect of the pain. Treatment should be immediate, aggressive, and directed toward restoration of full function of the extremity.

Various analgesic techniques may be necessary to permit the patient to comply with the rehabilitation program. This program is best carried out in a comprehensive interdisciplinary setting, with a primary emphasis on functional restoration.5

SMP/ Sympathetically Maintained Pain is one of the factors common to CRPS and is significant in that almost all patients will respond to sympathetic blockade (blockage of the sympathetic nerves supplying the area with local anesthetics).

The term sympathetically maintained pain describes a symptom that might accompany a variety of diseases (CRPS, post- herpetic and post-injury neuralgia), which might transform into sympathetically independent pain (SIP) after some time.

Patients with SMP present a bunch of disorders of the autonomic and sensory system, but the only reliable way to diagnose a pain as SMP is a positive response to an intervention at the sympathetic nervous system.6 Sympatholytic interventions are recommended only for the subgroup of patients with sympathetically maintained pain.

The sympathetic nervous system has been implicated in numerous pain syndromes while interruption of the sympathetic flow has been proven to relieve certain pain syndromes.

The term "sympathetically maintained pain" does not imply that the pains are due to the sympathetic system. It is not a matter of excessive or decreased sympathetic activity. The extreme sensitivity and hyperpathia are removed by blocking the sympathetic supply, also when the lesion is central to the blocked region.7

Sympathetically maintained pain syndrome is considered to be a clinical form of reflex sympathetic dystrophy. It develops usually after trauma, and consists of continuous, burning pain with sympathetic component. Previous studies have suggested that sympathetic sprouting in the periphery may contribute to the development and persistence of sympathetically maintained pain in animal models of neuropathic pain.8

The treatment recommendations in patients with SMP vary in dependence of the kind of disease. In SMP, invasive measures play an important, but only limited role within the comprehensive treatment concept.

This fact suggests that we are not concerned primarily with abnormal states induced by the sympathetic system, but with a general kind of abnormality of the total nervous system. This phenomenon may be relieved by removal of the sympathetic nerves to the relevant neurons of the periphery with sympathetic injections.

In CRPS patients with sympathetically maintained pain, a few temporary blocks of the sympathetic innervation of the affected extremity sometimes lead to long-lasting (even permanent) pain relief and to resolution of the other changes observed in CRPS.9

Sympathetic nerve blocks should be performed at least once to assess if sympathetically maintained pain is present. To the extent that peripheral somatosensory nerve blocks can diminish nociceptive input to the central nervous system, these techniques may help reduce the nociceptive sensitization of spinal neurons.

Neuropathic pain syndromes may be treated by intervention at the sympathetic nervous system. The pain in these syndromes is therefore called sympathetically maintained pain (SMP). Typical disorders with a SMP component are complex regional pain syndromes (reflex sympathetic dystrophy and causalgia), traumatic neuralgias and herpes zoster.10

Pain relief, however it is achieved and however temporary it is, is intended to facilitate participation in functional therapies to normalize use and to improve motion, strength, and dexterity.

Psychologic therapies, such as biofeedback and cognitive-behavioral techniques targeting pain, stress, and mood disorders, are valuable adjunctive treatments for pain control and can facilitate functional improvement.

Sympathetically maintained pain is one factor common to CRPS and causalgia in that almost all patients will respond to sympathetic blockade (blockage of the sympathetic nerves supplying the area with local anesthetics), which will take away their pain for a variable length of time. The term RSD was first used by Evans in 1946.

However, many patients do not present with the full-blown syndrome that includes all the signs listed above, but do respond to a sympathetic blockade. For example, a patient may come to a doctor with pain only. At the site of the precipitating event, pain occurs presenting with a glove-and-stocking anatomical distribution.

The sympathetic nervous system and inflammation interact: norepinephrine influences the immune system and the production of cytokines. There is substantial evidence that this interaction contributes to the pathophysiology and clinical presentation of CRPS.[4]

A previous study examined the effect of an intradermal injection of phenylephrine an adrenoceptor agonist in normal subjects, and patients with sympathetically-independent and sympathetically-maintained pain.

Normal subjects and patients with sympathetically-independent pain experienced only brief stinging pain, while subsets of both sympathectomized and non-sympathectomized SMP patients experienced an additional abnormal pain response accompanied by mechano-allodynia around the injection site.[11]

Abnormal pain response evoked by norepinephrine or phenylephrine injection in the ipsilateral symptomatic limb of SMP patients may be due to injury-evoked nociceptor responsiveness to catecholamines. However, such a response in contralateral asymptomatic limbs suggests an additional factor that more likely than not is of central origin and may or may not be related to sympathectomy and its success or failure to treat pain.

There are three stages of RSD. Stage I: Beginning within a few days or weeks of the precipitating event, this stage is characterized by pain, and often by burning, in the area of the injury. There is frequently hyperesthesia as well. Movement worsens pain, and immobility of the limb is obvious by its protected position. Stage II: As the RSD progresses, pain can increase or decrease or remain unchanged.

There may be beginnings of local hyperesthesia, abnormal sensations, or allodynia. Swelling spreads, local joints become stiff, muscle wasting in the region of the injury begins, and the skin may become cold, pale, cyanotic, and moist.

Stage III: This stage is marked by severe trophic changes and resistance to treatment. The pain is variable, with increased spreading allodynia and mistaken sense of sensation, e.g. soft touch feels like pin pricks. The pain is usually a burning discomfort, which is often aching or throbbing. Exposure to cold air or a draft may aggravate the pain, as may damp weather. Extreme immobility of the limb is present.

The skin is shiny, cold, and often damp. RSD can spread, usually to the opposite side limb. This occurs in 25% of cases. Some investigators report a fourth stage of CRPS. In the fourth stage, CRPS is resistant to many forms of treatment. Not all Doctors however agree on the existence of a Fourth Stage.

CRPS is an evolving and constantly changing disease. The symptoms you have today may not be Symptoms depend on how the body is reacts to the environment at a particular time. Triple phase bone scanning is a very sensitive corroborative test to confirm the clinical suspicion of CRPS during the initial stages, but not in late cases.12

Three current hypotheses that propose both a site and method for sympathetic-sensory coupling: (i) direct coupling between sympathetic and sensory neurons in the dorsal root ganglion; (ii) chemical coupling between sympathetic and nociceptive neuron terminals in skin; and (iii) the development of a-adrenoceptor-mediated super sensitivity in nociceptive fibers in skin in association with the release of inflammatory mediators.13

Another hypothesis is one that integrates the mechanisms of chemical coupling and a-adrenoceptor-mediated super sensitivity. A histological substrate suitable for sympathetic-sensory coupling exists in normal subjects. In the diseased state, the nociceptive fibers implicated in this substrate may be activated by both endogenous and exogenous noradrenaline.

Previous studies have suggested that sympathetic sprouting in the periphery may contribute to the development and persistence of sympathetically maintained pain in animal models of neuropathic pain.8

There may not be allodynia, swelling or muscle spasms or any of the other factors relevant to the diagnosis of RSD. However, a sympathetic blockade takes away the pain. In fact, patients can present with any of the symptoms of RSD on their own.

If patients respond to sympathetic blocks, they are then defined as having sympathetically maintained pain. Sensitized mechano-insensitive nociceptors can be activated by endogenously released catecholamines and thereby may contribute to sympathetically maintained pain.14

Sympatholytic interventions are recommended only for the subgroup of patients with sympathetically maintained pain. The classical targets for sympathetic blockade are the stellate (cervicothoracic) sympathetic ganglia (for the upper extremities) and the lumbar sympathetic ganglia for lower extremity RSD.

In the beginning nearly all CRPS pain is sympathetically-mediated. This type of pain is very responsive to local pain reduction efforts, most notably sympathetic nerve blocks, but also includes topical creams, massage, etc. Only a very small percentage of the pain is sympathetically independent.

As time passes, 6 to 9 months, the pain gradually changes. The percentage of sympathetically-mediated is decreased and the percentage of SIP is increased. As CRPS progresses, more and more of the pain becomes sympathetically independent. It becomes centered or generated in the brain. It actually becomes independent of the injury.

If one blocks the sympathetic nervous system and the pain goes away, but it doesn't go away with a placebo, then sympathetically-maintained pain is present. If the pain doesn't resolve, or if it disappears both with sympathetic blockade and with placebo, then it is sympathetically-independent pain.

Some CRPS Types I and II are sympathetically-maintained pain, some are sympathetically-independent pain and some have elements of both. The entire sympathetic maintained pain component is not constant in the course of the disease but decreases over time.15

Animal models establish an important role for the sympathetic nervous system in many forms of neuropathic and inflammatory pain. Damage to rats' sciatic nerves by tying them, and other damage, gives rise to a syndrome that we could recognize as a complex regional pain syndrome in humans.16

Sympathectomy is often effective. Sympathectomy is a surgical procedure that destroys nerves in the sympathetic nervous system. The procedure is done to increase blood flow. However, there are qualifications here. In some groups it is only effective during the first 10 days after surgery. In other groups, it affects only thermal hyperalgesia.

A therapy to avoid however, due to lack of efficacy or a high likelihood of adverse outcomes is a sympathectomy.17

Tactile allodynia and cold allodynia in the neuropathic pain model are not dependent on the sympathetic nervous system, and this model can be used to investigate sympathetically-independent pain syndromes. The practice of surgical and chemical sympathectomy for neuropathic pain and CRPS is however based on very little high quality evidence.

Sympathectomy should be used cautiously in clinical practice, in carefully selected patients, and probably only after failure of other treatment options.18

To diagnose CRPS, there has to have been an injury. There has to be pain out of proportion to that injury, perhaps accompanied by hyperalgesia. There has to be edema or skin blood flow changes, compared with the other side, or abnormal sweating. Investigations can show whether or not this is sympathetically-maintained. If a nerve has been damaged, and there is clinical evidence of this, this is a CRPS Type II. Sympathetic blocks are useful in the diagnosis of sympathetically-maintained pain. 19

However, their value is limited by the potential for false positives (unintentional sensory block) or false negatives (insufficient sensory block). Adequate monitoring of the sympathetic and somatosensory function for a minimum of 90 minutes after the intervention is essential to ensure that a valid diagnosis of sympathetically-mediated is made.

Sympathetically-maintained is diagnosable only by means of placebo-controlled sympathetic blockade. Thus a person cannot be said to have it unless this has been done.

Sympathetic nerve blocks should be performed at least once to assess if sympathetically maintained pain is present.20 To the extent that peripheral somatosensory nerve blocks can diminish nociceptive input to the central nervous system, these techniques may help reduce the nociceptive sensitization of spinal neurons.

Pain relief, however it is achieved and however temporary it is, is intended to facilitate participation in functional therapies to normalize use and to improve motion, strength, and dexterity.

Sensitized mechano-insensitive nociceptors can be activated by endogenously released catecholamines and thereby may contribute to sympathetically maintained pain.14

Psychologic therapies, such as biofeedback and cognitive-behavioral techniques targeting pain, stress, and mood disorders, are valuable adjunctive treatments for pain control and can facilitate functional improvement.

The understanding that sympatholysis per se is not a "diagnostic" test for CRPS, but rather a useful procedure that may facilitate treatment for pain that is sympathetically maintained.21

There is increasing evidence that inflammation in both the peripheral and central nervous systems follows some peripheral nerve injuries may be related to the clinical manifestations of CRPS. Chronic pain secondary to neuronal injury is actively and continuously modulated at multiple locations along the sensory neuraxis.22

Nociceptive fibers (the fibers that carry pain signals to the brain) have free nerve endings. The pain associated with the condition may be sympathetically maintained, sympathetically independent, or both. No evidence-based treatment regimens for CRPS/RSD are available. Treatment of the individual patient is empiric and uses symptomatic techniques that seem logical or that have been proven to be effective in other conditions.

The sympathetic nervous system makes an unknown contribution to CRPS/RSD, but it is not known whether this is a cause or an effect of the pain. Psychological and psychiatric changes are probably secondary rather than etiologic. Treatment should be immediate, aggressive, and directed toward restoration of full function of the extremity.5

These nociceptors usually respond only when a stimulus is strong enough to cause an injury to the body. These fibers all connect peripheral organs to the spinal cord. Some chronic pain conditions are maintained or enhanced by sympathetic activity. In animal models of pathological pain, abnormal sprouting of sympathetic fibers around large- and medium-sized sensory neurons is observed in dorsal root ganglia.

Large- and medium-sized cells are also more likely to be spontaneously active, suggesting that sprouting may be related to neuron activity. The sprouting could be reduced by systemic or locally applied lidocaine.23

Peripheral and central sensitization is a common feature in CRPS as in other neuropathic pain syndromes. One important mechanism is the sensitization of spinal dorsal horn cells via activation of postsynaptic NMDA-receptors by chronic C-fiber input.24

Sympathetic neural activity might contribute to pain and sensory disturbances in CRPS by feeding into nociceptive circuits at the site of injury or elsewhere in the CRPS-affected limb, within the dorsal horn, or via thalamo-cortical projections.25

The difference between the speeds at which the two types of nociceptive nerve fibers (A delta and C) conduct nerve impulses explains why, when you are injured, you first feel a sharp pain, which gives way to a more diffuse, dull pain.

Fast pain", which goes away fairly quickly, comes from the stimulation and transmission of nerve impulses over A delta fibers, while "slow pain", which persists longer, comes from stimulation and transmission over non-myelinated C fibers.

Chronic pain secondary to neuronal injury is actively and continuously modulated at multiple locations along the sensory neuraxis.22 The ascending pain pathways consist of A delta and C fibers and are called nociceptors. There are descending pain-control pathways in the brain and spinal cord.

These are neural pathways that descend from the central structures of the nervous system and diminish the pain signals travelling up the ascending pathways from the body to the brain. With CRPS, the pain impulses that travel to the brain are not diminished by the descending pathways for some reason.

Sympathetic afferent coupling takes place in the skin and in the deep somatic tissues, but especially in the acute stages of CRPS, the pain component that is influenced by the sympathetic innervation of deep somatic structures is more important than the cutaneous activation. The entire sympathetic maintained pain component is not constant in the course of the disease but decreases over time.15   The diagnosis of sympathetically maintained pain in posttraumatic complex regional pain syndrome with laser Doppler flowmetry.

Changes in regional cerebral blood flow appear to support the theory that the pathogenesis of CRPS is also related to the central nervous system. Multiple sympathetic nerve blocks in one study not only improved physical function but also reversed the CRPS symptoms, for which it was presumed that reduced nociceptive input signals led to cortical reorganization.26

Sympathetic nerve blocks should be performed at least once to assess if sympathetically maintained pain is present. To the extent that peripheral somatosensory nerve blocks can diminish nociceptive input to the central nervous system, these techniques may help reduce the nociceptive sensitization of spinal neurons.

Pain relief, however it is achieved and however temporary it is, is intended to facilitate participation in functional therapies to normalize use and to improve motion, strength, and dexterity.

Psychologic therapies, such as biofeedback and cognitive-behavioral techniques targeting pain, stress, and mood disorders, are valuable adjunctive treatments for pain control and can facilitate functional improvement.20

References

1.   Janig W, Baron R. Complex regional pain syndrome: mystery explained? Lancet Neurol. 2003;2(11):687-697.

2.   Stanton-Hicks M, Janig W, Hassenbusch S, Haddox JD, Boas R, Wilson P. Reflex sympathetic dystrophy: changing concepts and taxonomy. Pain. 1995;63(1):127-133.

3.   Baron R, Janig W. [Pain syndromes with causal participation of the sympathetic nervous system]. Anaesthesist. 1998;47(1):4-23.

4.   Schlereth T, Drummond PD, Birklein F. Inflammation in CRPS: role of the sympathetic supply. Auton Neurosci. 2014;182:102-107.

5.   Wilson PR. Complex Regional Pain Syndrome-Reflex Sympathetic Dystrophy. Curr Treat Options Neurol. 1999;1(5):466-472.

6.   Maier C, Gleim M. [Diagnostic and treatment measures in patients with sympathetically maintained pain]. Schmerz. 1998;12(4):282-303.

7.   Nathan PW. The sympathetic system and pain. Funct Neurol. 1989;4(1):11-15.

8.   Yen LD, Bennett GJ, Ribeiro-da-Silva A. Sympathetic sprouting and changes in nociceptive sensory innervation in the glabrous skin of the rat hind paw following partial peripheral nerve injury. J Comp Neurol. 2006;495(6):679-690.

9.   Janig W, Baron R. Complex regional pain syndrome is a disease of the central nervous system. Clin Auton Res. 2002;12(3):150-164.

10.   Wasner G, Baron R. [Sympathetic nervous system and pain--some open questions]. Schmerz. 1998;12(4):276-281.

11.   Mailis-Gagnon A, Bennett GJ. Abnormal contralateral pain responses from an intradermal injection of phenylephrine in a subset of patients with complex regional pain syndrome (CRPS). Pain. 2004;111(3):378-384.

12.   Pankaj A, Kotwal PP, Mittal R, Deepak KK, Bal CS. Diagnosis of post-traumatic complex regional pain syndrome of the hand: current role of sympathetic skin response and three-phase bone scintigraphy. J Orthop Surg (Hong Kong). 2006;14(3):284-290.

13.   Gibbs GF, Drummond PD, Finch PM, Phillips JK. Unravelling the pathophysiology of complex regional pain syndrome: focus on sympathetically maintained pain. Clin Exp Pharmacol Physiol. 2008;35(7):717-724.

14.   Jorum E, Orstavik K, Schmidt R, et al. Catecholamine-induced excitation of nociceptors in sympathetically maintained pain. Pain. 2007;127(3):296-301.

15.   Schattschneider J, Binder A, Siebrecht D, Wasner G, Baron R. Complex regional pain syndromes: the influence of cutaneous and deep somatic sympathetic innervation on pain. Clin J Pain. 2006;22(3):240-244.

16.   Han DW, Kweon TD, Kim KJ, Lee JS, Chang CH, Lee YW. Does the tibial and sural nerve transection model represent sympathetically independent pain? Yonsei Med J. 2006;47(6):847-851.

17.   Quisel A, Gill JM, Witherell P. Complex regional pain syndrome: which treatments show promise? J Fam Pract. 2005;54(7):599-603.

18.   Straube S, Derry S, Moore RA, Cole P. Cervico-thoracic or lumbar sympathectomy for neuropathic pain and complex regional pain syndrome. Cochrane Database Syst Rev. 2013;9:CD002918.

19.   Krumova EK, Gussone C, Regeniter S, Westermann A, Zenz M, Maier C. Are sympathetic blocks useful for diagnostic purposes? Reg Anesth Pain Med. 2011;36(6):560-567.

20.   Yung Chung O, Bruehl SP. Complex Regional Pain Syndrome. Curr Treat Options Neurol. 2003;5(6):499-511.

21.   Stanton-Hicks M. Complex regional pain syndrome. Anesthesiol Clin North America. 2003;21(4):733-744.

22.   Saab CY, Hains BC. Remote neuroimmune signaling: a long-range mechanism of nociceptive network plasticity. Trends Neurosci. 2009;32(2):110-117.

23.   Xie W, Strong JA, Li H, Zhang JM. Sympathetic sprouting near sensory neurons after nerve injury occurs preferentially on spontaneously active cells and is reduced by early nerve block. J Neurophysiol. 2007;97(1):492-502.

24.   Nickel FT, Maihofner C. [Current concepts in pathophysiology of CRPS I]. Handchir Mikrochir Plast Chir. 2010;42(1):8-14.

25.   Drummond PD. Sensory disturbances in complex regional pain syndrome: clinical observations, autonomic interactions, and possible mechanisms. Pain Med. 2010;11(8):1257-1266.

26.   Lin BF, Cherng CH, Fan YM, Wong CS, Huh BK, Yeh CC. Changes in regional cerebral blood flow and three-phase bone scan after repeated somatic nerve blocks for sympathetically independent pain. Clin Nucl Med. 2010;35(6):391-395.

24. Physical Therapy

Complex regional pain syndrome (CRPS) is a highly painful, limb-confined condition that usually arises after a trauma although its causes remain unknown. It is associated with a particularly poor quality of life, and considerable healthcare and societal costs.

Its distinct combination of abnormalities includes limb-confined inflammation and tissue hypoxia, sympathetic dysregulation, small fiber damage, serum autoantibodies, central sensitization and cortical reorganization, which place it at the crossroads of disciplines including rheumatology, pain medicine and neurology.[1]

There is currently no strong consensus regarding the optimal management of complex regional pain syndrome although a multitude of interventions have been described and are commonly used. CRPS can be classified into two types: type I (CRPS I) in which a specific nerve lesion has not been identified, and type II (CRPS II) where there is an identifiable nerve lesion. Guidelines recommend the inclusion of a variety of physiotherapy interventions as part of the multimodal treatment of people with CRPS, although their effectiveness is not known.[2]

There was low to very low quality evidence that tactile discrimination training, stellate ganglion block via ultrasound and pulsed electromagnetic field therapy compared to placebo, and manual lymphatic drainage combined with and compared to either anti-inflammatories and physical therapy or exercise are not effective for treating pain in the short-term in people with CRPS I. Interdisciplinary treatment includes physical, pharmacologic, and invasive interventional therapy, as well as stimulation techniques.[3]

Although its incidence is relatively low, the pain and suffering it causes can be severe and functionally debilitating. Early, accurate diagnosis permits initiation of appropriate therapeutic interventions and enhances the potential for successful treatment.[4]

Because CRPS 1 remains one of the most difficult pain syndromes, early diagnosis and treatment are important to have adequate functional results from physical therapy. Manipulation under general anesthesia may be an additional effective treatment tool to obtain functional improvement in some patients diagnosed with CRPS 1.[5]

Physical and/or occupational therapy can be important for the management of CRPS pain. Physical therapy is an important modality that are referred to as simply PTs. These individuals are healthcare professionals who diagnose and treat individuals of all ages, from newborns to the very oldest, who have medical problems or other health-related conditions, illnesses, or injuries that limits their abilities to move and perform functional activities as well as they would like in their daily lives. the effects of low level laser therapy and therapy with interferential current in treatment of CRPS I.6

Occupational therapists help patients improve their ability to perform tasks in living and working environments. They work with individuals who suffer from a mentally, physically, developmentally, or emotionally disabling condition. Occupational therapists use treatments to develop, recover, or maintain the daily living and work skills of their patients.

The therapist helps clients not only to improve their basic motor functions and reasoning abilities, but also to compensate for permanent loss of function. The goal is to help clients have independent, productive, and satisfying lives. A therapist will rehabilitate you following an injury.

The physical/occupational therapist will decide which treatment is best for a patient based on the overall health after an evaluation. The physical/occupational therapist will emphasize to a patient that a patient is a major component in the rehabilitation and in the management of the chronic pain. The physical/occupational therapist also will train you to avoid future re-injury and/or a recurrence of the pain problems.

Not only is a physical/occupational therapy evaluation a planned treatment course for the pain, you also will receive an education on future injury prevention. However, impairment percentages in RSD patients treated with PT or OT did not differ significantly from those treated with CT at 12 months after inclusion.7 Early diagnosis and prompt treatment with an epidural block, followed by intensive physiotherapy, are recommended.

A multimodal therapeutic concept, which includes all available possibilities, is absolutely necessary to avoid grave permanent disabilities caused by insufficient or failed therapy. Nevertheless, already established as well as new treatment modalities have to be critically observed by further randomized, prospective control trials.8

If a patient was injured in the workplace, the physical therapist will tell a patient how to avoid further injury in that environment. A patient may be placed in a work-hardening program to enable one to become maximally conditioned for the occupation. This program duplicates the regular work duties and helps increase the muscle strength and endurance so that you can return safely back to work, hopefully without further injury.

Physical therapy results in clinically relevant improvement in RSD. Costs associated with adjuvant treatment are moderate compared to other medical costs. The incremental cost-effectiveness ratios of physical therapy versus occupational therapy were moderate or even dominant.9 Pain relief and functional restoration are the primary goals of all therapeutic intervention and should start as early as possible.10

A therapist will attempt to get a patient back to normal daily activity as soon as possible in a safe manner. a patient does not want to return to activity too soon following the onset of sudden pain because of the possibility of reinjury.

When a patient sees the physical therapist on the first visit, the therapists will obtain a detailed medical history. To provide a patient with adequate treatment, the therapist will want to know the complete medical history as well as the pain history. The history that a patient telsl the therapist will give the therapist important information about the pain syndrome, the prognosis, and the appropriate time that a patient will need to be under the physical therapist's treatments.

The therapist also will assess the behavioral response to the pain associated with the injury if a patient was injured in an accident or at work. If the pain is worse in the morning and becomes progressively better during the day, this may be an indication that a patient has arthritis. Post traumatic arthritis is not uncommon after an injury to the arm or leg.

The therapist will need to know this information in order to prescribe the proper treatment. Providing a good medical history to the therapist will make it much easier for the therapist to do the proper method of treatmen. Physical therapy is widely recommended as a first-line treatment. The efficacy of local anesthetic sympathetic blockade on the other hand as treatment for CRPS I is questionable.11

The therapist will need to know if the pain is in the bones, muscles, nerves, or all of them together. If the pain is in the bones, the pain is usually confined to that particular area. If the pain is in a nerve, the pain will usually go down the arm or leg from where the therapist is pressing on the spine or neck. If the pain is in the muscles, the physical therapist will note increased contractility of the painful muscles. The therapist will examine the range of motion of the joints.

The color of the skin will be noted by the therapist. Sometimes if a patient has arthritis, there may be redness about the joints. With RSD, a patient's skin may have a bluish tint or be shiny. The hair pattern in the arms and legs will be evaluated. If a patient has decreased blood flow with the RSD, there may be a loss of hair on the skin. Movements of the joints, neck, and lower back will be done to see how flexible a patient is. Any movements that are painful will be recorded and then will be addressed during the therapy session.

The therapist will decide whether heat or cold could help a patient with the range of motion or decrease the muscle spasms, which in turn will help decrease the pain. The physical therapist's examination will emphasize the joints of the body as well as the muscles.

The examination by the therapist may be a thorough as the examination by the doctor with respect to joint movement. On examination, the therapist will try to determine what movements worsen the pain. The physical therapist will examine a patient for paralysis or a loss of the reflexes in the arms and legs.

Any shrinkage of the muscle in the arms and legs will be addressed. If a patient cannot use the arm or leg because of CRPS, the muscle will decrease in size. For example, if a patient has decreased muscle size in the thigh, the therapist will target this area to increase strength and muscle mass. The therapist will, furthermore, examine a patient for any loss of sensation in the arms and legs.

For example, if a patient has a loss of sensation in the right shoulder, the therapist will be careful not to apply heat on this area for any significant length of time. If a patient has limited range of motion about the arm or leg, the therapist will work with a patient to increase the range of motion.

A heating pad could cause a burn on the skin if a patient is unable to detect the sensation of heat about the shoulder. After the therapist has examined a patient, the therapist may call the doctor to recommend any further laboratory tests or x-rays.

After the history and physical examination has been completed, the physical therapist will determine what is causing the pain problem and will design a treatment program for you based on these findings. A patient will be treated as a complete individual, and not as just a pain symptom. If the assessment was not done thoroughly, the treatment regimen may not help you with respect to the pain syndrome.

The carefully chosen physical agents in combination with analgesic and non-steroidal anti-inflammatory drugs may benefit in patients with CRPS-1 on the upper extremity if the treatment starts as soon as possible.12 The following physical therapy regimen has been reported to be effective for the treatment of CRPS. Physical therapy management (1st three sessions) is initially focused on pain neurophysiology education with an aim to reduce kinesiophobia and reconceptualise pain perception.

Following this, pain modulation in the form of transcutaneous electrical nerve stimulation, kinesio tape application, "pain exposure" physical therapy and exercise therapy is carried out for a period of 7 weeks.13

The therapist may do a muscle and joint stabilization program to increase the strength and flexibility. A patient, on the other hand, must always feel that he/she is a main component in the rehabilitation. If the therapist gives you exercises to do at home you follow the instructions on how to do them and do them on the prescribed schedule.

The physical therapist will treat a patient with exercise and strengthening techniques, but also may complement the therapy with whirlpool baths, paraffin baths, or other methods such as using electrical current. The occupational therapist will evaluate and treat a patient with respect to function at home as well as in the workplace.

For example if you have RSD/CRPS of the hand, the therapist will teach a patient you how to use the painful hand to eat, dress etc.

Heat packs can provide a patient with surface heating, which may reduce the pain in some surface muscles in the back, arms, or legs. Ultrasound is a deep application of heat. This method can relax the deep muscles. Elastic exercise bands and medicine balls may be used to increase the arm and leg strength.

The elastic bands can be used to increase the strength, and medicine balls can be used to increase the range of motion and the flexibility as well as the strength. Some physical therapists use traction for the management of the pain. A patient should avoid ice on the affected extremity that has RSD. Cold can decrease blood flow to injured skin and muscle which will cause the RSD pain to worsen.

Electricity can be used to treat the pain syndrome as well. Over the years, many claims have been made for the therapeutic application of electrical current for the treatment of some pain syndromes. Electrical current is applied to the body by placement of electrodes, which are patches with adhesive that stick to the body. The current is directed over the painful areas of the body. Electrical current can vibrate the molecules of the tissues similar to ultrasound therapy.

The vibration produced by friction between the molecules of the tissues will increase the tissue temperature. As a result, heat is produced. As electrical current passes through the tissue, some nerves are excited while others are not. It has been shown that electricity can stimulate tissue growth and repair such as bone and is sometimes used by orthopedic surgeons to stimulate bone growth following bone surgery.

Sometimes stimulators can be placed following orthopedic surgery to enhance bone growth. Theoretically, the electrical current should speed up the healing time. A popular electrical current emitting device that is used frequently in pain medicine by conventional physicians, chiropractic physicians, and physical therapists is the transcutaneous electrical nerve stimulator (TENS).

A TENS unit applies electrical current to the body through electrodes that are adhered to the body. The TENS unit is used for pain control. The power source is battery operated. TENS unit therapy became popular in the late 1960s and early 1970s.

The use of a TENS unit for the treatment of the chronic pain syndrome if you have neck, back, arm, and leg pain is well documented. RSD pain can be controlled with a TENS unit. A TENS unit has an amplitude knob that lets the control the pain relief. These TENS units are about the size of a pager. The TENS unit patches can be placed over the muscles or nerves for the management of pain both in the muscles as well as the nerves in the arms and legs.

A patient can use a TENS unit for the control of the pain long term without any significant side effects. Some people have allergic reactions to the adhesive in the patches. Iontophoresis is another use of an electrical current to drive medications through the skin. Different medications can be applied through the skin to decrease the pain. Not only is electrical current used for pain relief, it can also speed up the tissue healing. Phonophoresis is another device that uses energy to drive medications into the body.

In addition, visiting a physical/occupational/therapist is often part of the treatment regimen. To take care of patients suffering from this condition, physical therapists often conduct electrical stimulation. The physical therapist may also perform manual techniques such as massage to decrease the pain associated with RSD. In addition, the physical therapist may prescribe desensitization techniques including sanding wood, scrubbing and carrying weights.

With early intervention and a commitment to physical therapy, the patient can reduce the pain associated with RSD. Physical therapy is primarily used to strengthen muscles (although it can also be helpful for building bone density, improving circulation, improving nerve function and endurance). Physical therapy can be "the cure" for some RSD patients while others have no response or negative responses to physical therapy.

Functional limitations should be identified. A therapist should define specific functional goals for treatment related to the affected extremity. All RSD treatment programs should include: A progressive active exercise program should include progressive weight bearing for lower extremity RSD. Progressive improvement of grip strength, pinch strength, and shoulder range of motion of the upper extremity RSD should be addressed as well.

A desensitization program using a rough texture may desensitize the painful nerve endings. For specific RSD / CRPS cases, additional treatment options may be indicated to enhance effectiveness of the above elements.

For example, bracing of the affected extremity may be necessary. Excessive exercise and physical therapy that causes fatigue, pain, and distress to any part of the body and may aggravate the inflammation and pain of RSD. On the other hand, bed rest and inactivity can worsen the symptoms of CRPS.

Because CRPS 1 remains one of the most difficult pain syndromes, early diagnosis and treatment are important to have adequate functional results from physical therapy. Manipulation under general anesthesia may be an additional effective treatment tool to obtain functional improvement in some patients diagnosed with CRPS 1.5

Prolonged bed rest results in aggravation of pain and insomnia in RSD patients. The RSD patients suffer from severe, chronic insomnia due to the constant allodynia pain as well as due to the aggravation of constriction of blood vessels secondary to inactivity.

On the other hand, too much exercise can worsen RSD pain. Before choosing a therapist, a patient should interview the therapist. A patient should ascertain if the therapist has experience in treating CRPS/RSD.

The pharmacological treatment of CRPS I is empirical and insufficiently effective. Further research is needed regarding the therapeutic modalities discussed in the guidelines. Physical therapy is widely recommended as a first-line treatment. The efficacy of local anesthetic sympathetic blockade as treatment for CRPS I is questionable.11

A patient should not be treated by a therapist who has no experience with RSD/CRPS. In summary physical/occupational therapy can benefit patients suffering from RSD. As a result, a patient with RSD may not need stellate ganglion or lumbar sympathetic injections, surgical sympathectomy, and numerous oral and topical medications, dorsal column stimulators or morphine pumps, all of which are frequently unsuccessful.

Available researches on efficacy of different treatment options are still insufficient to create precise therapy guidelines, so future researches are needed in order to promote better rehabilitation outcomes.14 There is currently no strong consensus regarding the optimal management of complex regional pain syndrome although a multitude of interventions have been described and are commonly used.15

The addition of transcutaneous electrical nerve stimulation (TENS) to the physical therapy program was seen to make a significant contribution to clinical recovery in CRPS Type 1.16

A therapist shouls his/her patients about the condition, sustaining or restoring limb function, reducing pain, and providing psychological support.1 Furthermore, laser therapy may provide small clinically short-term, improvements in pain compared to interferential current therapy in people with CRPS I.2

References
1.   Casale R, Atzeni F, Sarzi-Puttini P. The therapeutic approach to complex regional pain syndrome: light and shade. Clin Exp Rheumatol. 2015;33(1 Suppl 88):S126-139.
2.   Smart KM, Wand BM, O'Connell NE. Physiotherapy for pain and disability in adults with complex regional pain syndrome (CRPS) types I and II. Cochrane Database Syst Rev. 2016;2:CD010853.
3.   Baron R, Wasner G. Complex regional pain syndromes. Curr Pain Headache Rep. 2001;5(2):114-123.

4.   Bryant PR, Kim CT, Millan R. The rehabilitation of causalgia (complex regional pain syndrome-type II). Phys Med Rehabil Clin N Am. 2002;13(1):137-157.

5.   Celik D, Demirhan M. Physical therapy and rehabilitation of complex regional pain syndrome in shoulder prosthesis. Korean J Pain. 2010;23(4):258-261.

6.   Kocic M, Lazovic M, Dimitrijevic I, Mancic D, Stankovic A. [Evaluation of low level laser and interferential current in the therapy of complex regional pain syndrome by infrared thermographic camera]. Vojnosanit Pregl. 2010;67(9):755-760.

7.   Oerlemans HM, Goris JA, de Boo T, Oostendorp RA. Do physical therapy and occupational therapy reduce the impairment percentage in reflex sympathetic dystrophy? Am J Phys Med Rehabil. 1999;78(6):533-539.

8.   Kock FX, Borisch N, Koester B, Grifka J. [Complex regional pain syndrome type I (CRPS I). Pathophysiology, diagnostics, and therapy]. Orthopade. 2003;32(5):418-431.

9.   Severens JL, Oerlemans HM, Weegels AJ, van 't Hof MA, Oostendorp RA, Goris RJ. Cost-effectiveness analysis of adjuvant physical or occupational therapy for patients with reflex sympathetic dystrophy. Arch Phys Med Rehabil. 1999;80(9):1038-1043.

10.   Vacariu G. Complex regional pain syndrome. Disabil Rehabil. 2002;24(8):435-442.

11.   Bussa M, Guttilla D, Lucia M, Mascaro A, Rinaldi S. Complex regional pain syndrome type I: a comprehensive review. Acta Anaesthesiol Scand. 2015;59(6):685-697.

12.   Zecevic Lukovic T, Ristic B, Jovanovic Z, Rancic N, Ignjatovic Ristic D, Cukovic S. Complex regional pain syndrome type I in the upper extremity - how efficient physical therapy and rehabilitation are. Med Glas (Zenica). 2012;9(2):334-340.

13.   Anandkumar S, Manivasagam M. Multimodal physical therapy management of a 48-year-old female with post-stroke complex regional pain syndrome. Physiother Theory Pract. 2014;30(1):38-48.

14.   Nedeljkovic UD. How to treat complex regional pain syndrome in rehabilitation settings? Acta Chir Iugosl. 2013;60(1):69-75.

15.   O'Connell NE, Wand BM, McAuley J, Marston L, Moseley GL. Interventions for treating pain and disability in adults with complex regional pain syndrome. Cochrane Database Syst Rev. 2013(4):CD009416.

16. Bilgili A, Cakir T, Dogan SK, Ercalik T, Filiz MB, Toraman F. The effectiveness of transcutaneous electrical nerve stimulation in the management of patients with complex regional pain syndrome: A randomized, double-blinded, placebo-controlled prospective study. J Back Musculoskelet Rehabil. 2016;29(4):661-671.

25. Occupational Therapy

There are no adequate comparative studies on physical therapy (PT) versus occupational therapy (OT) in patients with complex regional pain syndrome I (CRPS I).Occupational therapists usually are responsible for introducing and maintaining a stress-loading program for patients with CRPS.1 PT, and to a lesser extent OT, were helpful for reducing pain and improving active mobility in patients with CRPS I of less than one year duration, localized in one upper extremity.1

CRPS therapy comprises medication, interventional therapies and non-pharmaceutical treatments like physiotherapy (PT), occupational therapy, PT with cognitive behavioral elements (mirror therapy, 'motor imagery', and 'graded exposure'), psychotherapeutic methods, local therapies and neurostimulation. 2 These treatments are mostly as successful as medical or interventional treatment.

One program involves active compression and distraction exercises that provide stimuli to the affected extremity without joint motion. The scrubbing technique requires use of a scrub brush. Scrubbing is performed by gradually increasing the weight on the patient's affected extremity as he/she scrubs in circles. Weight loading of the joints is completed with increasing weight as the scrubbing process continues.

The therapeutic management of the complex regional pain syndrome depends on its severity, and should take place in an interdisciplinary setting. Based upon the severity of the clinical presentation, a patient-tailored course of occupational therapy is designed and implemented.3

A previous study was published and the purpose of the study was to assess the value of combining occupational therapy with physical therapy for the rehabilitation of complex regional pain syndrome and to measure its effectiveness on activities of daily life. In CRPS, occupational therapy combined with physical therapy brings a real benefit in restoring the essential activities of daily life.

This strategy could be implemented as soon the diagnosis confirmed and continued for a very long time.4 Physical therapy and to a lesser extent occupational therapy , were helpful for reducing pain and improving active mobility in patients with CRPS I of less than one year duration, localized in one upper extremity.1

Recreational therapy can help the patient with chronic pain to take part in pleasurable activities that help to decrease pain. The patient finds enjoyment and socialization in previously lost or new recreational activities. Usually, patients with chronic pain are depressed. Recreational therapists may play an important role in the treatment process and enable the patient to become active.

Vocational therapy should be recommended and initiated early for all appropriate patients. Vocational therapy can provide work capacities and targeted work hardening, and the patient may return to gainful employment.

An assessment of hand function is obtained using a quantitative determination of pain levels, edema, and overall hand function, mobility and strength, and, subsequently, therapeutic goals are set. Based upon the severity of the clinical presentation, a patient-tailored course of occupational therapy is designed and implemented.3

It's important for patients to understand and embrace their role in the recovery process. The therapist can coach, mentor, and design treatment, but if patients are unable or unwilling to follow through with regular participation in treatment exercises and activities outside of designated therapy sessions, the results will be minimal. Empowering patients to understand their condition and take control of treatment minimizes apprehension and builds rapport.

The more actively patients participate in treatment planning and the more compliant they are with individualized home programs, the greater the chance they will regain function and manage pain. Engaging in or working toward functional activities that are most meaningful to patients can help them overcome fear of movement and distract them from the pain associated with the activity.

A stress loading procedure can be an effective tool for treatment and management of CRPS. Stress loading is comprised of two components: scrubbing and carrying. Each component engages the affected extremity in consistent weight bearing activities within a small range of movement for gradually increasing periods of time.

These activities "load" the affected joints or extremity. This, in turn, provides inhibitory proprioceptive input to the nervous system, through the use of deep pressure.

The key to stress loading is providing as much force or weight bearing as can be consistently tolerated during scrubbing and carrying, gradually increasing the frequency and duration of these activities throughout the day. Loading the affected area to tolerance and gradually increasing the frequency and duration of weight bearing activities enables the nervous system to acclimate to these stimuli.

This acclimation progressively desensitizes the heightened pain response and allows the nervous system to "remodel" itself; the nervous system shifts from recognizing the stimulus presented as threatening, to accepting it as a normal sensation once again.

Scrubbing applies constant force through the affected area for progressively increasing periods of time without a break. Scrubbing for the upper extremity may be done with a towel or a hand-held scrub brush. The towel or brush is moved back and forth against a solid surface, as if scrubbing a stubborn stain off that surface.

Scrubbing for the lower extremity may be done wearing a sock or by adding a strap to a deck brush to secure it to the foot. The sock foot or scrub brush is then moved back and forth against the floor from a standing or seated position.

In order for scrubbing to have the maximum effect, consistent pressure must be maintained while moving the brush in both directions and the weight bearing as tolerated. The initial protocol for scrubbing calls for three minute scrubbing sessions, three times per day, gradually increasing in frequency and duration over a period of days or weeks, until ten to fifteen minutes of scrubbing can be tolerated at least three times per day.

Carrying involves toting a weighted object for increasing periods of time with the affected extremity or on the affected side, in order to provide "loading" to the area. Carrying weighted objects in a handled bag or briefcase is effective for the upper extremity. Walking and weight shifting can be an effective means of loading for the lower extremity.

Creativity in treatment design can facilitate longer periods of carrying and distract from the painful task at hand (or foot!). Otherwise, inconsistent participation or frequent breaks during these activities can result in increased pain and lead to greater disuse of the affected area.

Desensitization techniques can be used to decrease hypersensitivity to cutaneous stimuli. Various textures or fabrics can be presented to the area, progressing from least noxious to most noxious, and consistent to intermittent application, to improve tolerance to light touch or pressure. The process may take several weeks or months to achieve tolerance of all stimuli. Desensitization to a particular texture or fabric may not mean that the stimulus that previously invoked pain now feels good. Desensitization typically enables a stimulus to be tolerated for longer periods with a lower pain response.

Success with desensitization may enable patients to be more flexible with choice of clothing items or to tolerate various bed linens during sleep. Temperature desensitization can be achieved by gradually varying air or water temperature to challenge tolerance to warm or cold. As with stress loading, these techniques should be performed for gradually increasing periods of time without a break.

Edema should be addressed with edema management garments and active range of motion. Passive retrograde massage and passive range of motion should be avoided initially as they can stimulate an inflammatory response resulting in greater pain and swelling, jeopardizing the trust between the patient and practitioner. Splinting may be necessary in severe cases of CRPS to maintain joint integrity and promote adequate circulation and nutrition to the tissues.

However, once patients are able to achieve some pain management with a medication regiment and the use of stress loading and desensitization techniques, they can often actively engage in range of motion activities that promote improved circulation, increased movement and decreased swelling, thus minimizing or eliminating the need for edema management garments or splinting.

Active range of motion activities should be geared toward improving function with the affected hand, such as drinking from a cup, turning a doorknob, or using a knife. With the affected leg, activities can include pushing off for reciprocal stair climbing or fast walking. As guarding is decreased or eliminated and range of motion is restored, initiate strengthening.

Continued support and reinforcement gives patients the confidence to challenge themselves consistently throughout the day. Finding the balance between enough and too much can enable patients to successfully resume activities in all areas of life: occupation, home, self, leisure, and community. Additional pain management techniques, such as biofeedback or relaxation and distraction, can also be useful in pacing activities and modulating pain response.

A comprehensive approach to CRPS treatment can facilitate restoration of function by empowering patients to manage their pain and understand their condition. Patients are able to stay motivated for treatment when they can maintain control of their own progress through collaboration with their therapists, when it comes to how much and how frequently to challenge their "comfort" zone to achieve their goals.

A goal of occupational therapy is to help patients continue to engage with the activities which are important to them as individuals after injury, the onset of illness, or working with elderly clients. It is such an important function in so many ways. The basic principle of keeping active is beneficial to mental health so can ward of depression and feelings of hopelessness that can sometimes be overwhelming. It can help prevent dependency on medication to treat these symptoms, by engaging and encouraging active participation which is a far more gratifying experience.

The therapeutic management of the complex regional pain syndrome (CRPS I) depends on its severity, and should take place in an interdisciplinary setting. In addition to medical and psychological intervention, occupational therapy plays a major role in the care of patients.

Following a case review and patient interview, an assessment of hand function is obtained using a quantitative determination of pain levels, edema, and overall hand function, mobility and strength, and, subsequently, therapeutic goals are set.

PT and, to a lesser extent, OT resulted in a significant and also more rapid improvement in the ISS as compared with controls.4 On a disability level, a positive trend was found in favor of OT. On a handicap level, no differences were found between the groups. PT had an advantage over OT regarding the cost-effectiveness ratio. In different ways PT and OT each contribute to the recovery from RSD of the upper extremity.

Therapeutic treatment can assist in decreasing sensitivity to the injured area through deep-tissue massage (as tolerated), scar mobilization, stretching, and strengthening and energy-conservation techniques to assist the patient in activities of daily living.

Therapists can apply many helpful treatment techniques for patients suffering with CRPS, including easing patients into joint range of motion, gentle joint mobilization, edema massage and soft-tissue mobilization with a very gentle, superficial approach, and muscle flexibility and strengthening exercises.

Aerobic exercise is very helpful to reduce sensitization of the central nervous system, so starting the patient on some low-grade exercise as early as possible should be a prominent goal of therapy. Patient education is the key to address guarding postures, and to allow gentle stimulation from a variety of sources in the affected area. Stress-relaxation techniques, diaphragmatic breathing and other activities to assist in nervous system relaxation can be helpful.

Therapy goals are focused on movement and function, not pain, as the typical CRPS patient is already quite focused on pain. The prognosis will be slow, especially in later stages of the disease, and depending on the co-morbidities the patient may have. It is important to fully explain to the patient what is happening, so he or she can understand the disease process and become more compliant with the home exercise program and suggested activities.

Typical therapy goals for this population include increased range of motion, decreased pain, increased strength, becoming independent with activities of daily living and home exercise programs. Physicians may also prescribe medications to assist in desensitizing the nervous system, such as Gabapentin, anti-depressants, NSAIDs, corticosteroids and pain medications, which may be helpful in easing the transition to more movement in early physical therapy visits.

Occupational therapy can be helpful in address the impact of CRPS on a patient's ability to work, as well as to deal with normal daily activities and to enjoy recreational opportunities. First, the therapist will work with the patient to determine the particular activities that produce an increase in pain levels.

This is following by identify alternate methods for achieving those activities in ways that will hopefully minimize any symptomatic worsening. This may include behavior modification and/or equipment that help the patient adapt to the activities.

All patients with chronic CRPS should receive a thorough psychological evaluation, followed by cognitive-behavioral pain management treatment, including relaxation training with biofeedback. Patients making insufficient overall treatment progress or in whom comorbid psychiatric disorders/major ongoing life stressors are identified should additionally receive general cognitive-behavioral therapy to address these issues.

The psychological component of treatment can work synergistically with medical and physical/occupational therapies to improve function and increase patients' ability to manage the condition successfully.5

Ultimately, this type of occupational therapy can help a patient achieve a new daily routine that accomplishes as many of the prior work and life activities as possible, while reducing those activities negative impact on pain symptom levels. This is helpful not only in physical terms, but psychological terms as well, by returning the patient as much normalcy in their daily activities and social interactions as possible.

Physical therapy is a complement to occupational therapy and the physical therapist will help the patient understand how their RSD symptoms are created and exacerbated so that the patient can minimize symptoms and increase physical capacity.

This treatment includes setting realistic goals and working with the patient to meet those goals. This is followed by gradual increases in activity designed to re-map the brain and bypass the pain signals being created in the affected limbs.

A rehabilitation program, with successive types of exercises, including limb laterality recognition, imagined movements and mirror therapy can be conducted in patients with CRPS I1. This graded motor imagery program, needs patients' participation, is educative, and improves edema, pain, and functional capacities.6

Physical therapy in association with occupational therapy plays an important role in functional restoration. The goal is to increase strength and flexibility gradually, beginning with gentle gliding exercises. Patients usually are reluctant to participate in PT because of intense pain. A self-directed or therapist-directed PT program is important and should be individualized to each patient's needs and goals. Treatment should be based on a multidisciplinary experienced team approach that is focused on functional restoration.7

Essentially exercise therapy, manual therapy, graded motor imaging, CO_2 baths and occupational therapy have a proven benefit for the patients. Although for many of the treatments reliable evidence-based data are lacking a treatment algorithm was established but there is a strong need for further investigations concerning the therapeutic effectiveness in the treatment of CRPS.8

As previously mentioned, a study was to assess the value of combining occupational therapy (OT) with physical therapy (PT) for the rehabilitation of complex regional pain syndrome (CRPS) and to measure its effectiveness on activities of daily life.4

The patients who received PT+OT had on average 10% better dressing and undressing function, 25% better for meal preparation, and 20% better on personal care than those who underwent PT only. In CRPS, OT combined with PT brings a real benefit in restoring the essential activities of daily life.

References

1.   Oerlemans HM, Oostendorp RA, de Boo T, Goris RJ. Pain and reduced mobility in complex regional pain syndrome I: outcome of a prospective randomised controlled clinical trial of adjuvant physical therapy versus occupational therapy. Pain. 1999;83(1):77-83.

2.   Kramer HH, Tanislav C, Birklein F. [Non-drug therapies for CRPS]. Handchir Mikrochir Plast Chir. 2012;44(3):142-146.

3.   Hugle C, Geiger M, Romann C, Moppert C. [The treatment of CRPS I from the occupational therapist's point of view]. Handchir Mikrochir Plast Chir. 2011;43(1):32-38.

4.   Rome L. The place of occupational therapy in rehabilitation strategies of complex regional pain syndrome: Comparative study of 60 cases. Hand Surg Rehabil. 2016;35(5):355-362.

5.   Bruehl S, Chung OY. Psychological and behavioral aspects of complex regional pain syndrome management. Clin J Pain. 2006;22(5):430-437.

6.   Winisdoerffer N, Leclercq MM, Muller A, Martin M, Pierrat M. Complex Regional Pain Syndrome type I (CRPS I) and self-rehabilitation: A health-related quality of life study. Ann Phys Rehabil Med. 2016;59S:e148.

7.   Doro C, Hayden RJ, Louis DS. Complex regional pain syndrome type I in the upper extremity. Clin Occup Environ Med. 2006;5(2):445-454, x.

8.   Korbler C, Pfau M, Becker F, Koester U, Werdin F. [Hand Therapy in the Treatment of Patients with CRPS]. Handchir Mikrochir Plast Chir. 2015;47(3):182-189.

This chapter presents the results of multiple studies emphasizing injections and/or medications administered intravenously for pain reduction. Pain relief in complex regional pain syndrome (CRPS) remains a major challenge, in part due to the lack of evidence-based treatment trials specific for this condition.

There is currently no strong consensus regarding the optimal management of complex regional pain syndrome although a multitude of interventions have been described and are commonly used.

In a pain clinic team the anesthetist has the knowledge and experience concerning the peripheral and central neural blockades. Patients with a chronic regional pain syndrome (CRPS) can find some relief with a series of somatic and sympatholytic blockades, which allow an aggressive physiotherapy.1

Pain-relieving effects of lidocaine/bupivicaine local anesthetic and saline block of sympathetic ganglia (stellate block, 4 patients; lumbar sympathetic block, 3 patients) were compared in complex regional pain syndrome (CRPS) patients on a double-blind crossover basis to evaluate the diagnostic and therapeutic value of local anesthetic sympathetic blocks. The combination of these results provides evidence that duration of pain relief is affected by injection of local anesthetics into sympathetic ganglia.2

Like most medical conditions, an early diagnosis and treatment increase the likelihood of a successful outcome. Accordingly, patients with clinical signs and symptoms of CRPS after an injury should be referred immediately to a physician with expertise in evaluating and treating this condition. Physical therapy is the cornerstone and first-line treatment for CRPS.3

With respect to injections for the treatment of CRPS, many physicians begin with a sympathetic nerve block (a stellate ganglion block, or a lumbar sympathetic block) for example and evaluate the patient's response.4

A long-term randomized, double-blinded active-control study to was done evaluate the efficacy of thoracic sympathetic block (TSB) for upper limb type I CRPS. The quality of life was only slightly improved by TSB. No major adverse events occurred.

Only some patients with nerve injury or CRPS respond to sympathetic nerve blockade, and it has been proposed that patients' pain be defined as sympathetically maintained or sympathetically independent according to their response to a temporary sympathetic nerve block.

As CRPS progresses, more and more of the pain becomes sympathetically independent, as it becomes centered or generated in the brain. It actually becomes independent of the injury. This explains why localized pain reduction techniques like sympathetic blocks no longer work after the first few months of the onset of CRPS.

A review raised questions as to the efficacy of local anesthetic sympathetic blockade as treatment of CRPS. Its efficacy is based mainly on case series. Less than one third of patients obtained full pain relief. The absence of control groups in case series leads to an overestimation of the treatment response that can explain the findings.5

If a patient's response to the initial sympathetic block is less than expected, the next step is to perform an intravenous lidocaine infusion. This modality is used to block the sodium channels in neuronal membranes, consequently stopping the initiation and conduction of impulses associated with neuropathic and inflammatory pain. The use of regional intravenous lidocaine has been well-documented in the literature with a successful decrease in pain symptoms.6,7

Repeated lumbar sympathetic blockade (LSB) with local anesthetics is generally used in CRP of the lower extremities if the initial block has been successful. However, the symptoms of CRPS may inevitably recur in spite of repeated LSB. Clonidine, an alpha2-adrenoceptor agonist, has both anesthetic and analgesic sparing effects, and when added to local anesthetics may enhance peripheral and central neural block due to its local or central analgesic effects.8

A complex regional pain syndrome of an extremity that has previously resolved can recur after repeat surgery at the same anatomic site. A study was done to evaluate preoperative and postoperative sympathetic function and the recurrence of complex regional pain syndrome type I (CRPS I) in patients after repeat carpal tunnel surgery.9 CRPS I can recur after repeat hand surgery. Preoperative sympathetic blockade may prevent the recurrence of CRPS.

Allodynia and hypoesthesia are negative predictors for treatment success in CRPS-1. There are no reported symptoms or signs of CRPS-1 that positively predicted treatment success. A majority of patients experience transient side effects such as headache, dysphagia, increased pain, backache, nausea, blurred vision, groin pain, hoarseness, and hematoma at the puncture site associated with sympathetic blockade.

The presence of allodynia and hypoesthesia are negative predictors for treatment success.10 The selection of sympathetic blockade as treatment for CRPS-1 should be balanced carefully between potential success and side effect ratio. The procedure is as likely to cause a transient increase in pain as a decrease in pain. Patients should be informed accordingly.

The block of sympathetic system with guanethidine is an important method in the therapy of the CRPS. It is less invading than the blocks of the stellate ganglion or of the lumbar sympathetic plexus.11 LBTX-B can produce an efficacious and durable sympathetic blocking effect on patients with CRPS. Serial intravenous regional blockade (IVRB) with 15 mg of guanethidine on the other hand does not improve the outcome of CRPS condition and may delay the resolution of vasomotor instability when compared with the placebo.12

Lumbar sympathetic block (LSB) is an effective method for relief of sympathetically mediated pain in the lower extremities. To prolong the sympathetic blockade, sympathetic destruction with alcohol or radiofrequency has been used. The pre-ganglionic sympathetic nerves are cholinergic, and botulinum toxin (BTX) has been found to inhibit the release of acetylcholine at the cholinergic nerve terminals.13 BTX-B can produce an efficacious and durable sympathetic blocking effect on patients with CRPS.

With respect to sympathetic blockade there however, remains a scarcity of published evidence to support the use of local anesthetic for CRPS. From the existing evidence it is not possible to draw firm conclusions regarding the efficacy or safety of this intervention but the limited data available do not suggest that local anesthetic sympathetic blockade is effective for reducing pain in CRPS.14,15

A positive correlation however, exists between stellate ganglion blockade (SGB) efficacy and how soon stellate ganglion blockade therapy is initiated. A duration of symptoms greater than 16 weeks before the initial SGB and/or a decrease in skin perfusion of 22% between the normal and affected hands adversely affects the efficacy of SGB therapy.16 Another study verified furthermore that stellate ganglion blockade successfully decreased symptoms in patients with CRPS type I.17 Further, the duration between symptom onset and therapy initiation was a major factor affecting blockade success.

The Stellate Ganglion Block (SGB) is performed by placing a small amount of local anesthetic and sometimes steroids around the stellate ganglion, for the sympathetic nervous system in the arm. The ganglion itself is in the neck. The SGB is performed with a patient lying supine, under fluoroscopy or ultrasound guidance, a needle is directed to the ganglion and the medication is injected.

Usually within minutes, relief of pain, increasing temperature and skin color, and a temporary Horner's syndrome are noted. Horner's syndrome is characterized primarily by drooping of the eyelid on the side of the face we injected. This syndrome resolves as the local anesthetic wears off.

A positive correlation exists between SGB efficacy and how soon SGB therapy is initiated. A duration of symptoms greater than 16 weeks before the initial SGB and/or a decrease in skin perfusion of 22% between the normal and affected hands adversely affects the efficacy of SGB therapy.16

The Lumbar Sympathetic Block is performed with a patient lying on the abdomen. Under fluoroscopic guidance, a needle is advanced to the lumbar sympathetic chain and a local anesthetic with or without steroid is injected. Usually within a short duration relief of the pain and increasing temperature and skin color are noted in the affected leg.

Continuous epidural anesthesia on the other hand may be effective in the treatment of CRPS as well. In a patient case report, pharmacotherapy and stellate ganglion block were ineffective, and continuous epidural anesthesia was commenced 14 days after the falling event.

The pain and accompanying symptoms completely disappeared within 5 days. Early treatment with continuous epidural anesthesia may be a promising option for the management of complex regional pain syndrome during childhood.18

Pain associated with Complex Regional Pain Syndrome (CRPS) is frequently excruciating and intractable. The intramuscular injection of botulinum toxin in the upper limb girdle muscles was beneficial for short term relief of pain caused by CRPS.19

A brachial plexus block (BPB) has been mentioned as a treatment modality for complex regional pain syndrome type I of the upper limb.20 The Brachial Plexus runs from the neck down under the collarbone to the armpit. The location of a patient's CRPS will determine where the block is performed. The block may be an interscalene block, or an infraclavicular block.

These blocks are performed with a patient lying supine. Ultrasound or fluoroscopy is used to guide the needle to the correct location and local anesthetic with or without steroid is injected. These injections may be effective when combined with physical therapy.

Nerve blocks may be useful in allowing patients with CRPS do physical therapy. By decreasing pain and thereby improving the ability to tolerate physical therapy, this method may have an advantage compared to other treatment modalities.21 Nerve block is a valuable diagnostic and therapeutic option in the management of joint stiffness caused by CRPS-1.22

The changes in regional cerebral blood flow seem to support the theory that the pathogenesis of CRPS is also related to the central nervous system. Multiple somatic nerve blocks (SNB) not only improved physical function but also reversed the CRPS symptoms, for which it was presumed that reduced nociceptive input signals led to cortical reorganization.23

The sympathetic nervous system makes an unknown contribution to CRPS/RSD, but it is not known whether this is a cause or an effect of the pain.24 Psychological and psychiatric changes are probably secondary rather than etiologic. Treatment should be immediate, aggressive, and directed toward restoration of full function of the extremity.

Various analgesic techniques may be necessary to permit the patient to comply with the rehabilitation program. This program is best carried out in a comprehensive interdisciplinary setting, with a primary emphasis on functional restoration. A Bier block with methylprednisolone and lidocaine in CRPS type I does not provide long-term benefit in CRPS, and its short-term benefit is not superior to placebo.25

Patients, aged between 33 and 72 years, suffering from CRPS type I of the hand received two series of intravenous regional sympathetic block (Bier's block) sessions with guanethidine and lidocaine. The above-described therapeutic protocol method resulted in excellent pain relief and full restoration of both function and range of movement of the affected extremity in each of the study patients suffering from CRPS type I of the hand.26

Intravenous magnesium significantly improved pain, impairment and quality of life and was well tolerated in patients with CRPS I. The results of this pilot study are encouraging and suggest that magnesium IV as a treatment in CRPS 1 should be further explored in a large size formal trial design.27

Intravenous phentolamine infusion is potentially a new significant option for the therapy of CRPS.28 A simple and easily tolerated method of treatment that includes intravenous regional anesthetic block with lidocaine and methyloprednisolone.29

Peripheral nerve pathology commonly results in symptoms that suggest a diagnosis of complex regional pain syndrome. The clinical entity of CRPS quite apparently encompasses symptomatology caused by peripheral nerve entrapment, irritative lesions, and neuroma.

Sometimes a diagnostic end point may overlook these treatable conditions. Peripheral nerve pathology may prove a diagnostic challenge and alternative techniques of investigation other than electrophysiologic studies are often helpful.30

References

1. Ingold O. [Pain management from the viewpoint of the anesthetist]. Praxis (Bern 1994). 1998;87(7):232-237.

2. Price DD, Long S, Wilsey B, Rafii A. Analysis of peak magnitude and duration of analgesia produced by local anesthetics injected into sympathetic ganglia of complex regional pain syndrome patients. Clin J Pain. 1998;14(3):216-226.

3. Rho RH, Brewer RP, Lamer TJ, Wilson PR. Complex regional pain syndrome. Mayo Clin Proc. 2002;77(2):174-180.

4. Rocha Rde O, Teixeira MJ, Yeng LT, et al. Thoracic sympathetic block for the treatment of complex regional pain syndrome type I: a double-blind randomized controlled study. Pain. 2014;155(11):2274-2281.

5. Cepeda MS, Lau J, Carr DB. Defining the therapeutic role of local anesthetic sympathetic blockade in complex regional pain syndrome: a narrative and systematic review. Clin J Pain. 2002;18(4):216-233.

6. Rickard JP, Kish T. Systemic Intravenous Lidocaine for the Treatment of Complex Regional Pain Syndrome: A Case Report and Literature Review. Am J Ther. 2016;23(5):e1266-1269.

7. Toda K, Muneshige H, Asou T. Intravenous regional block with lidocaine for treatment of complex regional pain syndrome. Clin J Pain. 2006;22(2):222-224.

8. Chen LC, Wong CS, Huh BK, et al. Repeated lumbar sympathetic blockade with lidocaine and clonidine attenuates pain in complex

regional pain syndrome type 1 patients--a report of two cases. Acta Anaesthesiol Taiwan. 2006;44(2):113-117.

9.   Ackerman WE, 3rd, Ahmad M. Recurrent postoperative CRPS I in patients with abnormal preoperative sympathetic function. J Hand Surg Am. 2008;33(2):217-222.

10.   van Eijs F, Geurts J, van Kleef M, et al. Predictors of pain relieving response to sympathetic blockade in complex regional pain syndrome type 1. Anesthesiology. 2012;116(1):113-121.

11.   Verre M, De Santis F, Glyronakis S, et al. [Pharmacological sympathetic block in complex regional pain syndrome]. Clin Ter. 2002;153(6):367-372.

12.   Livingstone JA, Atkins RM. Intravenous regional guanethidine blockade in the treatment of post-traumatic complex regional pain syndrome type 1 (algodystrophy) of the hand. J Bone Joint Surg Br. 2002;84(3):380-386.

13.   Choi E, Cho CW, Kim HY, Lee PB, Nahm FS. Lumbar Sympathetic Block with Botulinum Toxin Type B for Complex Regional Pain Syndrome: A Case Study. Pain Physician. 2015;18(5):E911-916.

14.   Stanton TR, Wand BM, Carr DB, Birklein F, Wasner GL, O'Connell NE. Local anaesthetic sympathetic blockade for complex regional pain syndrome. Cochrane Database Syst Rev. 2013(8):CD004598.

15.   O'Connell NE, Wand BM, Gibson W, Carr DB, Birklein F, Stanton TR. Local anaesthetic sympathetic blockade for complex regional pain syndrome. Cochrane Database Syst Rev. 2016;7:CD004598.

16.   Ackerman WE, Zhang JM. Efficacy of stellate ganglion blockade for the management of type 1 complex regional pain syndrome. South Med J. 2006;99(10):1084-1088.

17.   Yucel I, Demiraran Y, Ozturan K, Degirmenci E. Complex regional pain syndrome type I: efficacy of stellate ganglion blockade. J Orthop Traumatol. 2009;10(4):179-183.

18.   Saito Y, Baba S, Takahashi A, et al. Complex regional pain syndrome in a 15-year-old girl successfully treated with continuous epidural anesthesia. Brain Dev. 2015;37(1):175-178.

19.   Kharkar S, Ambady P, Venkatesh Y, Schwartzman RJ. Intramuscular botulinum toxin in complex regional pain syndrome: case series and literature review. Pain Physician. 2011;14(5):419-424.

20.   Wang LK, Chen HP, Chang PJ, Kang FC, Tsai YC. Axillary brachial plexus block with patient controlled analgesia for complex

regional pain syndrome type I: a case report. Reg Anesth Pain Med. 2001;26(1):68-71.

21.	Bredahl C, Kristensen AK, Christensen KS. [Treatment of reflex dystrophy with continuous peripheral nerve block]. Ugeskr Laeger. 2007;169(1):59-60.

22.	Muhl C, Isner-Horobeti ME, Laalou FZ, Vautravers P, Lecocq J. The value of nerve blocks in the diagnoses and treatment of complex regional pain syndrome type 1: a series of 14 cases. Ann Phys Rehabil Med. 2014;57(6-7):381-393.

23.	Lin BF, Cherng CH, Fan YM, Wong CS, Huh BK, Yeh CC. Changes in regional cerebral blood flow and three-phase bone scan after repeated somatic nerve blocks for sympathetically independent pain. Clin Nucl Med. 2010;35(6):391-395.

24.	Wilson PR. Complex Regional Pain Syndrome-Reflex Sympathetic Dystrophy. Curr Treat Options Neurol. 1999;1(5):466-472.

25.	Taskaynatan MA, Ozgul A, Tan AK, Dincer K, Kalyon TA. Bier block with methylprednisolone and lidocaine in CRPS type I: a randomized, double-blinded, placebo-controlled study. Reg Anesth Pain Med. 2004;29(5):408-412.

26.	Paraskevas KI, Michaloglou AA, Briana DD, Samara M. Treatment of complex regional pain syndrome type I of the hand with a series of intravenous regional sympathetic blocks with guanethidine and lidocaine. Clin Rheumatol. 2006;25(5):687-693.

27.	Collins S, Zuurmond WW, de Lange JJ, van Hilten BJ, Perez RS. Intravenous magnesium for complex regional pain syndrome type 1 (CRPS 1) patients: a pilot study. Pain Med. 2009;10(5):930-940.

28.	Niaki AS, Bagherzadi K, Momenzadeh S, Shahriyari H, Dori MM. Intravenous regional block with phentolamine in the treatment of complex regional pain syndrome. Acta Med Iran. 2011;49(8):523-526.

29.	Varitimidis SE, Papatheodorou LK, Dailiana ZH, Poultsides L, Malizos KN. Complex regional pain syndrome type I as a consequence of trauma or surgery to upper extremity: management with intravenous regional anaesthesia, using lidocaine and methyloprednisolone. J Hand Surg Eur Vol. 2011;36(9):771-777.

30.	Thimineur MA, Saberski L. Complex regional pain syndrome type I (RSD) or peripheral mononeuropathy? A discussion of three cases. Clin J Pain. 1996;12(2):145-150.

27. Electrical Therapy

Adjuvant therapies were shown to reduce pain and the severity of dysfunction in CRPS. Therefore, these non-drug therapies should be an essential part of any multimodal CRPS treatment.1   The addition of TENS to physical therapy program has been reported to make a significant contribution to clinical recovery in CRPS Type 1.2

Historically, in both adult and pediatric populations, a lack of knowledge regarding complex regional pain syndrome (CRPS) and absence of clear diagnostic criteria have contributed to the view that this is a primarily psychiatric condition. Stressful life events are more common in CRPS patients, which indicate that there may be a multiconditional model of CRPS.

The experience of stressful life events besides trauma or surgery are risk factors, not causes, in such a model. Stressful life events were experienced by 19 patients (79.2%) in the CRPS group and by 9 patients (21.4%) in the control group. This difference was significant.

Testing of psychological dysfunction (SCL-90) in CRPS patients and the control group demonstrated some significant differences: male patients were more anxious than male controls; female patients were statistically more depressed, had feelings of inadequacy, and were emotionally less stable than female controls.

Complex regional pain syndrome (CRPS) is a disabling pain condition poorly understood by medical professionals. Because CRPS is particularly enigmatic, and has significant impact on patient function, researchers have examined psychological processes present among patients with this diagnosis. However, research does not reveal support for specific personality or psychopathology predictors of the condition.3

Electrical neurostimulation is efficacious in chronic neuropathic pain and other neurological diseases. European Federation of Neurological Societies (EFNS) launched a Task Force to evaluate the evidence for these techniques and to produce relevant recommendations. They searched the literature from 1968 to 2006, looking for neurostimulation in neuropathic pain conditions, and classified the trials according to the EFNS scheme of evidence for therapeutic interventions. Spinal cord stimulation (SCS) is efficacious in failed back surgery syndrome (FBSS) and complex regional pain syndrome (CRPS) type I (level B recommendation).4

Spinal cord stimulation (SCS) is a neuromodulation technique using electricity, proposed for the first time by Shealy in 1967, as an alternative to neuroablation. With respect to spinal cord stimulation however, psychological characteristics play an important role in shaping individual differences in the pain experience and may influence responses to SCS.[5] SCS seems to improve notably pain control and quality of life in many of patients.[6]

A review of randomized controlled studies supports the use of SCS as an effective treatment modality for pain associated with FBSS, refractory angina pectoris, peripheral vascular disease, and CRPS Type I.[7]

Electrical stimulation of selected peripheral nerves for treatment of intractable pain has been used inconsistently over the past 30 years due to difficulties in clarifying appropriate indications, utilizing approved device technology, and standardizing the surgical techniques.

Circumferential electrodes treating mononeuropathies have given way to paddle electrode techniques and, most recently, the application of percutaneous wire electrode methods will allow for minimally invasive peripheral nerve stimulation for certain intractable CRPS and other painful monoeuropathies.[8]

If no response to conventional treatment (e.g., pharmacotherapy) is noted within 12-16 weeks from the onset of CRPS, a more interventional technique such as spinal cord stimulation (SCS) should be used. SCS has been shown to be highly effective in the treatment of CRPS type I, resulting in a significant, long-term reduction in pain and improvement in quality of life.

SCS is particularly effective at helping to restore function in affected extremities, especially if applied early in the course of the disease. SCS is also cost effective and improves health-related quality of life.[9]

Further controlled trials are warranted for SCS in conditions other than failed back surgery syndrome and CRPS and for MCS and DBS in general. These chronically implanted techniques provide satisfactory pain relief in many patients, including those resistant to medication or other means.[4]

Psychological and behavioral factors can exacerbate the pain and dysfunction associated with complex regional pain syndrome (CRPS) and could help maintain the condition in some patients. Effective management of CRPS requires that these psychosocial and behavioral aspects be addressed as part of an integrated multidisciplinary treatment approach.

There is little knowledge regarding the association between psychological factors and complex regional pain syndrome (CRPS) in children. Children with CRPS are not particularly prone to symptoms of anxiety or depression. Importantly, children with CRPS experienced more stressful life events than children with chronic headaches or abdominal pain.

Prospective long-term studies are needed to further explore the potential role of stressful life events in the etiology of CRPS.10

Anxiety, pain-related fear, and disability are associated with poorer outcomes in CRPS and could be considered as target variables for early treatment. The findings support the theory that CRPS represents an aberrant protective response to perceived threat of tissue injury. Even in the early stages of CRPS, a cycle of pain, disability, depression, and work absence can emerge.

All patients with chronic CRPS should receive a thorough psychological evaluation, followed by cognitive-behavioral pain management treatment, including relaxation training with biofeedback.

Patients making insufficient overall treatment progress or in whom comorbid psychiatric disorders/major ongoing life stressors are identified should additionally receive general cognitive-behavioral therapy to address these issues.

The psychological component of treatment can work synergistically with medical and physical/occupational therapies to improve function and increase patients' ability to manage the condition successfully.

Psychological and behavioral factors can exacerbate the pain and dysfunction associated with complex regional pain syndrome (CRPS) and could help maintain the condition in some patients.11

Management of CRPS is challenging, partly because of a lack of clinical data regarding the efficacy of the various therapies, and partly because successful treatment of CRPS requires a multidisciplinary, patient-tailored approach. In CRPS, disability and pain severity were more strongly associated with psychological factors than they were in low back pain.

The risk of CRPS type I is significantly increased in patients with high trait anxiety scores. Early traumatic experiences were reported in 87% of the CRPS-I patients and were found to be moderately related to somatoform dissociative experiences, indicating that early traumatic experiences might be a predisposing, although not a necessary factor for the development of CRPS-I-related dystonia.

Many CRPS patients with allodynia manifest clinical signs of special psychological distress. The high incidence of personality pathology in CRPS patients may represent an exaggeration of maladaptive personality traits and coping styles as a result of a chronic, intense, state of pain. Stressful life events are more common in the CRPS group, which indicates that there may be a multiconditional model of CRPS.

A previous study demonstrated that subjects with complex regional pain syndrome have asymmetric venous pool plasma concentrations of norepinephrine (NE) when affected and unaffected limbs are compared, with most demonstrating decreased NE levels in the affected limb.12

This study suggests that increased NE and epinephrine (E) levels in CRPS patients may result from the pain of CRPS, consequent affective distress, or both.

Alternatively, the findings from this study could reflect premorbid adrenergic hyperactivity caused by affective, endocrine, or other pathology, which might predispose these individuals to develop the syndrome.

There is controversy regarding the importance of psychological/psychiatric factors in the development of the Complex Regional Pain Syndrome. A study was done was to determine whether CRPS type I patients were psychiatrically different from other chronic pain patients, with particular attention to personality pathology.

The high incidence of personality pathology in both groups may represent an exaggeration of maladaptive personality traits and coping styles as a result of a chronic, intense, state of pain.13

CRPS in children and adolescents is underdiagnosed, although many of the epidemiologic features of pediatric CRPS are similar in different countries/cultures. Early recognition and management is the major factor in improving outcome and preventing resistant CRPS, but even children with delayed diagnosis still have a good outcome.

The management of this disease by an experienced multidisciplinary team is recommended. Because psychosocial factors play an important role, it is recommended to provide psychological evaluation and cognitive behavioral treatment as soon as possible.14

Historically, in both adult and pediatric populations, a lack of knowledge regarding complex regional pain syndrome and the absence of clear diagnostic criteria have contributed to the view that this is a primarily psychiatric condition.

As a group, clinic-referred children with CRPS may be more functionally impaired and experience more somatic symptoms compared with children with other pain conditions.15

However, overall psychological functioning as assessed by self-report appears to be similar to that of children with other chronic pain diagnoses. Comprehensive assessment using a biopsychosocial framework is essential to understanding and appropriately treating children with symptoms of CRPS.

CRPS is comorbid with depression, anxiety, and insomnia, but this relationship is not psychopathological. Medical and health professionals should not dismiss symptoms related to CRPS as caused by emotional distress.16 When CRPS sufferers are grouped as mentally ill, serious consequences follow.

Primarily, CRPS patients will not have access to treatment interventions such as pharmacotherapy and physical rehabilitation that could improve quality of life, daily functioning, and thwart disease progression.

There may be decreased cortical thickness in the prefrontal cortex and neurocognitive dysfunctions in patients with CRPS.17 These findings may contribute to the understanding of pain-related impairments in cognitive function and could help explain the symptoms or progression of CRPS.

Animal and human studies indicate that electrical stimulation of dorsal root ganglion (DRG) neurons may modulate neuropathic pain signals. Results have shown that DRG stimulation provided a higher rate of treatment success with less postural variation in paresthesia intensity compared to SCS.18

Neurostimulation of peripheral nerves should be considered as an established concept to treat surgically failed peripheral nerve lesions.

Neuromodulation of the DRG appears to be a promising option for relieving chronic pain and other symptoms associated with CRPS. The capture of discrete painful areas such as the feet, combined with stable paresthesia intensities independent of body position, suggests this stimulation modality may allow more selective and consistent targeting of painful areas than traditional SCS.8

As these therapies evolve, so too will their placement within the pain care algorithm grounded by a foundation of evidence to improve patient safety and management of patients with difficult neuropathic pain.

References

1.   Kramer HH, Tanislav C, Birklein F. [Non-drug therapies for CRPS]. Handchir Mikrochir Plast Chir. 2012;44(3):142-146.

2.   Bilgili A, Cakir T, Dogan SK, Ercalik T, Filiz MB, Toraman F. The effectiveness of transcutaneous electrical nerve stimulation in the management of patients with complex regional pain syndrome: A randomized, double-blinded, placebo-controlled prospective study. J Back Musculoskelet Rehabil. 2016;29(4):661-671.

3.   Lohnberg JA, Altmaier EM. A review of psychosocial factors in complex regional pain syndrome. J Clin Psychol Med Settings. 2013;20(2):247-254.

4.   Cruccu G, Aziz TZ, Garcia-Larrea L, et al. EFNS guidelines on neurostimulation therapy for neuropathic pain. Eur J Neurol. 2007;14(9):952-970.

5.   Campbell CM, Jamison RN, Edwards RR. Psychological screening/phenotyping as predictors for spinal cord stimulation. Curr Pain Headache Rep. 2013;17(1):307.

6.   Costantini A. Spinal cord stimulation. Minerva Anestesiol. 2005;71(7-8):471-474.

7.   Lee AW, Pilitsis JG. Spinal cord stimulation: indications and outcomes. Neurosurg Focus. 2006;21(6):E3.

8.   Van Buyten JP, Smet I, Liem L, Russo M, Huygen F. Stimulation of dorsal root ganglia for the management of complex regional pain syndrome: a prospective case series. Pain Pract. 2015;15(3):208-216.

9.   Stanton-Hicks M. Complex regional pain syndrome: manifestations and the role of neurostimulation in its management. J Pain Symptom Manage. 2006;31(4 Suppl):S20-24.

10.   Wager J, Brehmer H, Hirschfeld G, Zernikow B. Psychological distress and stressful life events in pediatric complex regional pain syndrome. Pain Res Manag. 2015;20(4):189-194.

11.   Bruehl S, Chung OY. Psychological and behavioral aspects of complex regional pain syndrome management. Clin J Pain. 2006;22(5):430-437.

12.   Harden RN, Rudin NJ, Bruehl S, et al. Increased systemic catecholamines in complex regional pain syndrome and relationship to psychological factors: a pilot study. Anesth Analg. 2004;99(5):1478-1485; table of contents.

13.   Monti DA, Herring CL, Schwartzman RJ, Marchese M. Personality assessment of patients with complex regional pain syndrome type I. Clin J Pain. 1998;14(4):295-302.

14.   Kachko L, Efrat R, Ben Ami S, Mukamel M, Katz J. Complex regional pain syndromes in children and adolescents. Pediatr Int. 2008;50(4):523-527.

15.   Logan DE, Williams SE, Carullo VP, Claar RL, Bruehl S, Berde CB. Children and adolescents with complex regional pain syndrome: more psychologically distressed than other children in pain? Pain Res Manag. 2013;18(2):87-93.

16.   Hill RJ, Chopra P, Richardi T. Rethinking the psychogenic model of complex regional pain syndrome: somatoform disorders and complex regional pain syndrome. Anesth Pain Med. 2012;2(2):54-59.

17.   Lee DH, Lee KJ, Cho KI, et al. Brain alterations and neurocognitive dysfunction in patients with complex regional pain syndrome. J Pain. 2015;16(6):580-586.

18.   Deer TR, Levy RM, Kramer J, et al. Dorsal root ganglion stimulation yielded higher treatment success rate for CRPS and causalgia at 3 and 12 months: randomized comparative trial. Pain. 2016.

28. Non-conventional Therapy

Complementary and alternative medicines are not researched extensively to date. However practitioners of alternative medicine do treat patients with the complex regional pain syndrome and it therefore mentioned in this book for completeness. The management of patients with chronic pain is a nearly daily challenge to rheumatologists, neurologists, orthopedic surgeons, pain specialists and indeed an issue in nearly every clinical practice including chiropractic therapy.

Among the numerous causes of pain there is often included a unique syndrome, generally referred to as complex regional pain syndrome type I (CRPS). Unfortunately CRPS I has become a catch all phase and there are serious questions on whether it exists at all.1

"Conventional medicine" is considered to be practiced by individuals who have a medical doctor degree (M.D.) or a doctor of osteopathy degree (D.O.). Conventional medicine also includes methods practiced by allied health-care professionals such as physical therapists, occupational therapists, psychologists, and registered nurses. Other terms for conventional medicine include allopathy, mainstream medicine, and orthodox medicine.

In contrast, complementary and alternative medicine are referred to as unconventional or nonconventional medicine as well as unproven health care. Practitioners of alternative medicine hold to the theory that germs can cause illness only if there is an imbalance in various body systems allowing the germs to thrive. They believe that the body's internal environment is healthy and must be kept healthy, and that everyday exposure to germs does not result in illness.

The following is a definition for alternative medicine specialties by the National Center for Complementary and Alternative Medicine. "Complementary and alternative medicines are practices and products that are not currently considered to be part of conventional medicine."

Complementary and alternative medicine practices change and update continually. Those therapies that have been thoroughly investigated and that are proven to be safe and effective eventually do become adopted into the conventional health-care system. Complementary and alternative medicines, unlike many conventional medicine therapies, are designed to help you develop control over your overall health.

If a patient is going to use any of these methods, one is encouraged to learn the side effects of some of these medications as well as learn about drug interactions with medications that a patient currently may be taking. Inasmuch, do not be afraid to tell a physician what complementary medicines you are taking.

Complementary and alternative medicine practices may help a patient control complex regional pain syndrome (CRPS) pain on occasion and should be considered as a form of treatment as an alternative to narcotic medications.

The purpose of this chapter is not to condemn or advocate the utilization of nonconventional medicine practices and substances but to educate a patient that he/she can have some control over the overall health as well as control over the pain. Medical professionals are beginning to recognize the benefits of alternative medicine.

As an example, the National Institute of Health Office of Alternative Medicine was established in 1992. In addition, there has been a significant increase in professional interest in the area of alternative medicine. Approximately 30 medical schools are currently offering at least one elective course on alternative medical therapies. The attitudes of medical school faculty toward the use of complementary medicine practices are important.

A bone scan, radiographs, and clinical examination led to the diagnosis of complex regional pain syndrome (CRPS). Following chiropractic care, the patient had improved grip strength, functional abilities, and pain reduction.2 The primary characteristics of CRPS include motor, trophic and sensory changes, usually in a peripheral limb following some form of trauma.

Due to the varied symptom presentation, it may be unclear which conservative therapies will be most beneficial in the treatment of CRPS. A multidisciplinary approach to treatment should be pursued with these patients. More investigation of therapies such as chiropractic care as it relates to the pathophysiology of CRPS is needed.

Recent research calls into question the predominant theories that view excessive sympathetic nervous system activity as the cause of CRPS. No evidence of an increase in sympathetic nervous system activity has been found, and new theories suggest that an increase in the sensitivity of neurotransmitter receptors may be the cause of CRPS.

Alternatively, other research has suggested that a local inflammatory process may in fact cause CRPS. Although no research has been completed examining the role of chiropractic care in the treatment of CRPS, there is reason to believe that spinal manipulation may be beneficial to patients with CRPS.3

Some health plans have announced their intention to incorporate payment for some alternative medicine practices into their insurance coverage. Some managed care corporations have revealed their intentions to include alternative medicine practices for payment.

Some state governments are considering legislation pertaining to the practice of alternative medicine by health-care professionals. If you are going to use a natural substance or therapy, you are responsible for your own care.

A patient must not self-diagnose and should discuss the symptoms of pain with the physician before taking any nutritional supplement. There are risks and benefits that you should be aware of when using alternative medications and therapies to manage your pain. In addition, the alternative medications you take could react with the prescription medications your doctor has given you and cause you even more problems.

If in doubt, consult the Physician's Drug Reference for herbal medicines. This will advise you about safe doses and any precautions and drug interactions that you may need to be aware of.

There was a study published previously in the New England Journal of Medicine in 1993 that was a survey of individuals. More than 30 percent of those surveyed chose alternative medicine over conventional medicine methods to prevent and treat disease.

In 1994, Congress passed the Dietary Supplement Health and Education Act. In passing this act, Congress recognized that many individuals believed that dietary supplements offered health benefits. The bill gave dietary supplement manufacturers freedom to produce more products and to provide information about their products' health benefits.

The Food and Drug Administration (FDA on the other hand, is responsible for overseeing any claims by the dietary supplement manufacturers to the truthfulness of these claims.

The Federal Trade Commission regulates the advertising of all of the dietary supplements. A patient should be aware that the quality control standards for natural substances are a problem within this industry. Some of the manufacturers of these products will not have the amount of substance in the natural medication as stated on the container label.

A patient must do his/her own research to determine whether the natural substance that he/she is taking has an accurate dosage as stated on the container label for the product. Remember the drug can be actually less than what the label states.

A good rule of thumb for you to consider is that if one product is much cheaper than an identical product, you may want to consider purchasing the more expensive product. The reason for this is that companies that follow appropriate standards usually have their own quality-control systems in effect.

As a result, they will have a higher overhead and will have to charge more for the natural medication. It should be emphasized that the FDA has no control over alternative substances that are categorized as "supplements," and that this has huge quality implications when these agents are compared with conventional drugs.

In an Atlanta medical school, 200 full- and part-time medical school faculty were given a survey concerning alternative medicine practices. The 24-item survey was given to each medical school faculty member.

Three of the 24 items requested participants to respond to a list of 30 specific alternative medical therapies, which included the following: Whether they saw alternative medicine as a legitimate medical practice. Whether they have had personal experience with alternative medicines and felt that they were effective. Whether they have had training in alternative medicine science

Eighty-five of the responders said they have had training in at least one alternative medical therapy. Fifty-seven percent of the responders said they had training in five or more alternative medicine therapies.

More than 80 percent had a personal experience with at least one alternative medical therapy and close to 50 percent of the responders reported personal experience with five or more different alternative medical therapies.

Almost 90 percent of these alternative medicine experiences were rated effective. Only 3 percent were rated not effective. Less than 1 percent of the medical school faculty felt that these therapies were potentially harmful. The results of this Atlanta medical school study demonstrated that the medical school faculty had a positive exposure to alternative medical therapies. This study is important because medical school faculty members have the responsibility for the education and training of future physicians.

The NIH does award grants for the study of research in complementary as well as alternative medicines. Clinical trials are being done throughout the United States with respect to complementary and alternative medicines. You may want to participate in one of these trials. Trials with respect to herbal medicines are an important part of the medical research process. The results from clinical trials can define better ways to treat your painful conditions.

A clinical trial is a research study in which a therapy is tested on individuals like yourself to ensure that the what is being tested is safe and effective. Always remember that clinical trials have risks. Before participating in a clinical trial, discuss this trial with your primary care physician.

To find out about ongoing clinical trials for example, studies on arthritis and neurological disorders such as RSD/CRPS go to www.nccam.nih.gov. You also may want to access the National Library of Medicine online (www.pubmed.com). Complementary medicine on PubMed is available that contains citations to articles on recently published research.

Homeopathic specialists prescribe dilutions of natural substances from plants, minerals, and animals. Homeopathy has been around for more than 200 years. About 500 million people around the world receive homeopathic treatment. The World Health Organization has recommended that homeopathy is a system of traditional medicine that should be integrated with conventional medicine, which is considered the traditional approach to medicine.

It is important to know that the U.S. Food and Drug Administration recognizes homeopathic remedies as official drugs and regulates their manufacture. This is unlike the herbs used for medicinal use. Homeopathy qualities of medicine are used frequently by conventional physicians in Europe. In Britain, homeopathy is a part of the national health system.

The basic principles of homeopathy are that a disease can be destroyed and removed by a type of medicine that is able to produce the disease in humans. In other words, a substance that in large doses would produce symptoms of a disease can be used in very minute doses to cure it.

In conventional medicine, this is called the theory of antibiotics. Homeopathic practitioners adhere to the fact that the more a substance is diluted, the more potent it is. In conventional medicine, it is believed that a higher dose of the medicine will lead to a greater effect.

The purpose of diluting out substances in homeopathic medicineis to avoid side effects. Homeopathic practitioners adhere to the fact that illness is different for every person. Homeopathic treatments are unique for each patient. Homeopathic medicine emphasizes that patients are individuals and have individual signs and symptoms of an illness and should be treated only on an individual basis. The entire individual is treated, which includes the physical, psychological and spiritual portions of each person.

Naturopathic medicine treats disease by using the body's natural ability to heal itself. Naturopathic practitioners invoke healing processes by using a variety of treatment options based on your particular needs. In naturopathic medicine, disease symptoms are a sign of the body's attempt to heal itself naturally. Naturopathic medicine gets its data from Chinese, Native American, and Greek cultures.

Naturopaths recommend healing of the person and not the disease. Naturopathic medicinal treatments will include doses of natural substances that are much higher than those used by practitioners of homeopathic medicine.

Even though a primary care physician may not "believe" in complementary and alternative medications, one should not be afraid to approach the doctor with the fact that one is taking herbal medications. This is important not only because of possible drug interactions, but because some substances such as garlic and gingko can decrease the blood's ability to form a blood clot normally. This could result in excessive bleeding.

It is extremely important if a patient is about to have a surgical procedure that the patient let the surgeon know the patient is taking an herb that can thin the blood. The surgery may need to be delayed until the blood's ability to form a normal clot has been restored.

Be aware that when one is are using alternative medicines that these medicines are not strictly controlled with respect to dosage and the amount of drug in a pill, capsule, or tea. All plants have different amounts of substances in them. A true dose of a medication is unknown in many instances.

A patient should look carefully at the label before taking one of these substances and not take more than the label recommends. The overall drug interactions of herbal substances have not been established because they are not required to be strictly studied by the FDA.

To best choose a natural product to decrease the pain, one should know which chemicals in the body produce pain. With this knowledge, a patient can pick the analgesic best suited to relieve the pain. If a patient has joint pain, for instance, one will want to use an alternative medicine that has anti-inflammatory properties.

If a patient is injured or has inflammation, ther body makes a variety of chemicals that transmit pain impulses to a pain-processing center in your brain. These chemicals include the prostaglandins, cytokines, substance P, glutamic acid, and nitric oxide. Nitric oxide is a gas that is a pain chemical transmitter in the nervous system. This should not be confused with nitrous oxide, which is used for pain control in dental procedures.

The following remedies are anti-inflammatory substances that a patient may want to use as a prostaglandin inhibitor to relieve the pain: Tumeric has anti-inflammatory and antioxidant effects and has been shown to inhibit prostaglandin formation. This drug should not be used if you have gallbladder disease.

No significant health risks or side effects with use of this drug have been reported to date. The average dose is 3 grams of turmeric per day. This dose can be divided up into 1-gram doses and be taken 3 times per day with meals. For example, a patient may take 1 milligram with each meal for a total dose of 3 grams.

Ginseng has anti-inflammatory effects and is used in homeopathic medicine for the treatment of rheumatoid arthritis. A patient should not use this medicine if a patient has hypertension. Do not use ginseng with caffeine. Exercise caution if a patient use ginseng along with any antidiabetic medicine or insulin.

A patient should not use ginseng with MAOI inhibitors, which are used to decrease a patientr blood pressure. Do not use ginseng in combination with diuretics. Side effects include sleep deprivation, nosebleeds, headaches, nervousness, and vomiting. The average daily dose of this root is 1 to 2 grams. Do not take more than 2 grams per day. The 2 grams can be divided up and taken 3 times a day.

Resveratrol is an antioxidant and a COX-2 inhibitor that some believe prevents heart disease and cancer. It is largely found in the skin of red grapes. Therefore, many people obtain resveratrol by drinking red wine. This substance can prevent clot formation, whereas the conventional COX-2 inhibitors do not prevent clot formation. The usual dose is no more than 600 mg per day. There are no known side effects or drug interactions for resveratrol itself.

Fish oils contain the omega-3 fatty acids and can decrease prosta-glandins. Fish oils are used for the treatment of rheumatoid arthritis. One also may use fish oils for the control of joint pain. The most common side effect that a patient may experience with fish oil supplementation is mild stomach upset. The fish oils can decrease the blood's ability to clot. If one is taking blood-thinning drugs, he/she should not take fish oils, because it will give you an increased risk of bleeding. A patient may take up to -10 grams of fish oil per day.

N-acetylcysteine is an amino acid produced by the body that will decrease prostaglandin N-acetylcysteine formation. It can help prevent some diseases and boost one's immune system. One should not take this drug if yhe/she is taking carbamazepine (Tegretol).Side effects include headaches, nausea, vomiting, and stomach upset. The recommended dose is 200 milligrams 3 times a day.

Cayenne is an anti-inflammatory medication that is helpful for the treatment of muscle pain and arthritis. This drug may be helpful for inhibiting the release of substance P as well. Cayenne side effects include diarrhea and intestinal colic. It can decrease your body's ability to form a normal blood clot.

It also can reduce the effects of aspirin, so a patient should not use this drug for more than two days in a row. After two weeks one a patient may use it again for two days. The daily dose of cayenne should not exceed 10 grams.

Ipriflavone can be used as a prostaglandin inhibitor. Women also use it to decrease the incidence of osteoporosis. This medicine can actual-ly stop bone loss. It can decrease the risk of fractures in bone pain in females. This drug, like the other drugs that are prostaglandin inhibitors, can increase the blood-thinning activity of other drugs that you may be taking, such as Coumadin.

It also can increase the effects of some asthma drugs such as theo-phylline, so avoid taking ipriflavone if you are using such medications. Side effects are mostly stomach upset. The average dose is 200 milligrams 3 times a day.

Procyanidolic oligomers are natural substances extracted from grape seeds. They are useful for their antioxidant effects. They can decrease arthritis pain. However, another important effect of this medicine is that it can decrease the effects of nitric oxide. Nitric oxide is released from cells in your bloodstream. Nitric acid essentially exists in a gas form to transmit pain impulses. There are no significant side effects associated with this drug. The daily dose of this drug ranges from 150 to 300 milligrams per day.

Cytokine inhibitors include the fish oils, as previously mentioned. Cytokines are chemicals produced in the bloodstream that enhance pain impulses. They contribute to the formation of substances that can destroy joint linings if one has rheumatoid arthritis. Substance P inhibitors include cayenne and ginseng. Substance P is a neurotransmitter chemical that can be associated with nerve pain, such as shingles. If one has shingles, he/she may want to consider using a substance P inhibitor.

Histamine also can provide a patient with pain relief. Histamine released from certain cells in your body can cause one to develop a rash, a headache, and itching all over the body. However, in extremely small doses, histamine may relieve pain. There have not been any placebo-controlled studies to date that compare a histamine cream to a placebo cream. However, one animal study did conclude that morphine may exert its pain-relieving effect in the brain and spinal cord by releasing histamine into the central nervous system.

Hydroxytryptophan is an amino acid that naturally occurs in your body. It has been found to significantly decrease substance P formation. Because substance P may be involved in fibromyalgia, this medicine can improve your fibromyalgia pain. It also may helpful for the treatment of headaches, shingles, and neuropathic pain entities such as carpal tunnel syndrome or RSD.

Nausea is a common side effect of this drug. A patient also may experience drowsiness, dry mouth, and stomach pain. In 1989, some people taking this drug developed joint pain, high fever, weakness in their arms and legs, and had shortness of breath.

The Center for Disease Control concluded that the drug came from a Japanese manufacturer and was contaminated. Drug interactions reveal severe effects if a person is taking an antidepressant medicine from their doctor. A patient should not take this drug if a patient have Parkinson's disease and are not taking the drug Sinemet. Do not use this drug if one has scleroderma. This drug also may interfere with the effects of drugs that a patient may be taking for migraine headaches. Adults should take no more than 50 milligrams 3 times a day.

Cannabinoids are another natural substance for the control of pain. State legislation throughout the United States will eventually make a decision on the use of cannabinoids for medical purposes. Marijuana has been used since antiquity. In 1942, marijuana was reported to be a dangerous, harmful, and addictive drug. In 1970, marijuana was classified as a highly addictive drug with no accepted medical use.

However, in 1996, voters in Arizona and California passed referenda to legalize marijuana for medicinal use. To date, doctors are prohibited from prescribing marijuana for medical conditions. There has been a recent discovery of two cannabinoid receptors, CB-1 and CB-2. Now the scientific medical community is interested in this substance.

Cannabinoids are now reported to have therapeutic value as pain relievers. This means that marijuana could help a patient with a patient's pain in many situations. There have not been any controlled clinical trials for the use of this drug. Cannabinoids do exhibit some anti-inflammatory properties. However, they are no more effective than the current anti-inflammatory medications available.

If a patient suffers from pain involving nerves, such as shingles or reflex sympathetic dystrophy, a patient may be able to note some pain relief with the use of marijuana. To date the safety and efficacy of marijuana has not been found. In 1997, the American Medical Association House of Delegates recommended adequately designed controlled studies with respect to pain as well as other illnesses.

The normal human endocannabinoid system is important in the understanding of such issues as normal physiology, cannabis use disorder, and the development of medications that may act as agonists or antagonists to CB1 and CB2.4

By understanding the endocannabinoid system, it may be possible to enhance the beneficial effects of cannabinoid-related medication, while reducing the harmful effects. Cannabinoids have a favorable drug safety profile, but their medical use is predominantly limited by their psychoactive effects and their limited bioavailability.5

Cannabis-based medicinal extracts used in different populations of chronic nonmalignant neuropathic pain patients may provide effective analgesia in conditions that are refractory to other treatments.6 Overall there is evidence that cannabinoids are safe and modestly effective in neuropathic pain with preliminary evidence of efficacy in fibromyalgia and rheumatoid arthritis.7

The use of cannabis has been described in classical and recent literature for the treatment of pain, but the potential for psychotropic effects as a result of the activation of central CB (1) receptors places a limitation upon its use.8 There are, however, a number of modern approaches being undertaken to circumvent this problem, and this review represents a concise summary of these approaches, with a particular emphasis upon CB (2) receptor agonists.

Selective CB(2) agonists and peripherally restricted CB(1) or CB(1)/CB(2) dual agonists are being developed for the treatment of inflammatory and neuropathic pain. Clinical studies largely affirm that neuropathic pain patients derive benefits from cannabinoid treatment.9

A growing body of evidence that cannabis may be effective at ameliorating neuropathic pain, and may be an alternative for patients who do not respond to, or cannot tolerate, other drugs.10   The analgesia obtained from a low dose of delta-9-tetrahydrocannabinol in patients, most of whom were experiencing neuropathic pain despite conventional treatments, is a clinically significant outcome.11

Acupuncturists practice alternative medicine methods. Acupuncture is used in traditional Chinese medicine. It involves inserting fine needles into the body at specific points that have been found to be effective in the treatment of specific health problems. The purpose of acupuncture is to balance the body's flow of energies. Acupuncture can relieve pain, and those who perform acupuncture say it is able to restore health. Sometimes acupuncturists will burn herbs around a specific acupressure point for added relief.

Chiropractic medicine has been around since 1895. It is the second largest health profession in the world and one of the fastest growing. Chiropractors are aware of the possible dangers posed by conventional medical procedures. Chiropractors have found the nonmedical approach to body ailments that uses the body's own healing abilities to restore health.

Chiropractic medicine emphasizes individual well-being, including having a healthful diet and using natural medicines. Chiropractic therapy can be extremely effective in the management of painful conditions of the spine. Chiropractors do not prescribe conventional medicines, but do recommend natural substances that can promote healing of the body and prevent illnesses.

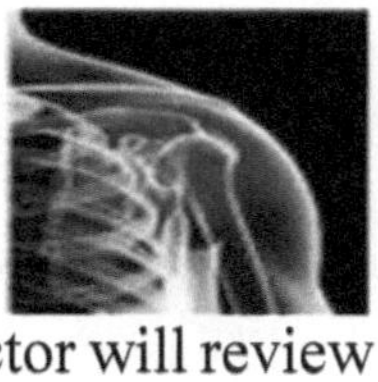

Figure 1. A chiropractor will review imaging studies rays and do a thorough physical examination before initiating treatment.

Although no research has been completed examining the role of chiropractic care in the treatment of CRPS, there is reason to believe that spinal manipulation may be beneficial to patients with CRPS.3 Due to the varied symptom presentation, it may be unclear which conservative therapies will be most beneficial in the treatment of CRPS.

A multidisciplinary approach to treatment should be pursued with these patients. More investigation of therapies such as chiropractic care as it relates to the pathophysiology of CRPS is needed.12

A case study reported that following chiropractic care, the patient had improved grip strength, functional abilities, and pain reduction. The primary characteristics of CRPS include motor, trophic and sensory changes, usually in a peripheral limb following some form of trauma.

Due to the varied symptom presentation, it may be unclear which conservative therapies will be most beneficial in the treatment of CRPS. A multidisciplinary approach to treatment should be pursued with these patients. More investigation of therapies such as chiropractic care as it relates to the pathophysiology of CRPS is needed.12

In summary, although the symptoms may be devastating and the medical prognosis poor at best, there are very specific chiropractic neurological protocols that can be followed to afford these patients some relief. Isolation of the initial nociception must be accomplished first and foremost, to assure that we eliminate any further nociceptive barrage into the nervous system and IML.

If it is a chronic patient, many times the initial causative factor has long since healed and may not even be associated with the present condition. The next step to address by chiropractic therapy is to promote large-diameter afferent barrage into the apical internuncial pool through some stimulus of the system.

This could be accomplished by any of the means mentioned previously, with the possibilities of treatment too numerous to address specifically in this chapter. The final factor to address is treatment of the opposite side of pain, to promote thalamic-hypothalamic-reticulo-spinal pathways and inhibit nociception suprasegmentally. When all of these factors are brought into play efficaciously, there are positive and long-standing results that cannot be underestimated in the eyes of a suffering patient.

CRPS symptoms may be managed with a combination of painkillers and cold-laser treatment; cold-laser treatment is used to treat both chronic and acute pain, and may be an effective mode of therapy for CRPS sufferers. Cold-laser therapy does not emit any heat, but does emit low-power light waves over the treatment area to reduce inflammation.

Cold-laser therapy uses a combination of electrical stimulation and cold-laser beams to increase serotonin levels in the body and allow the body to heal naturally.

Cold-laser therapy has been proven effective for the treatment of chronic and acute pain in more than 100 successful randomized double-blind clinical trials. Cold-laser therapy for RSD works by emitting electromagnetic energy directly into the skin tissues. These energy waves are absorbed by the mitochondria in the cell, and are converted to chemical energy. This stimulates the cells at a deep level and encourages healing, thereby reducing the sensation of pain, and triggering the natural healing process.

Cold-laser therapy for CRPS sufferers can be used on nearly any area of the body, including the knees, elbows, upper back, neck, shoulders and other inflamed joints. Some of the key benefits of cold-laser therapy for CRPS sufferers are: reduction of pain without medication, non-invasive treatment, and improved rate of tissue repair for natural healing, enhanced sense of well-being, no medication needed to complement treatment, reduction of skin sensitivity in the treated area and progressive results.

Recent research calls into question the predominant theories that view excessive sympathetic nervous system activity as the cause of CRPS. No evidence of an increase in sympathetic nervous system activity has been found, and new theories suggest that an increase in the sensitivity of neurotransmitter receptors may be the cause of CRPS.

Alternatively, other research has suggested that a local inflammatory process may in fact cause CRPS. Although no research has been completed examining the role of chiropractic care in the treatment of CRPS, there is reason to believe that spinal manipulation may be beneficial to patients with CRPS.3

It can be concluded that complimentary medicine can be an adjunct to conventional medicine for the treatment of RSD/CRPS in some instances.

References

1.   Borchers AT, Gershwin ME. The clinical relevance of complex regional pain syndrome type I: The Emperor's New Clothes. Autoimmun Rev. 2016.

2.   Meshkin B, Lewis K, Kantorovich S, Anand N, Davila L. Adding Genetic Testing to Evidence-Based Guidelines to Determine the

Safest and Most Effective Chronic Pain Treatment for Injured Workers. Int J Biomed Sci. 2015;11(4):157-165.

3. Muir JM, Vernon H. Complex regional pain syndrome and chiropractic. J Manipulative Physiol Ther. 2000;23(7):490-497.

4. Schrot RJ, Hubbard JR. Cannabinoids: Medical implications. Ann Med. 2016;48(3):128-141.

5. Abrams DI, Guzman M. Cannabis in cancer care. Clin Pharmacol Ther. 2015;97(6):575-586.

6. Boychuk DG, Goddard G, Mauro G, Orellana MF. The effectiveness of cannabinoids in the management of chronic nonmalignant neuropathic pain: a systematic review. J Oral Facial Pain Headache. 2015;29(1):7-14.

7. Lynch ME, Campbell F. Cannabinoids for treatment of chronic non-cancer pain; a systematic review of randomized trials. Br J Clin Pharmacol. 2011;72(5):735-744.

8. Anand P, Whiteside G, Fowler CJ, Hohmann AG. Targeting CB2 receptors and the endocannabinoid system for the treatment of pain. Brain Res Rev. 2009;60(1):255-266.

9. Rahn EJ, Hohmann AG. Cannabinoids as pharmacotherapies for neuropathic pain: from the bench to the bedside. Neurotherapeutics. 2009;6(4):713-737.

10. Wilsey B, Marcotte T, Tsodikov A, et al. A randomized, placebo-controlled, crossover trial of cannabis cigarettes in neuropathic pain. J Pain. 2008;9(6):506-521.

11. Wilsey B, Marcotte T, Deutsch R, Gouaux B, Sakai S, Donaghe H. Low-dose vaporized cannabis significantly improves neuropathic pain. J Pain. 2013;14(2):136-148.

12. Shearer HM, Trim A. An unusual presentation and outcome of complex regional pain syndrome: a case report. J Can Chiropr Assoc. 2006;50(1):20-26.

Orofacial pain disorders are relatively uncommon and pose a substantial diagnostic challenge. Reflex sympathetic dystrophy (RSD) of the face is an infrequently reported clinical pain syndrome characterized by dysesthesia, hyperalgia, hyperpathia, and allodynia. Treatment strategies, extrapolated from RSD and causalgia of the extremities, remain variable and poorly defined.

Sympathetic blockade is generally the diagnostic and therapeutic treatment of choice; however, the frequency, timing, and duration of injections; need for neurolytic blocks; and role of sympathectomy are not well understood. Complex regional pain syndrome is an infrequently reported differential diagnosis that can be considered in patients with persistent facial pain.

CRPS is a pathology that has been described as occurring almost always in a limb, but a published review reported cases that were found that met the International Association for the Study of Pain criteria for the disease.

The clinical characteristics were similar to those of CRPS elsewhere in the body, with the main features being burning pain, hyperalgesia, and hyperesthesia starting after a trauma to the craniofacial region.2 Physical signs were reported less frequently. The treatment of choice was seen to be a series of stellate ganglion anesthetic blocks.

Findings demonstrate an infrequent association of vasomotor and sudomotor changes with facial RSD, and lack of progression to a dystrophic or an atrophic stage, in contrast to extremity RSD. Furthermore, treatment response to sympathetic blockade is durable and less critically dependent on timing. The authors conclude that facial RSD has a favorable prognosis and should be managed conservatively with nonneurolytic stellate ganglion blocks, even when initiated as a delayed and repetitive injection series.3

A case report described a 65 year-old man with severe facial pain after extended maxillectomy due to carcinoma of maxillar sinus. He had been suffering from pain at rest, on mastication, or at treatment of surgical wound. Various kinds of analgesics had been tried, but his pain did not respond.

Because his pain was thought to be due to reflex sympathetic dystrophy stellate ganglion blocks were performed. After 5 administrations of stellate ganglion blocks, the pain was reduced markedly but the pain at treatment of wound persisted. It was thought that persistent pain would need a trigeminal nerve block.

A Gasserian ganglion block was subsequently performed directly through an open wound after the operation. After the the Gasserian ganglion block, the pain was diminished remarkably. He could tolerate procedures for facial a prosthesis. Pain control after the operation in this patient was very efficient to improve his quality of life.4

The complex regional pain syndrome is a debilitating neuropathic pain condition that has been extensively reported in the extremities following variable degrees of nerve trauma. CRPS has rarely been reported in the orofacial region. A previous study reported two orofacial pain patients whose clinical phenotypes fit the criteria for CRPS. Two cases of orofacial complex regional pain syndrome are described, both of which began following trigeminal nerve trauma.5

In case 1 the patient presented with redness of the ipsilateral ear during painful episodes, pain that extended into the ipsilateral arm and was associated with variations in the appearance of the ipsilateral hand. Symptoms also included "electric-burning pain" of the right side of the head, including the ear, teeth, jaw, eye, neck, and cheek.

In case 2 the patient presented with intractable pain of the upper left face, head, and neck accompanied by color changes in the painful areas, which increased with exposure to cold.

Spontaneous allodynia that is not limited to peripheral nerve distribution and is not proportionate to the inciting event may occur in the head and neck. One may present with an abnormal sudomotor activity, skin blood flow abnormality, edema, or other autonomic symptoms. Furthermore, there may be exclusion of other conditions that may otherwise contribute to the extent of the symptoms.

Only 13 cases of CRPS involving sympathetically maintained pain in the head and neck region have been described, and all reported trauma as the identifiable etiologic factor. Another case has been presented with the occurrence of sympathetically maintained pain in the head and neck region, but without nerve injury as a clear initiating factor.6

It has been suggested that central nociceptive processing is disrupted in CRPS, possibly due to disturbances in the thalamus or higher cortical centers.7

A case report described a patient as a 68-year-old man who suffered from inveterate pain with trophic changes of the right face and tongue and vasomotor dysfunction on the right side of the face after ipsilateral trigeminal nerve block. Allodynia and hyperalgesia were observed on the affected side of the face.

Pain initially improved after sympathetic nerve block, but similar pain returned that was unresponsive to the same procedure. Repeated intravenous administration of low-dose ketamine preceded by intravenous midazolam alleviated the pain, but trophic changes of the tongue persisted.8

Distinct cases of CRPS involving the orofacial region are rare. Thorough observations and documentation of signs and symptoms may lead to future standardization of diagnostic criteria and treatment strategies for this disorder.9 CRPS involving the facial region in children are rare. One case report described a 13-year-old girl with CRPS involving the face, which developed after being struck by a snowball.10

The clinical characteristics were similar to those of CRPS elsewhere in the body involving burning pain, hyperalgesia, and hyperesthesia. This was later accompanied by skin edema, fluctuating color, and temperature changes, as well as loss of eyebrow hair. Following detailed but inconclusive investigations, a clinical diagnosis of CRPS was made in line with Budapest diagnostic criteria. Over the next year, her condition gradually improved with ongoing comprehensive multidisciplinary input.

References
1.   Parkitny L, Wand BM, Graham C, Quintner J, Moseley GL. Interdisciplinary Management of Complex Regional Pain Syndrome of the Face. Phys Ther. 2016;96(7):1067-1073.
2.   Melis M, Zawawi K, al-Badawi E, Lobo Lobo S, Mehta N. Complex regional pain syndrome in the head and neck: a review of the literature. J Orofac Pain. 2002;16(2):93-104.
3.   Arden RL, Bahu SJ, Zuazu MA, Berguer R. Reflex sympathetic dystrophy of the face: current treatment recommendations. Laryngoscope. 1998;108(3):437-442.
4.   Iwade M, Fukuuchi A, Kawamata M, et al. [Management of severe pain after extended maxillectomy in a patient with carcinoma of the maxillary sinus]. Masui. 1996;45(1):82-85.

5.   Heir GM, Nasri-Heir C, Thomas D, et al. Complex regional pain syndrome following trigeminal nerve injury: report of 2 cases. Oral Surg Oral Med Oral Pathol Oral Radiol. 2012;114(6):733-739.

6.   Giri S, Nixdorf D. Sympathetically maintained pain presenting first as temporomandibular disorder, then as parotid dysfunction. Tex Dent J. 2007;124(8):748-752.

7.   Drummond PD, Finch PM. Sensory changes in the forehead of patients with complex regional pain syndrome. Pain. 2006;123(1-2):83-89.

8.   Sakamoto E, Shiiba S, Noma N, et al. A possible case of complex regional pain syndrome in the orofacial region. Pain Med. 2010;11(2):274-280.

9.   Drummond PD, Finch PM. Persistence of pain induced by startle and forehead cooling after sympathetic blockade in patients with complex regional pain syndrome. J Neurol Neurosurg Psychiatry. 2004;75(1):98-102.

10.   Goenka A, Aziz M, Riley P, Vassallo G. Complex regional pain syndrome involving the face following snowball injury. Eur J Pediatr. 2014;173(3):397-400.

It is a sad fact that the typical Complex Regional Pain Syndrome patient sees an average of seven physicians before they're even diagnosed, and subsequently treated. The possibility of curing the illness falls off quickly with time (around the first six months), and relies on fast and aggressive diagnosis and treatment, so quickly finding expert medical resources is vital.

Treatment is complicated, involving medications, physical and occupational therapy, psychological treatments, and neuromodulation and is often unsatisfactory, especially if delayed CRPS, formerly known as RSDS, was also known many years ago as the "Suicide Disease" because of the number of patients who took their life. This was mainly because it was so difficult to get diagnosed, physicians didn't believe their pain was real, and in the end very little relief was offered and patients suffered far greater and longer and in much greater silence than they do today.

Many anesthesiologists, neurologists and physical medicine and rehabilitation specialists treat CRPS. One should be aware that pain medicine as an entity is a sub classification and certification awarded by the American Board of Anesthesiology. An anesthesiologist, physical medicine rehabilitation specialist, neurologist, orthopedic surgeon, or neurosurgeon can all call themselves pain specialists, as can psychiatrists, psychologists, and chiropractors. Alternative medicine specialists such as acupuncturists can call themselves pain management practitioners as well. A qualified pain physician will be listed in ABMS.org.

Some practitioners have completed fellowships in pain medicine. These individuals have had comprehensive training at a medical center. These doctors have had training in reading a MRI, CT scan, and so on and training in how to decide whether a patient needs physical therapy, psychological evaluation, medications, or injections therapies to manage pain.

A fellowship-trained individual is one who has had special training in his or her specialty, whether it is anesthesiology, physical medicine, rehabilitation, or neurology. These specialty-trained individuals are equipped with the proper tools to treat a patient as a whole individual. This is not to say that the other individuals are not doing an adequate job for managing pain.

Some entities such as reflex sympathetic dystrophy are more complex and require the expertise of someone who has a more in-depth knowledge of a patient's disease. This individual may be affiliated with a university pain-management program. Most anesthesiology departments at university medical centers throughout the country have comprehensive pain-medicine programs. This ensures patient that patient may be evaluated by a physical therapist, occupational therapist, or psychologist. These types of programs offer a patient multiple methods.

A problem is that some insurance plans advise a patient to stay away from multidisciplinary pain centers because they can be expensive. If a patient has been involved in a motor vehicle accident or have sustained a work-related injury, and develop RSD/CRPS a case may end up before a court. When choosing a pain-management practitioner, one may want someone who not only can treat pain but also who can be an expert witness in a court of law.

No matter what type of individual a patient chooses to manager patient's pain, remember that individual is ultimately being paid by a patient. Even if the insurance company is paying the individual, remember that patient or employer is the one who pays the insurance premiums. Because most chronic pain syndromes require long-term care with a health-care provider, patient needs to ask the health-care provider for a curriculum vitae.

A curriculum vitae will show the qualifications of a potential health-care provider. Most individuals are proud of their accomplishments and will readily furnish patient with a resume or curriculum vitae. If the potential health-care provider does not have this information readily available, one must ascertain the educational background of the health-care provider.

A patient needs to know what schools that individual has attended. A patient may want to know the major areas of study during college and the major areas of study during professional training. A health-care provider should provide one with any additional courses attended as well as the dates of completion.

Some individuals have attended no additional courses in pain management. Some individuals have attended no additional courses for several years. However, most state medical boards now require individuals to meet continuing medical education courses to keep their licenses. Other health professions also have this continuing education rule. A patient needs to know if a health-care provider has done a fellowship in pain medicine. This fact is important because remember that anyone can place a shingle outside of his or her office claiming a specialty in pain management.

Most individuals keep a list of the education courses that they have attended in the past 10 years. To be a member of an HMO or certain insurance plans, health-care providers must update their curriculum vitae each year (and submit it to the HMO or insurance company). A health-care provider should, therefore, have a curriculum vita that lists what education courses he or she has taken in the past 10 years.

A patient needs to know if the health-care provider has been the subject of any disciplinary actions. Sometimes a health-care provider license will not be renewed for various reasons. A common reason is that the individual forgot to pay his or her dues. This is a much different disciplinary action than a disciplinary action for someone who has injured a patient because of medical negligence.

State medical boards can revoke a doctor's license if the doctor has been accused of improperly prescribing narcotic medications or other medications. For example, if a doctor has been accused of overprescribing narcotic medications to patients and if these patients have either died or have had to be admitted to hospitals, the doctor may not be allowed to practice. Patients need to know if a health-care provider has ever had his or her license suspended or revoked. A doctor may have practiced in another state, and lost his or her license there. Sometimes that individual will apply for a license in other states.

If he or she is able to obtain a license, the doctor will move to that state. A patient therefore, needs to know if the health-care provider has ever had a suspended or revoked license anywhere. Some practitioners have been suspended from practicing because they were taking drugs. However, most individuals are able to return back to their respective health-care practice after going through a rehabilitation program. A patient should not hesitate asking what the health-care provider's grades were.

The institution that the pain-management specialist attended should also be considered. A patient, furthermore, needs to know whether a health-care provider has had any gaps in his or her education. In other words, was he or she in school for continuous education or was his or her education interrupted. If that individual was in a four-year program and did not finish until 1999, that individual has a gap in education. A patient should not be embarrassed to ask why. Some individuals have to interrupt their education because of money or because they had to fulfill military obligations. Other individuals may have had drug problems or personal family problems.

Furthermore, they may have had some problem in doing the course work. If a patient detects a gap in an individual's education, ask why there is that gap. A patient should also examine curriculum vitae for the dates of each doctor that the health-care provider held. Are they chiefs of their departments? On the other hand, were they fired repetitively from positions? Health-care providers who are repeatedly dismissed from positions may have had problems with their patients or with their peers.

Examine a health-care provider's curriculum vitae to see how many positions that individual has held. One may discover that the ar health-care provider may have been a medical director of a pain center somewhere or was head of a physical therapy or occupational therapy department. A chiropractor may have practiced at a pain center. A psychologist, for example, may have been on staff at a multidisciplinary pain center. Review the positions that the potential health-care provider may have had.

Teaching at medical schools usually involves more expertise than nonteaching professionals. A patient should ask if a health-care provider taught at any educational facility. A patients need to know where and when they did teach. If a pain-care provider taught anatomy at a reputable university medical school, this individual should be an expert in doing nerve blocks. This individual can also be an expert in determining what anatomic site is the cause of the pain. Check the curriculum vitae or ask the health-care provider if he or she has been on the faculty of any seminars, conferences, or workshops.

Again, someone who has recognition in his or her field is usually asked to be a faculty member at a local or national seminar or local or nation conference. Some individuals are asked to help with workshops. Workshops are hands-on teaching experiences for health-care providers. For example, pain-medicine doctors can go to a workshop to learn how to do radiofrequency ablation of nerves in facet joints. These are hands-on courses with faculty who are well experienced in these procedures.

Did a health-care provider speak on reflex sympathetic dystrophy or post-herpetic neuralgia? The subject matter they spoke on usually indicates that they have some expertise in these particular fields. If a patient has a certain pain syndrome, he/she will probably want to go to an individual who has special expertise in treating this syndrome.

If a patient has been injured on the job or was injured in a motor-vehicle accident or in a fall in a store, it is helpful to know if a health-care provider usually sees patients referred by insurance companies, by attorneys, or by other doctors. If a patient has obtained a bodily injury, he/she may think that discovering this information is ridiculous.

However, many doctors have their referrals come primarily from insurance companies. If this happens, there is the chance that bias could be introduced into a patient's pain management. For example, if a patient sustained a RSD/CRPS injury in the course of a patient's employment, the employer may want to send a patient also to a doctor who they routinely use for their examinations.

Furthermore, a workmen's compensation insurance company may want a patient to see one of their doctors. Unfortunately, in some instances the company wants a patient to see a health-care provider who will find nothing wrong with patient. This is an instance where bias is introduced into pain management.

If a doctor consistently finds objective evidence to substantiate an employee's pain, that doctor may not be referred to again by the insurance company. These health-care providers are rare, but they do exist. So beware! A patient should, therefore, ask a potential health-care provider if he or she sees a significant number of patients referred by insurance companies.

If a patient anticipates that a CRPS case will go to court, he/she will want someone who has testified 50 percent for an insurance company and 50 percent for their patients. This information usually indicates to a jury or judge that the health-care provider is not biased.

Because there is essentially no real state or federal requirements for an individual to be a pain-management provider, a patient are ultimately responsible for choosing the correct individual. It is also important to know if a health-care provider did publish articles, book chapters, or reviews on certain pain conditions that a patient may be experiencing. More specifically, did the health-care provider research and do an article on a patient's particular pain syndrome? Advertisements are not the place to discover new revolutionary treatments.

Remember that if this particular treatment was safe and efficacious, the local university pain center would be utilizing this procedure. If one is in doubt about the efficacy of a procedure, do not hesitate calling a university pain center to see whether anyone has heard of the procedure and if they recommend the procedure.

A patient should not be misled by false claims from sometimes unscrupulous practitioners. Unfortunately, health care is a business like any other business. This is the reason why patient need to find a health-care practitioner who is knowledgeable as well as ethical.

Patients frequently seek treatment for chronic nonmalignant pain in primary care settings. Compared with physicians who have completed extensive specialization (eg, fellowships) in pain management, primary care physicians receive much less formal training in managing chronic pain. While chronic pain represents a complicated condition in its own right, the recent increase in opioid prescriptions further muddles treatment.

It is unknown whether patients with chronic pain seeking treatment in primary care differ from those seeking treatment in tertiary care settings. Primary care physicians care for a complicated group of patients with chronic pain that rivals the complexity of those seen in specialized tertiary care pain management facilities.[1]

Chronic pain management by Swiss specialist physicians with the primary hypothesis that pain clinic practitioners conform better to good practice (interdisciplinary, diagnostic/therapeutic routines, quality control, and education) than other specialists treating chronic pain was surveyed. Pain clinic practitioners were found to be more interdisciplinary and use more pain diagnostics than other specialists.[2] Pain clinic practitioners bring particular-differing-skills to chronic pain management compared to other physicians.

Patients who have complex pain problems such as RSD/CRPS patients sometimes require the skills of several health-care providers to manage their pain. Pain-management techniques are now being taught in some medical schools. It is anticipated that this training will increase at least to where medical students can take an elective in pain medicine.

Hopefully someday pain medicine will become a separate specialty that is recognized as a true specialty by the American Medical Association. It is unreasonable to expect one individual to know and comprehend the entire range of knowledge associated with pain medicine without extra training in pain medicine. This is the reason why a multidisciplinary approach to pain management has evolved. This type of approach utilizes the expertise of various disciplines that are brought together in an effort to provide patient with optimum pain management care.

A patient must do his/her homework when evaluating any method for pain-relieving medicines and devices sold over the counter that range from scientific nonsense to fraud. Some companies will include testimonials from patients in their advertisements. There is no way of knowing whether these individuals actually exist.

Testimonials can be a marketing tool not only for health-care products but for almost any type of product. Most of the time, a patient can take the testimonials that appear in advertisements with a grain of salt. If patient are evaluating a medicine or a product, look for studies on the Internet or in the library.

Although guidelines discourage the use of imaging, over one-quarter of patients were referred for imaging. Guidelines recommend that initial care should focus on advice and simple analgesics, yet only 20.5% and 17.7% of patients received these treatments, respectively. Instead, the analgesics provided were typically nonsteroidal anti-inflammatory drugs (37.4%) and opioids (19.6%).

This pattern of care was the same in the periods before and after the release of the local guideline. The usual care provided by GPs for LBP does not match the care endorsed in international evidence-based guidelines and may not provide the best outcomes for patients. This situation has not improved over time. The unendorsed care may contribute to the high costs of managing LBP, and some aspects of the care provided carry a higher risk of adverse effects.3

The medical board of the state of Ohio determined that pain physicians in Ohio for example come from many medical backgrounds and use different medical boards to claim board certification in the field of pain medicine. The names of Ohio physicians designating themselves as pain physicians were collected from the State Medical Board of Ohio and the American Medical Association.4

The directories of the American Board of Medical Specialties (ABMS), the American Board of Pain Medicine, the American Academy of Pain Management, and the American Board of Medical Acupuncture were referenced for certification in pain medicine, pain management, or medical acupuncture. The requirements for these credentials vary widely, yet they have all been used to claim "board certification."

Board certification in medicine implies recognition by an ABMS member board as having completed the required training, met the standards, and then passed an examination that validates qualifications, and knowledge in a specific medical field. In 2002, there were 335 Ohio physicians designating themselves as pain physicians. Two-hundred-eighteen (65%) had at least one pain board certification.4

Ninety-six (29%) of the Ohio pain physicians were certified in pain medicine by the American Board of Anesthesiology, the American Board of Physical Medicine and Rehabilitation, or the American Board of Psychiatry and Neurology, which are all member boards of the ABMS. One-hundred-seventeen (35%) of the self-declared Ohio pain physicians held no pain-related board certification. Anesthesiologists comprise the majority of all pain physicians and are the majority in all four pain boards.

References

1.	Fink-Miller EL, Long DM, Gross RT. Comparing chronic pain treatment seekers in primary care versus tertiary care settings. J Am Board Fam Med. 2014;27(5):594-601.

2.	Wilder-Smith OH, Mohrle JJ, Dolin PJ, Martin NC. The management of chronic pain in Switzerland: a comparative survey of Swiss medical specialists treating chronic pain. Eur J Pain. 2001;5(3):285-298.

3.	Williams CM, Maher CG, Hancock MJ, et al. Low back pain and best practice care: A survey of general practice physicians. Arch Intern Med. 2010;170(3):271-277.

4.	Buenaventura RM, McSweeney TD, Benedetti C, Severyn SA, Gravlee GP. The qualifications of pain physicians in Ohio. Anesth Analg. 2005;100(6):1746-1752.

Index